101

GREAT WAYS
TO IMPROVE
YOUR HEALTH

Selected and Introduced by

DAVID RIKLAN AND DR. JOSEPH CILEA

A PRODUCT OF
SELFGROWTH.COM

101 Great Ways to Improve Your Health
By David Riklan and Dr. Joseph Cilea

Published by
Self Improvement Online, Inc.
http://www.SelfGrowth.com
20 Arie Drive, Marlboro, NJ 07746

Cover Design:
Peri Poloni
Knockout Design
http://www.knockoutbooks.com

This book is dedicated, in loving memory, to our fathers, Dr. Manuel Riklan and Joseph C. Cilea. Each of these men lived a life dedicated to helping and serving others. We hope that we can continue this tradition by helping to serve in our respective fields. May their spirits and love live on forever.

Acknowledgements

Each and every one of us wants to live a life of optimum health. In our journey towards optimum health, we frequently find that attaining it is a team effort. We rely on others to provide quality foods for us to eat, quality information for us to learn and quality care when we are in need.

Similarly, the writing of this book was also a group effort. This book was truly created through a team effort that took countless hours of writing, revisions and updates. It could not have been created alone.

We'd like to acknowledge each and every author that contributed to this book – in fact, there would be no book without the inspiring wisdom and words of each of our contributing authors. Thank you to Dr. Joseph Mercola, Gary Craig, Dr. Susan Lark, Dr. Stephen Sinatra, Dr. Julian Whitaker, Dr. Marcus Laux and the other authors that made this book a powerful tool to help improve our health.

In addition to all of the contributors to the book, there are three people involved that deserve a very special thanks. Jerry Kimbrough, Stephanie Anastasio and Kristina Kanaley made the creation of this book possible. This three-person team worked closely together to create this powerful health book – and, in many ways, was more responsible for the completion of this book than we were.

We would also like to thank many other members of our team. We would like to thank Kevin McManemin, one of the newest members of the SelfGrowth.com team. He jumped right into this new project with both energy and focus.

There are many other members of our team involved with the creation and promotion of all of our products, including: Jamie Albert, Joe De Palma, Maryann Matera, Adriene Hayes, Todd Lesser, Greg Aronne, Iagia Mason, Alexa Wachstein, Gary Dong, Douglas Pak and Dr. Scott Beck. They have all helped to expand our self-improvement message around the world.

Many special thanks are due to our friends and family, who have provided much-needed support and encouragement throughout the process. A special thanks to our wives, Michelle and Maryann, who are a continual source of motivation for everything that we do.

Table of Contents

Table of Contents

Table of Contents

By David Riklan and Dr. Joseph Cilea

We live in an age of contradiction. Never has such a wonderfully diverse wealth of information about health been so easily accessible. Never have we known more of the secrets of the human body. And yet, never have so many Americans been making so many bad decisions about their health.

Today, according to the National Center for Health Statistics, about two-thirds of U.S. adults are overweight or obese – 133.6 million people in all. A new study completed by the National Cancer Institute indicates that 40.93% of men and women born today will be diagnosed with cancer at some time during their lifetime. Someone dies of heart disease every 34 seconds. One in six Americans is either pre-diabetic or diabetic. Over ten million Americans are taking anti-depressants. One in six Americans suffers from an anxiety disorder. And incidence rates of conditions like childhood diabetes, sleep disorders, Alzheimer's, anxiety and depression are spiraling upward with shocking speed.[1]

Why are so many of us so unhealthy?

When my co-author Dr. Cilea lectures about health, the first question he frequently asks is "How many people are interested in achieving a higher level of health?" Ninety percent of the audience usually raises their hands, but only a small percentage of these people are taking any action.

Health awareness is the first step on the path. We need to be more aware of the risk factors of our food choices, our sedentary lifestyles, the toxins in our environment, etc. When people understand that they need to work in alignment with the natural laws of health, good health will exist. It's not about good luck, optimal health comes from good living and good habits. It has little to do with going to the doctor and more to do with how we live our lives on a daily basis.

The decisions we make ultimately determine our levels of health. Are we going to exercise or lounge around? Will we eat good foods or bad? This is not to discount important preventative tests to screen for certain conditions at different phases of our life. We just think it's more important to be PROACTIVE with a healthy lifestyle rather than wait for a disease and then make drastic changes.

PROACTIVE HEALTH

Dr. Cilea is not a fan of the term "preventive medicine." He feels that it's an oxymoron. He believes "proactive health" is more appropriate. It implies that we take responsibility for our own health. This is not to discount the value of important preventative tests recommended for different age groups. People in their 30s should go

---

[1] CDC National Center for Health Statistics – http://www.cdc.gov/nchs.

check their sugar, insulin and cholesterol levels; 40s, their prostate; 50s, their colon and cardiovascular system. Early detection may in certain instances save or prolong lives.

Let's think of health as a bank account. We should make more deposits than withdrawals in our lifetime. A deposit would be getting up early and going to the gym. A withdrawal would be smoking cigarettes and eating processed foods. There are no shortcuts in health. Some people can get away with a less-than-healthy lifestyle and live to 100, while others with good health habits and poor genes can be afflicted with serious diseases at young ages. We would not gamble and hope for the good genes, or rely on them for that matter. It's more important to discipline yourself to health-promoting habits, including diet, exercise, and a positive frame of mind.

With the vast assortment of health books and information available, it's important to understand today's major principles of health and wellness. We believe we should all read up on the latest health issues. For instance, the issue Dr. Cilea is most concerned about is type 2 diabetes. This is on the rise in children. Type 2 diabetes was once an adult-dominated problem, but now it's showing up in all people because of our Standard American Diet (S.A.D.). Processed and refined sugars are the culprits, and our kids are ingesting them in record amounts. In 1900, the average American consumed 10 pounds of refined sugar per year. Today, that number is 110 pounds per year. The message needs to get out on the dangers of these foods. When it comes to nutrition, we need to eat more foods in their natural state.

There's no substitute for a good, balanced, wholesome diet that is free of hormones and pesticides. It's tough to get all our nutrients from food. Vitamins do a great job at supplementing the voids that may be created from our diet. They serve to fill in the cracks, so to speak. We can also look to other sources like spirituality to help improve our health naturally. There is a definite link between health and spirituality. And although spirituality helps mostly with our mental health, it can ultimately have a positive effect on every system in our body.

In the long run, improving our health is not only about physical and mental wellness. In a topic as broad as "health," we also need to talk about healthcare. Something is wrong with our healthcare system and our philosophy. Only two percent of the over $2 trillion Americans spend on healthcare is spent on education and prevention. Unfortunately, the vast majority of our spending is to treat chronic illness. Doctors need to put more responsibility on the patients to take care of themselves. Again, we need to stress PROACTIVE HEALTH. Patients will always look for the quick fix, and it is the responsibility of doctors to educate and hold patients accountable.

101 GREAT WAYS TO IMPROVE YOUR HEALTH

In this book you'll find 101 different authors with 101 different viewpoints on your health. The authors come from every branch of the medical and healing professions – from family physicians to psychologists, nurses to nutritionists, osteopaths to optometrists. We included such a broad array of specialists and ideas because we don't believe that there is one single path to better health, and no one expert with all the answers. Rather, our approach is to present you with a smorgasbord of interesting ideas from some of the best minds in their respective fields, and leave you to integrate them into your life as you see fit.

Our book is broken into nine sections - Better Health through Self Improvement, Diet and Nutrition, Energy Healing and Other Unique Techniques, Fitness & Exercise, Holistic Health, Hidden Health Dangers, Physical or Mental Disorders/Problems, Stress and Mental Health, and Vitamins, Minerals, and Nutritional Supplements. While there will be some overlap in the categories the articles cover, we feel this categorization will best help the reader in processing the incredibly varied information contained within. Here's what you'll find in each section.

Better Health through Self-Improvement: Our first section works from the premise that the body part most vital to your overall health and well-being may be your brain. Through constructing a proper mental attitude, building a life of balance and a mindset of harmony, you can achieve dramatic improvements in your bodily health. Chapters detail the healing properties of laughter, the importance of forgiveness and gratitude, and other ways you can think your way to better health.

Diet and Nutrition: Everyone knows the timeworn old maxim "you are what you eat," but recent scientific studies have proven that this line is far more profound than your grandmother ever knew. Our basic biochemistry is altered by the foods we choose – or neglect – to ingest, and making smart, healthy food choices is a necessary part of a healthy life. Our chapters on antioxidants, "good" fats, organic foods and living foods will give you fresh perspectives on the foods and nutrients your body needs to operate at its full potential. And for those worried that "healthy eating" is going to mean bland bean sprouts and tasteless wheat grass concoctions, look no further than the chapter entitled "Chocolate, Chocolate, Chocolate!"

Energy Healing and Other Unique Techniques: What is the true cutting edge in medicine? While some may think the cutting edge is ever-grander and ever-more-expensive technologies, some of the most revolutionary areas in the science of healing involve very old and very simple methods. From ancient techniques like acupuncture and Qigong to newer methods like halotherapy and bioelectromagnetic medicine, this section will acquaint you with modern medicine's true vanguard.

Fitness & Exercise: Far too often, exercise is thought of and discussed as an activity with a single goal; i.e., exercise = burning fat, period. And while exercise is key to this goal, a good fitness regimen can provide your body with a wealth of other benefits. Proper exercise can help you balance your hormones, look younger, and improve your mental functioning. Well tailored regimens can even tackle specific diseases and conditions. This section will show you how.

Holistic Health: Your body is the sum total of a bewildering variety of parts, pieces, reactions and relationships. Holistic healing proceeds from the belief that it is impossible to single out one aspect of the self and effect lasting changes without a firm understanding of the whole. From naturopathy (using natural methods to boost your body's innate abilities to ward off diseases) to trigger point therapy, this section will help you take a holistic approach to your health.

Hidden Health Dangers: Turn on the local news any given night and you're likely to be bombarded with the latest health scares. But beyond the hype and the headlines, what are the real dangers you and your family need to look out for? This section tackles eleven under-the-radar health concerns and gives you the information you need to stay healthy.

Physical or Mental Disorders/Problems: In recent years, a sea change has happened in the clinical understanding of topics like drug addiction and depression. Once viewed through the lens of Western medicine's hardwired concept of a mind/body duality, we are coming to see that disorders of the mind and disorders of the body are in fact oftentimes one in the same. This section details new approaches you can take to treat conditions as disparate as chronic pain and postpartum depression.

Stress and Mental Health: Stress not only strains the mind, but manifests itself in our bodies. Stress acts as an insidious catalyst, making bad conditions worse and bringing underlying diseases to raging new heights. This section details some simple, effective approaches you can take to help build a balanced, stress-reduced life.

Vitamins, Minerals, and Nutritional Supplements: This section will take you beyond the basics in the vitamin field. You'll learn of the importance of nutrients like fulvic acid, hudor, and dietary indoles. We'll also discuss herbal supplements that provide the essentials your body needs to stay fit and ward off potential problems.

CLOSING THOUGHTS

Finally, a few words on what the book is and is not meant to be.

It is not meant as a list of 101 things you MUST do to improve your health. (We don't expect you to find the time, money and willpower to follow all of these paths!) It is not meant to replace, reject or rebut your regular doctors, nutritionists, trainers, etc.

Rather, this book is here to make you an energized and active consumer of health information. By bringing you articles on a hugely diverse list of topics from some of the top experts in their respective fields, we hope you will be motivated to start to ask the right questions about your health. We want you to explore new healing methods, approaches or techniques and find out what works for you – because no one has more invested in your health than you do.

In closing, we hope this book becomes your bridge to a better, healthier, happier life.

PART ONE

Better Health through Self Improvement

Every day, in every way,
I am getting better and better.

-- Emilé Coué

1

The Paradox of Forgiveness

Anna Barbosa, MA, CHt

If you devote your life to seeking revenge, first dig two graves.
—Confucius

To forgive or not forgive?

Your decision could affect your health and the quality of your life. Studies prove that people who choose not to forgive have more stress-related illnesses, lower-functioning immune systems, and increased likelihood of heart disease than people who forgive.

A study by Kathleen Lawler, PhD, at the University of Tennessee measured noticeable differences in the increases of blood pressure, heart rate, and muscle tension between forgivers and nonforgivers when participants were asked to tell a story of betrayal. Results showed that the forgivers had a lower resting blood pressure and smaller increases in blood pressure than low forgivers or nonforgivers. High forgivers also reported fewer visits to their physicians for physical ailments.[1]

In his book *Forgive for Good*, Dr. Frederic Luskin states that unresolved anger resets the internal thermostat. This low level of anger begins to feel normal, but it actually burns out the body.[2] Anger is a secondary emotion that masks hurt feelings. Forgiving helps us give up the hurt and allows us to heal.

Let's take a moment for a quick experiment. Focus on someone or some event that has caused you hurt or pain. Close your eyes for about fifteen seconds, and feel what is happening in your body as you maintain that focus. Do your muscles tighten up? Do your heart beat and breathing rate increase? Does your body feel like it is on alert? Now imagine how that physical response plays out over and over again anytime you have an experience that is similar to or reminds you of that event or person.

---

[1] University of Tennessee, "UT study shows forgiveness linked to lower blood pressure," news release, March 1, 2000, http://www.psychosomatic.org/media_ctr/press/annual/2000/017.html.
[2] F. M. Luskin, *Forgive for Good: A Proven Prescription for Health and Happiness* (San Francisco: Harper, 2001).

To forgive does not mean that the offense is condoned. Whether the offense was done (1) with malicious intent (the violator was abusive), (2) with unintentional harm (the violator was unaware of the harm caused by his or her actions or words), or (3) by inappropriate positive intent (the violator criticizes or hurts to teach a lesson), it is not minimized with forgiveness. Forgiveness does not mean weakness. It does not mean surrendering to defeat or avoiding justice. In fact, it takes strength to truly forgive from your heart.

Often the greater the hurt, the more difficult it is for the injured person to want to forgive. However, there is no offense that is so great that it cannot be healed by the gracious act of forgiveness. A life of forgiveness is available to all of us.

The paradox of forgiveness is that the true beneficiary is the forgiver. Forgiving can enhance the immune system, lower blood pressure, and reduce secreted cortisol. A study by the Duke University Medical Center demonstrated that those who have forgiven experience lower levels of back pain and less associated problems such as depression.[3]

The emotional well-being of the forgiver is enhanced. Forgiveness returns the control of your emotions to you. Thinking becomes clearer because the mind is not clouded over with thoughts of anger, hate, or revenge. You live life in a proactive manner, rather than a reactive manner.

The benefits of forgiveness are far-reaching. According to research compiled by A Campaign for Forgiveness, a nonprofit organization, forgiveness affects health, marriages, businesses, relationships, communities, and nations.[4]

Forgiveness and Hypnosis

Forgiveness work can be done with various therapeutic modalities. One of the more powerful methods of doing this work is through hypnosis. The subconscious mind, which is considered the seat of emotions, is easily accessible in hypnosis. This direct connection to the emotions makes hypnosis a very efficient therapy.

In hypnosis, the forgiveness work is done without any interpersonal exchange between the injured and the violator because the violator is not present. This work is especially beneficial when the violator expresses no remorse or willingness to right the wrong, when the injured chooses not to interact with the violator, or when the violator is deceased. None of these possibilities have any effect on the forgiveness work once the decision is made to forgive. The purpose of this process is to free the injured from his or

---

[3] J. W. Carson et al., "Forgiveness and chronic low back pain: A preliminary study examining the relationship of forgiveness to pain, anger, and psychological distress," *Journal of Pain* 6 (2005): 84–91.

[4] See http://www.forgiving.org.

her internal prison of anger and hurt, thereby opening the heart to a new level of love and freedom.

During hypnosis, the injured creates a setting where he or she is able to address the violator with the understanding that the violator cannot interrupt, give excuses, or cause any more harm. The ability to verbalize everything that needs to be said to the violator, including expressions of painful feelings of hurt, disgust, or embarrassment, is a necessary step in the forgiving process. Typically, a great amount of emotional energy is spent during this time. When the injured feels that he or she has expressed every available hurt or emotion, the injured switches roles and becomes the violator.

In the role of the violator, the injured has the opportunity to perceive the event through the eyes of the violator. He or she may come to believe that the violator also had pain and was lashing out at someone more vulnerable. Maybe the violator didn't know a better way. As the injured continues to speak as the violator, he or she may begin to feel compassion for the violator. It is possible that this may take a few turns of switching roles. It is also possible to forgive when the injured can find no logical or fathomable reason for the offense. The work is near completion when the injured, while in the role of violator, is able to ask for forgiveness.

Forgiveness is a healing gift that you give to yourself, and the benefits are far-reaching. By doing forgiveness work through hypnosis or with any other modality, healing happens, and your health as well as your relationships with yourself and your loved ones can improve significantly and forever.

About the Author

Anna Barbosa, MA, CHt, is in private practice at the Healing Nexus in Houston, Texas. She utilizes hypnosis and Emotional Freedom Technique in assisting her clients through the forgiveness process and with other issues. Visit http://www.thehealingnexus.com.

2

Creating Better Health from the Inside Out with Gratitude

Katherine Scherer and Eileen Bodoh

Most of us become anxious when we are not feeling well. Our stability and security are threatened, and we become fearful. "What if I have to take off from work again?" or "How will I manage if I get sick?" are questions we may ask ourselves while feeling our anxiety build. Whether we are dealing with a serious illness or just an off day, it is important to eliminate stress as much as possible. A good way to do this is to tune in to gratitude. Gratitude, like other positive emotions, has an undeniable positive effect on our health and well-being.

"A distinguished emotions researcher recently commented that if a prize were given for the emotion most neglected by psychologists, gratitude would surely be among the contenders," says Emmons of the University of California at Davis, a psychologist and leading figure in the new field of gratitude research.[1] Along with Michael E. McCullough of the University of Miami, he edited the recently published book *The Psychology of Gratitude.* They report that grateful people are more optimistic, more satisfied with life, and have higher levels of vitality and lower levels of depression and stress. Gratitude research is beginning to suggest that feelings of thankfulness have tremendous positive value in helping people cope with daily problems, especially stress. In "Highlights from the Research Project on Gratitude and Thankfulness," they found that "in a sample of adults with neuromuscular disease, a 21-day gratitude intervention resulted in greater amounts of high energy positive moods, a greater sense of feeling connected to others, more optimistic ratings of one's life, and better sleep duration and sleep quality, relative to a control group."[2] It's no secret that stress can make us sick, and it has even been suggested that it can kill. Stress has been linked to heart disease and cancer, and 90 percent of all doctor visits include some form of stress-related illness. Researchers in the field

---

[1] Robert A. Emmons and Michael E. McCullough, eds., *The Psychology of Gratitude* (New York: Oxford University Press), 3.

[2] Robert A. Emmons and Michael E. McCullough, "Highlights from the Research Project on Gratitude and Thankfulness" (working paper).

of positive psychology are finding that positive emotions are far more important to mental health and physical well-being than scientists had ever realized.

When we are experiencing illness and discomfort, we do what we believe will help in our healing. We follow our doctors' advice, take the prescribed medications, eat well, get plenty of rest, and try other nontraditional alternatives that promise to promote good health. But have we ever considered how important our thoughts are?

Keeping our thoughts as positive as possible is critical because, generally, our thoughts precede our feelings. Positive emotions come from positive thoughts. When we think about what we are grateful for and it is something we truly value, we feel the positive emotion of gratitude. A mother may think of her newborn baby and feel gratitude; a father who has just been promoted at work may feel grateful for new opportunities; a child who gets exactly what she wanted for her birthday may feel gratitude.

Choosing to focus on the blessings in life and being grateful for them will help us stay positive. This doesn't mean that we won't ever have negative thoughts to deal with, but choosing to lift our thoughts higher with gratitude will help remove us from our victim status and empower us. Making the practice of gratitude a habit, even before we are under the weather, will help us stay well and get well sooner when we become ill.

There are always good reasons to be thankful, even if we don't feel like it. At first, we may have to fake it until we make it. By deciding to say thank you enough, we may even find troublesome thoughts occurring less often for an added benefit. Gratitude is an antidote for depression.

There are many simple and enjoyable ways to practice gratitude. Waking up to gratitude by immediately giving thanks before we throw off the covers is a great way. This action alone can set the tone for the entire day. Another way is to begin a gratitude journal. Keeping a gratitude journal is as easy as starting a notebook in which we write down five things a day that we are grateful for. It helps us achieve a grateful state of mind. It shifts our focus away from what we don't have to what we do have. It takes us from negative thinking to positive thinking in an instant, and we may be surprised at how much we find to be grateful for. According to Emmons and McCullough, "In an experimental comparison, those who kept gratitude journals on a weekly basis exercised more regularly, reported fewer physical symptoms, felt better about their lives as a whole, and were more optimistic about the upcoming week compared to those who recorded hassles or neutral life events."[3]

---

[3] Ibid.

When we stop for a moment, look at our surroundings, and focus on our gifts, we realize how much we have to be grateful for. The gifts of hearing, sight, and clear thinking are invaluable, yet we often take them for granted. Family members and friends, nature and its beauty, and positive actions that improve our world are good examples of things to be grateful for. Other examples include getting a clean bill of health from your doctor, finding the theater tickets you thought you had lost, arriving safely at your destination after a bumpy plane ride, finding shelter in a sudden downpour, smelling the sweetness of apple blossoms in the air, and having a shoulder to cry on. The list of things we have to be grateful for is endless, and the more we are grateful for, the more we will notice how much we have to be grateful for.

Because we have a natural tendency to focus on the negative, it is important to make a conscious effort to stay positive, and cultivating gratitude is one way to do this. The practice of gratitude has the power to turn our focus from our logical minds to the positive feelings we carry in our hearts. Why not practice gratitude until it becomes a habit?

- Make a commitment to be grateful every day.
- Find at least one person to say thank you to every day.
- Give thanks and praise for your loved ones every day.
- Send thank you notes more often.
- See the beauty in nature and be grateful for it.
- Look for the good in everything.
- Find a gratitude partner and share positive moments of gratitude.
- Take great care of yourself and choose to be grateful for all the gifts in your life.

About the Authors

Katherine Scherer and Eileen Bodoh are the authors of *Gratitude Works: Open Your Heart to Love*, an inspirational book that helps readers access the healing power of gratitude, and the e-books *Gratitude Works Journal* and *Gratitude Works Prayer Book*. Their mission is to touch lives with the spirit of gratitude. Katherine's and Eileen's diverse backgrounds include owning and operating a business, chairing nonprofit community groups, facilitating self-improvement groups, developing a holistic health conference, hospice training, and training in parent education. Their writing appears in publications and Web sites in the United States and Canada. Visit http://www.gratitudeworks.com.

3

Your Golden Hour: How to Jump-Start Your Day in a Positive Way

Dennis Collins and Dr. Donna Goldstein

How do you spend your precious first waking hour? If you find yourself checking your e-mail, gulping your coffee, reading the paper, or watching the news, you are not alone—this has become standard for many harried workers today. We believe that your first waking hour of each day is your Golden Hour[1], your opportunity to set your course and direction for the day. To a large extent, the way you spend this time determines the outcome of the rest of your day.

Here are some helpful hints for making the most of the first hour of your day, every day. Perhaps you already do some of these. If so, keep up the good work and expand to do more. If these are unfamiliar, try just one or two of these positive habits, and see how much of a difference it will make!

Positive Golden Hour Habits

1. Determine your intention for the day, and clarify your most important goals and outcomes.
2. Maintain a notebook with your personal mission and short-term and long-term goals handy. Review these each morning to ensure that your thoughts and activities of the day move you in the right direction.
3. Read something uplifting or inspirational such as poetry or a daily spiritual prayer or passage; some people like to do this out loud, others, silently. You might like to sit in a nearby park or garden or at least look out a window or focus on something beautiful in your home.
4. Take a few moments (or more) for meditation, or breathing and centering exercises, or to reflect on your life and all you have to be grateful for. Some

---

[1] Emergency medical professionals believe that trauma victims' chances of survival are greatly increased if they are delivered to trauma care within the first sixty minutes of an accident. They call this the "golden hour."

people keep a gratitude journal and find this to be a very helpful morning practice.

5. Stretch your body as well as your mind and spirit. Try some yoga or Tai Chi, a gentle Asian form of martial arts that energizes the body and mind. In certain Asian countries, workers do Tai Chi together in groups prior to the start of the workday to ensure that they maintain focus and achieve optimum performance.

6. Try some form of aerobic exercise, especially outside, where, climate permitting, you can breathe some enlivening fresh air while you jog or walk your dog, bike or swim or garden. This is the perfect way to jump-start your day!

7. Immediately on waking, drink a mixture of half natural juice diluted with half water. Many people experience low blood sugar in the morning, and this is an excellent way to get your body and brain in gear and ready to go.

8. As you are showering or getting dressed, how about some uplifting or "get me going" music? Whether it's golden oldies or gospel or eighties dance music, you know what helps put you in a great mood for the day.

There are also some things you can avoid if you want peak productivity in your day. Many of these may be hard habits to break, but once you start seeing your Golden Hour as something special or even sacred, perhaps you will want to make some different choices. Try reducing or eliminating these morning behaviors, and notice the difference you will feel.

- Avoid immersion in the radio, TV, computer, or newspaper when you first awake. While there is a place for morning news, try not to let fires, floods, scandals, and violence be the first thing to enter your consciousness in the morning. Search for a medium that also focuses on good news in your community or our world.

- Avoid the e-mail imperative. Whether you have an office at home or away, we have all had the experience of stopping to check just one e-mail and emerging hours later from urgent (or not so urgent) matters in cyberspace. Curb your urge to check your e-mail during your Golden Hour—you'll be glad you did!

- Consider that food is the fuel that runs your body, and don't skip breakfast because you are in a hurry. Instead, make yourself something you'll enjoy for breakfast the night before, or buy individual sizes of yogurt or oatmeal and always keep fresh fruit and nuts handy.

- Avoid the coffee and donut/junk food trap, which just revs up your body and then causes you to crash a few hours later. If you find you are addicted to your morning java, start gradually mixing decaf and regular coffee, or better yet, try a delicious cup of herbal, green, or white tea. Talk to a nutritionist about what food and food combinations are right for you.

Nobody can do all these things every day—it's not practical, or even necessary. Start with a few small changes, and note how your relationships and productivity improve. Begin tomorrow morning, then reward yourself after a week of consistent new practice. When you use your Golden Hour consciously and appropriately, expect a fruitful and successful day, week, and life!

About the Authors

Dennis Collins makes excellent use of his Golden Hour with study and both physical and mental workouts. Currently, he is the senior vice president and general manager of the Lincoln Financial Media group of radio stations in Miami. During his thirty-year, industry-leading career in advertising, communications, and marketing, he has trained thousands of record-breaking, unstoppable salespeople. Reach him at DPCWiz@bellsouth.net.

Dr. Donna Goldstein, the managing director of Development Associates International, uses her Golden Hour for journaling, meditation, and a walk or workout. A respected corporate psychologist and success coach, she has helped thousands of individuals worldwide to reduce their stress and burnout and enhance their productivity and sense of purpose. She has contributed to 26 books. Visit http://www.DrDonnaGo.com, or call her at (954) 893-0123 to arrange a complementary thirty-minute phone consultation.

4

Disease: Plague or Teacher?

Jacob Griscom

What kind of question is that anyway? Why would I even suggest that disease could be a teacher? This may seem strange, and yet, as I see it, this is the most important distinction that I draw between the current holistic and allopathic approaches to medicine.

The allopathic mind-set is one of eliminating or "destroying" disease. This is reflected in the language that is used when addressing disease: *the war on cancer or the fight against HIV*. On the upside, this approach has made Western medicine incredibly effective at managing acute and dangerous diseases. But on the downside, it really doesn't do much to address the roots of a condition and can instead create an ongoing struggle with numerous chronic diseases.

Western medicine isn't alone, of course, as this mind-set extends into just about every challenge we face in modern Western life, be it a war on terrorism, the fight against poverty, or the war on drugs. The war list goes on and on, and why shouldn't it? Indeed, when was the last time you had a battle with somebody that improved things?

The holistic approach to medicine, on the other hand—ideally, the approach of holistic health practitioners—is focused on supporting health by

1. addressing the unique physical, psychological, and spiritual needs of the individual
2. taking a radically different approach to disease, where instead of viewing disease as the enemy, the holistic practitioner and patient choose to view disease as a teacher.

What an incredible shift! Instead of wondering what drug or supplement will get rid of certain symptoms, they ask, "What do these symptoms have to *teach* me?"

This new question encourages looking within. It encourages personal growth and evolution. It encourages a compassionate understanding of the body and self, instead of aggravation. The symptoms (physical, psychological, or spiritual) can be seen as the best attempt to adapt to unfavorable circumstances, and they can be heard as the voice of Nature declaring that something is out of harmony.

The more you adopt this new consciousness, the more you will notice an increasing sensitivity and respect for this voice because you'll begin to understand that when we don't listen to Nature's whisper, she screams instead!

And what does Nature's scream sound like? It is our experience of increased and overwhelming stress, the epidemics of heart disease, cancer, diabetes, and many other chronic and debilitating diseases. It is devitalized and toxic food, massive environmental pollution and destruction, and startling global climate changes.

And yet these are all just branches on the Tree of Disease; the roots lie in our consciousness, lifestyles, and food choices. If the roots are not addressed, it won't matter what wonder drug or supplement comes along or how enthusiastically we chop away at the branches because new ones will continue to grow. But by affecting the roots, we can change the entire tree.

The roots in consciousness are reflected in our experiences of relationships and work. Are we engaged in battle or harmony? Do we feel deep significance and purpose in life, or are we confused, lost, or frustrated? Feeling connected to our source and seeing the importance of our contributions is essential for health.

The roots in our lifestyles relate to how we live each day. When and how do we eat, sleep, exercise, and have sex? Do our habits support us feeling alive and energized? A healthy lifestyle generates health!

And finally, the roots of disease or health lie in our food choices. Truly healthy people eat whole, organic, nutrient-dense food, with respect for the land and animals that nourish them and regard for the season, climate, and their constitutional needs. They eat real foods that have been valued for health for many generations, instead of our modern processed, packaged, low-fat invention foods. They also feed their senses with Nature's sunlight, sounds, and beauty, instead of just staying trapped inside with the television on.

Let's take the example of the common cold, which is something that we've all experienced. It can come at an entirely inconvenient time, or you may notice that sometimes you get a cold right *after* a really stressful period. It's almost as if you were waiting for the right time to allow yourself to get sick. Regardless, being sick, especially when it comes with a fever and heavy sinus congestion, really knocks us out of our ability to work and run around doing things.

It's at this point that we have a decision to make: will we take the time to rest and recuperate, or will we power through the cold with the aid of some over-the-counter cold medicines?

If we power through the cold, we won't have addressed the underlying reasons that we got the cold in the first place. This is the war model attempting to annihilate the symptoms. The trouble with this approach is that the battlefield (our body and mind) ends up in a worse state than before the cold. Nothing has really been done to strengthen the body or reduce stress, so now we're even more likely to get another cold, feel more stressed, and lay the foundation for other symptoms and disorders.

Our other option is to approach the cold as a teacher and to listen to what it is telling us about our state of health. Colds are essentially a request for rest and rejuvenation. They alert us that our immune system is not functioning optimally. The more quickly and fully we can satisfy these needs, the more quickly we will get well.

Recently, two days before I was scheduled to fly to Los Angeles for an important presentation to six hundred people, I got a sore throat and started feeling a little under the weather. I *had* to be well for this event!

So I decided to listen to what this cold had to teach me and followed my own recommendations for colds. I avoided solid food, meat, and eggs and switched to an all liquid diet with bone broth, coconut milk, vegetables, and lots of coconut oil, which has fantastic antimicrobial properties. I drank plenty of beet kvass, a lacto-fermented beverage that supports detoxification and immunity, and took extra cod liver oil, which is rich in fat-soluble vitamins. I also took some of my favorite immune support herbs: Echinacea, elderberry, and amalaki. This approach gives the digestive system and body both rest and nourishment so that the body can dedicate its energy to a quick recovery.

Then I was sure to get plenty of rest and spent some time viewing a special television program on inspiration by a speaker that I thoroughly enjoy. Stress is an immune depressant, whereas inspiration and joy stimulate and strengthen the immune system. When the time for my presentation arrived, I had fully recovered and delivered an excellent performance.

It is essential that each individual take personal responsibility for his or her health and world. A total reliance on a *passive* medical system that relies on drugs and miracle interventions is disabling, whereas an adoption of the principles of an active holistic health care system is positively life transforming!

I'm sharing a tremendous vision for the holistic health care movement. The vision is that as more and more people begin to relate to disease in their immediate bodies and minds as a teacher instead of an enemy, I believe we will see that same consciousness extend into our larger bodies and minds: our communities, our countries, our planet— and beyond.

About the Author

Jacob Griscom is a clinical Ayurvedic specialist and founder of Peaceful Living Holistic Healthcare Center. He is on the teaching faculty for the California College of Ayurveda and is a graduate of the Bay Area Nonviolent Communications Leadership Program. He offers classes, teleclasses, Compassionate Communication training, and in-person or online holistic health care consultations with an improved health guarantee. Jacob is the author of *Dietary Supplements for Enlightenment: Guidance for Inner Peace and Self-Realization.* His articles have been published nationally and internationally, and he has been a featured speaker at T. Harv Eker's Master of Influence seminar. Visit his Web site at http://www.peacefullivinghhc.com.

5

Balance and Well-Being through the Seven Dimensions of Health

Shawna Hansen, Linda Hartmann, and Benson Brown

A tool that helps bring awareness to all the areas of our lives that contribute to wellness are the Seven Dimensions of Health™. The premise is that every area of our lives contributes to our health and needs to be given the same amount of energy.

What Are the Seven Dimensions of Health and How Do We Use Them?

Physical

This dimension focuses on the body. It is about the degree of efficiency in the systems of the body. In the physical dimension, we bring attention to our nutrition, our cardiovascular health, and our strength, flexibility, and balance. We also look at our ability to deal with stress, the quality of our sleep, and the amount of quiet/meditative time we spend. The human body actually gains energy and vitality from use. There are many options available designed to provide balanced physical fitness. Some examples are Pilates, yoga, Tai Chi, and strength training as well as running, walking, and hiking. It is not so important what we do to exercise the body as that we are consistent in the practice and that we bring a joyful attitude.

Mental

The mental dimension refers to how we take in, process, and communicate information. It is based on the belief that all people are unique in this regard. What we think springs from what we believe. Our beliefs form how we view the world. It is important to be aware of our unique style of processing information. We can learn about the ways other people operate so we can be more harmonious with the people in our lives. Some ways to access this dimension are through meditation, reading books, and attending specialized workshops designed to enhance our understanding of how we process and communicate information. One example is Emergenetics®, a workshop that focuses on the blend of genetics and learned experiences expressed as a behavior and a way of thinking. Rapport Leadership International is a company that offers several courses on personal development that are also excellent tools for evolving our mental dimension of health. The key is education. We must embrace our unique way of living, while celebrating the differences in all the people around us.

Social

Our social health is really about who we choose to spend our time with. It cannot be understated how important the company we keep is to our health. When we have surrounded ourselves with people who enhance us, we feel energized in their presence. The opposite is also true. It is important to remember that like energy attracts. We draw to us people who are vibrating with the same energy we are putting out into the universe. The best way to make a change in our social atmosphere is to place a focus on being the person we want to be.

Occupational

Our occupational dimension includes all the roles we choose to occupy during our waking hours. Many people spend around half of their day working, yet we overlook how that time affects our wellness. Many elements of our occupation alter our ability to maintain balance. It is important to bring awareness to the amount of passion we have for our work. Can we pursue our full potential in our current situation? Do we stifle parts of our personality at work?

Awareness in this dimension can have a tremendous effect on our overall health. If our current situation is not working for us, we have choices. We can change our attitude or focus our energy in a new direction. We are always facing a choice about how we feel regarding our life circumstances.

Environmental

Let's consider the spaces we occupy. We begin by bringing awareness to our immediate surroundings, such as our homes, our vehicles, and our work spaces, and work outward to include larger spaces such as our communities, our countries, and our planet. Often, the condition of our overall well-being is reflected in our personal space. When we look at our surroundings, we can get clear about whether they express who we are and who we want to be. Often, all that is necessary is to give attention to a space. It can be as simple as painting a room or adding a plant to a cubicle. It may be as large an undertaking as replanting a burned forest. Our spaces provide a wonderful opportunity to express our passion and personality.

Emotional

This dimension is centered around the emotions we attach to the events in our lives. Everything that happens can be labeled as an event. It is natural for us to have emotional reactions to events. Each emotion we attach has a result that can directly affect every other dimension. We move toward balance once we take ownership over the emotions we feel in response to the events in our lives. Things happen all day, every day that are out of our control, from wars between nations to the mood of a loved one or coworker. Once we are able to confidently say to ourselves, "I am in control over how I feel about any event," we can maintain balance in our emotional dimension, no matter what happens.

Spiritual

The spiritual dimension deals with our awareness of the piece of us that makes us unique, an awareness of something larger than ourselves. The focus is on becoming clear about what we believe in down to our core and connecting (or reconnecting) with those beliefs. This dimension is the culmination of working toward balance in all the other dimensions of health. When we are doing the things necessary to pursue balance in the other six dimensions, we free up more energy for the pursuit of spiritual balance. For some the avenue is through their religion. Others find that a simple activity such as meditation provides a very deep spiritual experience. A consistent practice in meditation is one of the most widely accepted methods by which one can work on the spiritual dimension of health. Physical activities exercise the body and quiet the mind, helping us rid ourselves of the multitude of distractions that keep us from spirit. No matter what practice we choose, the connection (or reconnection) with our spirit is the most important thing.

Conclusion

Thinking of well-being in terms of the Seven Dimensions of Health is an effective way of breaking a large challenge into smaller, manageable pieces. Seeking balance in terms of health and well-being is a lifelong journey without a final destination. The only constant in life is change, and we must continually stay active in our pursuit of balance. In focusing on each dimension, the key is cultivating self-awareness. We must accept and take ownership of our current circumstances. Once we are cognizant of where we are, we can plan our journey. The Seven Dimensions of Health are a wonderful planning tool.

About the Authors

Shawna Hansen received her BS in health ecology at the University of Nevada, Reno, and has extensive experience in the health and fitness industry. Shawna has been a certified personal trainer for over nine years.

Linda Hartmann brings with her over twenty years of experience in business and management to the Sanctuary family. Linda has taken over 144 hours of leadership training, including a master graduate honor with Rapport Leadership International.

Benson Brown received his BS in English literature from the University of Nevada, Reno. He has an extensive background in teaching martial arts and self-development programs. He is co-owner of Elite Performance, LLC, which provides leadership training for corporate and youth sports programs.

For more information on the Seven Dimensions of Health and the Sanctuary, please visit our Web site at http://www.thesanctuaryreno.com, or call (775) 853-7007.

6

Humpty Dumpty Syndrome – Getting Yourself Together

Dr. Gerard Hefferon

Remember the old nursery rhyme?

> Humpty Dumpty sat on a wall.
> Humpty Dumpty had a great fall.
> All the King's horses and all the King's men
> Couldn't put Humpty together again.

If you are old enough to recall this childhood rhyme, you are old enough to have had a few great falls of your own. Many people in our society today feel fractured and torn, pressured by the strains of everyday living, overwhelmed by the amount of pressure and speed of change in our modern world. Stress in one form or another is behind all the major killers of our time, and we simply don't know what to do about it. After all, if Humpty Dumpty couldn't be put back together again, even with all the king's horses and all the king's men to help him, what chance do we have?

Recognizing that all the king's horses and all the king's men have been replaced by the ever-expanding personal development and self-help industries, you realize that there are many guides and gurus to consult and a plethora of how-to books filling the bookstore shelves. There are groups and gatherings, programs and protocols, principles and practices all designed to help you "be all you can be." There is helpful advice all around you, enlightenment is at hand, but still, you fall in greater numbers than ever before.

Access to the multimedia world of motivation is often not enough. So how do you live your life to the fullest? How can you convert good advice received into dynamic action taken? How do you manifest your true intentions and align with your highest purpose?

To do this, you must convert from the temporary, state-dependent world of external motivation and embrace the constant, enduring world of internal transformation.

Emergent research in the field of neuroscience holds the key. According to neuroscientific research from the last fifty years, much of which was done at the

National Institutes of Health, the organ in our head we call the brain is a multifaceted entity and actually represents our development as a species and as individuals. Scientists have discovered that the heart directly influences the activity of the brain and that the brain itself is not a single neural control center, but a minimum of three distinct yet interrelated centers. These are each encoded with specific biological functional capacities and are progressively distinguished from each other in evolution and embryology.

The most primitive component, the reptilian brain, is found in all animal species and is largely concerned with survival. This part develops in the human embryo in the first trimester and comprises the autonomic tools for health maintenance and survival. This is also where you find the sensory motor system for coordinating movement, posture, and balance. It is the main focus of the developing infant in the early months.

As species progress in complexity, as the embryo enters its second trimester, these events are paralleled by the emergence of the old mammalian brain, a center containing, among other things, the limbic system, which is responsible for emotions and feelings.

As the embryo develops into the third trimester, as the moving, feeling child begins to think for itself, the new mammalian brain appears. This is where the human species distinguishes itself from the rest, with the neocortex representing the faculties and function of logic, reason, creativity, and imagination.

Each area of neural function has its specific tasks as well as an integrated role in the whole system. Each level develops when it is needed, building on and adding to those that preceded. Eventually, a complete and coordinated organic system emerges to facilitate the individual in all aspects of his being. At least, that is the theory!

Surely three brains would be better than one; after all, isn't that what elevates us to the top of the food chain? Don't we outperform the reptiles and other mammals because of our cranial complexity? Didn't our big brains give us electricity and cell phones and iPods?

The problem is that this complexity can cause conflict and that chaos ensues when there is a lack of coherence. Think about it: these three brains, the paleo-, meso-, and neocortex, secure your survival, govern your emotions, and endow you with the capacity for rational thought, imagination, and creativity. While your primitive brain might tell you that you simply must survive, your thinking brain can encourage you to recognize your own divinity. Who should you believe? Who should you listen to?

When you try to apply the methods of manifestation you have learned, where should you apply them, and which area do they address? Before you know what will work for you, you need to determine where you are operating from. Are you coming from a place of deep insecurity, operating mainly from survival mode? Are you missing out on fulfilling relationships because you are still suffering from a previous emotional hurt? Are your interactions with your team based solely on logic and lacking in interpersonal connectivity and depth? Where you are relating from indicates which brain is in play and determines which modalities will be most useful to you at that time.

Understanding addiction provides an excellent template for this concept. Programs that focus on logical processes are usually not as effective as those that incorporate emotional and spiritual aspects of recovery. Changing behavior through a rational grasp of the prevailing situation and circumstances of your life is a difficult, slow and laborious process but is more rapidly achieved when you feel and believe what you need and want to be necessary in your life.

When you seek to rise above, to change the circumstances without, it is necessary to first create coherence within. Coherence is the difference between a lightbulb and a laser. Coherence converts diffuse, scattered photons into powerful, energetic beams. Coherence enables focused waves of light to cut through metal, to heal injured tissue, and to carry energy and information across the universe. To create coherence, you must reflect inwardly, harness the power of you, and direct focused attention toward creating and achieving your desired and intended outcome. You must create coherent action between all three brains to design the lifestyle you deserve.

Becoming coherent in yourself, entraining your entire system to your highest purpose, will turbo charge any and all attempts to reach your highest goals. You must think, feel, and act in alignment to fulfill your potential and transform any life situation from chaos to coherence.

Look within to your inner world; learn to meditate, resonate, and attract; and remember how to pray. Put your head in the clouds, and keep your feet on the ground.

Remember that the way to a whole, healthy, and happy life is to let your heart decide what to do, let your mind figure out how to do it, and allow your spirit govern the whole process.

When asked who he would like to have been if he had the choice of being anyone from any time in history, George Bernard Shaw said he would like to have been the man he could have been. Coherent entrainment of thoughts, feelings, and actions allows us all to be all we can be.

About the Author

Dr. Hefferon is a chiropractor and sports physician who teaches and trains students and practitioners internationally in the SynerChi Systems (SCS) concept. SCS focuses on the "seven brains," the "four elements," and the "Coherent Entrainment" model of health, well-being, and personal development. Visit http://www.synerchisystems.com.

7

Being Alive

Colleen Miller, JD, CPCC

Where would you rate your aliveness this minute on a scale of one to ten (one being "I am surprised I still have a pulse" and ten being "I am so excited to be alive that I can hardly wait to take my next breath")? Do you remember a time when most of your days were lived at a nine or ten? For most of us, this was when we were small children of three or four. Remember when you could imagine you were a superhero or a princess and connect so completely with all your senses that, for a time, you became whatever you imagined? Do you remember how it felt to be a child? One minute you were happy and laughing, engrossed in your play, then something would happen that felt like the end of the world, and you were sobbing inconsolably—life was over. Then, miracle of miracles, life did go on, your tears ended, and you quickly moved on to a new set of feelings, engrossed in something else. You completely experienced whatever feeling occurred in the moment, released it, and then focused on whatever showed up in the next moment. The smallest new discovery was awe inspiring and wonderful. The world was filled with laughter and magic. At the age of three, you stated the truth of how you really felt. You laughed out loud, you yelled at the top of your lungs, you sang, you danced, you made messes and became one, you played full out until the game got called, and sometimes you fell asleep in your dinner.

Then what happened? You were taught to behave appropriately, in a socially ordered manner, that pleased the people around you, and in doing, so you learned to suppress and perhaps even be afraid of that intoxicatingly thrilling, but unpredictable spontaneity of being present, feeling everything, and expressing how you felt, fully, completely aware and engaged, living as if each moment were all that existed. As your socialization, education, and societal programming continued, you learned to suppress more and more of your feelings as being inappropriate.

Many of us grew into adults who have suppressed and shut away so much of our vitality and vigorous aliveness that we are no longer capable of fully experiencing ourselves, our aliveness, or our creativity. No wonder as adults many of us are prone to feelings of depression and alienation. *Just talking about this is depressing the hell out of me!*

But here's the deal: this is not the worst of it. Psychoneuroimmunology is the scientific study of the interaction among emotions, the brain, and the immune system. Led by the work of Candace Pert, these scientists see the emotions as the doorway into the body-mind interaction. Their studies have demonstrated that different emotions produce different chemicals in our bodies. Positive, happy, joyous feelings produce greater concentrations of such feel-good chemicals as serotonin, dopamine, and endorphins, while negative, angry, stress-related feelings produce more cortisol-type chemicals that suppress the immune system and cause general havoc in the body.

However, just working to churn out as many feel-good chemicals as possible is not going to be of much benefit to us if we are also denying our negative feelings. The real damage to our bodies occurs when the body's freely flowing emotional juices are blocked by buried thoughts and feelings, which interrupt the natural flow of the body's autonomic processes, which, in turn, interferes with the body's normal healing and regenerative responses. These studies indicate that we must acknowledge and claim all our emotions, not just the positive, more socially acceptable ones. Emotions like anger, grief, and fear are essential to survival. When these feelings are denied and suppressed and are not processed, they can become toxic to the body. In other words, stuffing our feelings or denying we even have negative feelings creates interruptions in the flow of energy in the body down to the cellular level and lays the groundwork for disharmony and disease in the body-mind.

Well, just great! What are we supposed to do about this? We were all able to do this once, be in the moment, feel every emotion fully and completely and then release it and move on. Remember? What would it be like to live life the way we did when we were three years old? That kid holds much of our power, our spontaneity, and our ability to respond in the moment. He or she can also freely access our creativity and the vast power of our imagination. When we grew into adulthood, most of us mistakenly put away all the things of childhood, including all these powers. We began the process of slowly—or, for some of us, not so slowly—killing ourselves by taking life more and more seriously, suppressing more of our authentic selves and our passionate aliveness and the glorious panoply of all our diverse emotions in the belief that we must make these sacrifices to be responsible, successful adults. *Ugh!*

No wonder we are going around depressed, disillusioned, burned out, and popping antidepressants like popcorn at the movies. When we put away our toys and quit playing and forgot that life is only a game, we lost access to the best part of ourselves.

Reclaim the power of that three-year-old! Start to play again. Restart the flow of your emotions by playing in your life as if it were the game it really is. Plato said, "Life must be lived as play." Playing reconnects us to others and helps us lighten up, instantly reduces stress, reestablishes our emotional flow, and easily moves us into present time, heightening our awareness and reconnecting us to our creativity.

Attitude is very important to healing and remaining well. Being interested, curious, and playful is a proven formula for living longer. Surround yourself with people who honor these values. I require my dentist to give toys. Kids shouldn't be the only ones being rewarded. I insist that they provide good ones, too—no cheesy fake vampire teeth.

Your three-year-old could also be counted on to tell the truth, most especially about how he or she felt about things. By acknowledging and being present with all your feelings as they appear, expressing them, then releasing them, you honor yourself, your right to feel, and ultimately, you free yourself to become the full expression of your authentic self.

One Sunday, when our children were small and I was still invested in being the perfect mommy, I was going to make waffles in our new waffle iron. I'd had problems with it sticking before but was sure I had the problem solved. After picking out all the stuck-on dough with a toothpick and carefully oiling it, I was sure I'd make perfect waffles. The dough stuck everywhere. I cleaned it again, which took forever, while the kids were carrying on about being so hungry they could die, making noise and being generally obnoxious. This time, under severe pressure, I pulled out all the stops, put more oil in the batter, used cooking spray on the grids, made sure the temperature was exactly right. It was going to work for sure . . . when it stuck this time, it triggered something in me. I unplugged that waffle iron and took it out to the back deck, grabbed it by the handle, and threw it like a discus as far as I could throw it. It hit the back fence and broke into a hundred pieces. I felt such joy and freedom. Woman versus stupid machine! We had pancakes for breakfast, and the back fence became the graveyard for crappy appliances that didn't work. It was great! My inner three-year-old was cheering up a storm, and the kids thought it was awesome!

Recapturing the power of our inner child invites us to view the world with that sense of wonder and possibility that makes every day exciting and worth exploring. Engaging with the world from a child's honest willingness to tell the truth, feeling all that is there to feel, then moving on may be the most powerful gift you can give to your life and your health.

About the Author

After receiving a BA in psychology, Colleen A. Miller, JD, CPCC, went on to obtain a law degree and practice personal injury and family law for twelve years. Colleen is an entrepreneur, having created three successful businesses, and is now working as a certified life and relationship coach. As a transformational speaker and facilitator, she has helped people and organizations all over the country rediscover their vision and passion, reconnect with their power, and realize that they have all the tools they need, right now, to build the life, business, and relationships of their dreams. Visit her Web site at http://www.lightenupconsulting.com.

8

Enthusiastic Affirmations for Glowing Health

Betsy B. Muller, MBA, CEC, C.EHP

Be not lax in celebrating. Be not lazy in the festive service of God. Be ablaze with enthusiasm.
—Hildegarde von Bingen

When you embrace the connection of body, mind, and spirit as the foundation for creating optimal health, enthusiastic affirmations are a powerful way to take action.

Why would positive words and thoughts make such a positive difference to health? Affirmations mobilize emotions of optimism, which in turn keep unhealthy stress responses in check. Clinical studies have correlated optimism to the strength of our hearts, long-term cancer survival, a slowed pace of aging, a stronger immune response, and faster postsurgical recovery.[1]

Take a look at the Law of Attraction, a simple reminder that like attracts like. Affirmations are an incredible way of putting healthy energy into motion by creating an "attractor field" that becomes a magnet for attracting more health. It is all so simple—just practice a minute or two of affirmation time each day, and you initiate the process to attract radiant health to your physical body.

You can coach and empower yourself with affirmations through all sorts of life challenges, including health issues. Just follow the four simple steps on the following page.

---

[1] Charles S. Carver, "Optimistic Personality and Psychosocial Well-Being during Treatment Predict Psychosocial Well-Being among Long-Term Survivors of Breast Cancer," Health Psychology 24 (2005): 508–16; Glenn V. Ostir, "Onset of Frailty in Older Adults and the Protective Role of Positive Affect," Psychology and Aging 19 (2004): 402–8; M. F. Scheier and C. S. Carver, "Effects of Optimism on Psychological and Physical Well-Being: Theoretical Overview," Cognitive Therapy and Research 16 (1992): 201–28.

1. *Accept and Appreciate the Now*

Find something about your health to appreciate right now. Be grateful for the present situation. Even if you are dealing with a significant challenge, surgery, physical pain, or treatment, search deeply, and you will find something good. Speak words of appreciation *aloud* to express your acceptance for the present state.

Here are some affirmations appropriate for someone recovering from surgery or undergoing cancer treatment:

- I enjoy having enough energy to walk today.
- My digestive system is comfortable and efficient.
- I appreciate feeling rested when I awaken.
- I can comfortably push my body to do a little bit more today than yesterday.
- I enjoy experiencing my surroundings through my senses.
- I am alert and appreciate the people who are caring for me.

2. *Create Affirmations That Express Your Wildest Wishes*

Here's where you can have enormous fun. Develop a list of affirmations that express how you really wish things were. As you create these statements, allow your positive emotions to amplify. What would it feel like to actually feel twenty years younger? Get in touch with the joy and enthusiasm you hold for the possibility of something better. Make yourself a visually beautiful list, and post it for easy reference. Leave space to add new thoughts as these come up.

Here are a few of my favorite affirmations for people longing to feel younger, healthier, and more energetic:

- I am blessed to live in a body that feels as if it was twenty years younger.
- My body responds in wonderful ways when I make healthy choices.
- I am an example of health that inspires everyone I meet.
- I respond remarkably well to natural treatments.
- I am in tune with my body at all times, and it feels great!
- My skin radiates a healthy glow.
- I am passionate about my own health and the health of others.
- I believe health miracles happen all the time—even for me!
- I believe that a healthier body starts with my positive thoughts.
- My health radiates, even as I get older.

3. *Set Aside Time Each Day to Say Your Affirmations Out Loud with Emotion and Enthusiasm*

When I say out *loud*, that's exactly what I mean. Say affirmations *boldly*, with excitement. Use emphatic speech. Give your affirmations positive energy through positive emotion. Sprinkle in a bit of laughter if this seems too silly—that's healthy, too. Emphasis and positive emotion will launch these affirmations as targets for attraction.

Amp it up by tapping on meridians as you speak. I love to tap on the Emotional Freedom Techniques (http://www.emofree.com) meridian points while I say each affirmation for a powerful jolt of uplifting energy. Try it, and you'll be hooked.

4. *Return to Step 1—and Notice the Good Things That Emerge*

Create new statements to recognize your progress. Celebrate your success openly with others. Be your own healing coach. You are a creator with amazing power to attract positive change. Have fun setting your health into motion as you enjoy building an optimistic vocabulary to support and sustain your health. Don't forget to share these secrets with everyone you meet! We all deserve radiant health.

About the Author

Betsy B. Muller, MBA, CEC, C.EHP, is a holistic business coach, certified energy health practitioner, and speaker based in northeast Ohio. After decades working in a variety of traditional business and health care management settings, life changed in 2001 when she discovered energy psychology techniques at a conference in Switzerland. Since then, her passion has been to help others enjoy balanced and purposeful lives by integrating energy modalities into life and business applications. Her company offers individual coaching by phone and in person, training programs, and events. Ms. Muller holds a BA in chemistry and a MBA in systems management. Contact Betsy at http://www.TheIndigoConnection.com or (440) 238-4731.

9

Laugh, Don't Laugh

Jeff Niswonger

When was the last time you really laughed?

I am not referring to a giggle or a chuckle. What I am talking about is side-splitting, jaw-aching, tears-running-down-your-face, all-out, roll-on-the-floor laughing. If you are like most of us, it has been longer than you can remember.

The truth is that we need to laugh, we want to laugh, and we always feel better after we have a good laugh. *So why not just laugh?* Because life has become too serious. In our busy, hectic, stressed out schedules, we have lost the time and ability to laugh.

I say that now is the time to rediscover the joys and benefits of this contagious emotion called laughter.

We have always placed a tremendous amount of focus on this universal language of humor, comedy, and laughter. From as far back as the ancient Greek god of mischief, Dionysus, we have been seeking this emotional release and feeling. We have comedy movies, comedy television, comedy radio, and more recently, laugh coaches, laugh yoga, and laugh e-mail. We have more outside sources of comedy and humor than at any time in history.

Why All This Focus on Making Us Laugh?

Because it's good for you, it's healthy, it's fun, and it has no known side effects, except that it can easily be shared with others. Laughter lifts our spirits, gives us a better outlook on our day, and improves our behavior toward others by connecting with them in a natural way. Laughing lowers blood pressure, reduces stress hormones, and boosts immune function by raising levels of infection-fighting T-cells and disease-fighting proteins called gamma-interferon and B-cells, which produce disease-destroying antibodies. Laughter also triggers the release of endorphins, our natural painkillers, and produces a general sense and feeling of well-being and connectedness to others and ourselves. These findings have been published in several studies by Dr. Lee Berk and Dr. Stanley Tan of Loma Linda University in California over the past twenty years.

It has even been reported that laughter can provide an excellent source of cardiac exercise. When you monitor your pulse after a good side-splitting belly laugh, you find that your heart is racing, and your pulse will continue to be elevated for three to five minutes after the laughter is over. This type of cardiac conditioning has been called "internal jogging" by some researchers and can be as beneficial as aerobic exercise if done several times throughout the day.

On the emotional side, laughter can strengthen the bond of most relationships and can establish a positive emotional climate and a sense of connection, a feeling of togetherness. Most of us are naturally drawn to others who exhibit a good sense of humor because they make us feel good. We often take a lighter approach to our own problems when we see others laughing at theirs. When we can laugh at a problem or situation, it gives us a sense of superiority and control. Laughter can help create a positive outlook to what could be a negative situation. We are less likely to feel helpless in a situation if we can laugh at what is troubling us.

While all these benefits of laughter are great, the most important is that it just feels good. We sense a feeling of emotional relief, a sense of relaxation and calm, after we have experienced a good laugh. While what actually causes these effects may not be totally understood, we can certainly appreciate them and use them to improve our emotional state, relationships, health, and well-being.

Laughter is a muscle like any other: it can be strengthened and improved with regular, positive use and exercise, or it can grow weak and useless if not used. We all know someone who never laughs. He takes everything seriously, always seems grumpy, and feels disconnected from everyone. Laughter's most important attribute is creating a sense of connectedness. Most women have said that the first and most important trait they look for in a mate is a good sense of humor because a good sense of humor shows that you can connect with others in a loving way. It reveals that a person can connect with another in a lighthearted, emotional way, which will lead to more open communication in most other areas of any relationship.

Laughter is more about social and emotional relationships than it is about the humor itself. We know that the moods and emotions we experience have a direct effect on our feelings of connectedness with others in any relationship. Now we realize that by building up the muscle called our sense of humor, we can learn to laugh at the curve balls that life may throw at us and take a lighter approach to the people and obstacles in our life.

Does Having a Good Sense of Humor and an Ability to Laugh More Often Prevent Illness?

While very limited research has been done to substantiate this claim, it may be true. People that have a happy, more joyous outlook on life will naturally turn on the immune system metabolically and increase its ability to do what it is designed to do: protect and promote healing when external and internal threats to the body occur. To gain the full benefits, emotionally and physically, it may be necessary to change the perspective you have of your life. If you currently subscribe to the idea that something outside yourself needs to change for you to become the lighthearted, joke-telling, full-of-laughter person you want to be, you may need to take a look at the internal changes that would make the difference. Begin by changing your internal dialogue from one of stress and problems to one of joy and opportunities. Look for the opportunities to laugh, to smile, and to connect with another. Seize the moment—be the difference to make the difference.

You Can Decide to Laugh or Not Laugh: The Choice Is Yours

It is suggested that to maintain a healthy physical and emotional state, we should laugh fifteen to twenty minutes each day. Find new ways to laugh. Build a laugh library of all your favorite comedians and jokes. Subscribe to one of the joke of the day e-mail services. Learn to see life in a more joyous, nonstressful way. Observe children playing and laughing. Whatever works for you, find it and use it daily to create a better, lighter sense about you and life, and don't take everything so seriously.

As Groucho Marx said, "A clown is like an aspirin, only he works twice as fast."

About the Author

Jeff Niswonger is a professional life coach, mentor, author, and business consultant. With over twenty-five years' experience in personal and professional development through books, articles, seminars, coaching, consulting, and hands-on experience, he has helped many individuals and businesses realize their full potential. He is currently promoting his book, *Reflections to Feelings: A Coach's Journal,* which gives the reader an inside out approach to many years of wisdom, education, and practical experience. Books, articles, and services are available through http://www.YourLifeYourDreams.com. Jeff can be reached at jnis@centurytel.net or (509) 209-1431.

10

Your Brain in the Modern World

Alessandro Tamborrino

The stress that accompanies our lives can, at times, overwhelm us. Sadly, we are coping with stress by becoming a nation of addicts. According to a 2002 survey conducted by the Substance Abuse and Mental Health Services Administration, there are nineteen million drug users, sixteen million heavy drinkers, and seventy-one million smokers in the United States.[1] These numbers don't reflect those addicted to shopping, gambling, cybersex, video games, MP3 players, and caffeine. There are centers for Internet addiction and recovery, and establishments like Starbucks seem to be sprouting up all over the country like tulips in springtime.

The Pleasure Chemical

Scientists studying the neurochemistry of addiction found greater levels of dopamine and adrenaline in the brains of addicts.[2] Dopamine is a brain chemical associated with feelings of pleasure, well-being, and motivation. But stress lowers dopamine levels, in addition to serotonin, another neurotransmitter. In attempting to restore homeostasis, the brain transmits signals to increase these neurochemicals. Dopamine, with its powerful ability to form triggers with anything that is pleasurable, motivates us to seek satisfaction. Little surprise that the greatest surges of dopamine are caused by sex, drugs, and food.

---

[1] Substance Abuse and Mental Health Services Administration, *Results from the 2002 National Health Survey on Drug Use and Health: National Findings* (Washington, DC: U.S. Department of Health and Human Services, 2002).

[2] N. D. Volkow, J. S. Fowler, A. P. Wolf, D. Schlyer, C. Y. Shiue, R. Albert, S. L. Dewey, J. Logan, B. Bendriem, D. Christman, R. Hitzemann, and F. Henn, "Effects of Chronic Cocaine Abuse on Postsynaptic Dopamine Receptors," *American Journal of Psychiatry* 147 (1990): 719–24; N. D. Volkow, J. S. Fowler, G. J. Wang, R. Hitzemann, J. Logan, D. Schlyer, S. Dewey, and A. P. Wolfe, "Decreased Dopamine D2 Receptor Availability Is Associated with Reduced Frontal Metabolism in Cocaine Abusers," *Synapse* 14 (1993): 169–77.

Neuroplasticity

Research on the effects of long-term stress found that adults with elevated cortisol, the stress hormone, had, on average, a 14 percent smaller hippocampus.[3] The hippocampus is the brain region critical to the formation of new memories, and although prolonged stress can wreak havoc on the hippocampus, the brain is not defenseless.

One of the most important adaptive mechanisms we have is that our brain is not hard-wired with a predetermined number of neuronal circuits. The brain has a remarkable ability to remodel neuronal connections in response to the acquisition of new information and experience, a function known as neuroplasticity. About 90 percent of brain cells are composed of a type of cell known as glias. These cells stimulate the growth of neurons and appear to guide them to the exact place to form synapses. Glial cells also help in the repair of damaged synapses. In a fascinating analysis completed after dissecting Einstein's brain, researchers found that he had 73 percent more glial cells in comparison to the number observed in the brains of average people. The researchers concluded that Einstein's high percentage of glial cells is the result of greater connectivity between neurons and synapses.[4]

Creating the Twenty-first-Century Mind

Managing Stress

Reducing stress is one of the best things you can do for the health of your brain. Integrating these proven stress busters into your daily regimen will have a beneficial effect on brain function.

- *Laughter, humor, and play.* These lead to the formation of new neural connections, increase activity in the nucleus acumbens, and stimulate dopamine and GABA production, thus promoting creativity, relaxation, and alertness.
- *Visualization.* Alternately known as guided imagery, visualization consciously directs your imagination and creates a sense of well-being and relaxation.
- *Deep breathing.* We tend to take shallow breaths when feeling stress. One way to ensure deep breathing is with the practice of yoga. There is a breathing technique called "pranayama" (breath control), and one of its purposes is to bring more oxygen to the blood and brain.

---

[3] Bruce S. McEwen, "Plasticity of the Hippocampus: Adaptation to Chronic Stress and Allostatic Load," *Annals of the New York Academy of Sciences* 933 (2001). 265–77.

[4] M. C. Diamond, A. B. Scheibel, G. M. Murphy, and T. Harvey, "On the Brain of a Scientist: Albert Einstein," *Experimental Neurology* 88 (1985): 198–204.

- *Meditation.* This can provide proven benefits for the mind and body, reduce stress, lower blood pressure, and promote greater focus and concentration.
- *Physical activity.* Exercise or any vigorous movement will result in greater blood flow to the brain, promote neurogenesis, and increase dopamine, serotonin, norepinephrine, and endorphin levels. Exercise is a natural antidepressant.
- *Brain wave training.* Creative thinking occurs best when your brain is in a state called "alpha and theta." However, accessing an alpha and theta state is not all that easy. But with a brain wave machine, you can easily glide into alpha and theta states. It's like a digital drug, allowing you to access parts of your mind that are usually activated during peak experiences.

Raw Energy

Quite possibly the healthiest diet to detoxify, cleanse, and rejuvenate the brain is a raw food diet. I know firsthand about the amazing power of raw foods for it became the catalyst to a remarkable transformation in my life. During my tenure as a raw food chef at Hippocrates Health Institute, I stood witness to the miraculous healing properties of living foods in others.

The basic raw and living food diet consists of uncooked fruits, vegetables, and nuts; sprouted seeds, legumes, and grains; fermented foods and green drinks. Whole foods that are raw and alive are packed with enzymes that accelerate our metabolic processes. This is one of the reasons why raw foods are so healing. These enzymes provide tremendous vibrational energies, and the transfer of this energy into our bodies cleanses the blood and lymph system and removes toxins from the brain and other major organs.

There is a subset of the population that may not thrive in the long run on a raw food diet. And yet, even for those individuals, raw foods can still offer important health benefits.

Supplements for a Super Brain

It would be ideal to obtain concentrated amounts of brain-building nutrients from natural food. In truth, it is very difficult. The next best thing, however, is to take high-quality supplements to ensure optimal amounts of these valuable nutrients. Following are some of my favorites for maximizing brain power.

1. Acetyl-L-carnitine (ALC) prevents brain cells from deteriorating with its powerful antioxidant properties. ALC protects against the loss of receptors in brain cells as we age. It also strengthens the mitochondria, the power plants inside each cell, and increases acetylcholine levels, a neurotransmitter critical to memory.

2. Nicotinamide adenine dinucleotide (NADH) is the coenzyme form of vitamin B$_3$ and is needed by cells to produce energy. NADH boosts levels of adenosine triphosphate (ATP), which powers the activity in every cell. NADH stimulates brain activity by facilitating the turnover of tyrosine to dopamine, thus supporting mood, energy, and drive.
3. Omega-3 fatty acids play a crucial role in the structure of the brain and help optimize its function. The two most important omega-3 fatty acids are docosahexaenoic acid (DHA) and eicosapentaenoic acid (EFA). In the brain, DHA is found at the cell membrane and the synapse, facilitating the transmission of signals between neurons. DHA is also found in glial cells, assisting in their functions. Both DHA and EFA help inhibit inflammatory prostaglandins and promote blood flow in the brain through vasodilation. Some of the best food sources for omega-3s are wild Atlantic salmon, herring, mackerel, sardines, and flax oil.
4. DHEA is a hormone that acts as a neuroprotector and counteracts the effects of cortisol. It has been shown to inhibit the accumulation of beta-amyloid plaque, which is commonly found in persons with Alzheimer's disease. DHEA declines with age, particularly after forty.
5. Phosphatidylserine (PS) is present in every cell of the body and heavily concentrated in the membranes of brain cells. PS maintains the fluidity of cell membranes, promoting cell-to-cell communication. In the brain, PS protects dendritic connections in the hippocampus, promotes the availability of acetylcholine, stimulates the release of dopamine, lowers levels of cortisol, and increases the uptake of glucose.
6. L-theanine is an amino acid naturally found in green tea. Research has shown that L-theanine increases production of alpha brain waves, the brain waves responsible for relaxed wakefulness. L-theanine also heightens mental acuity and concentration, while reducing stress and anxiety. These seemingly contradictory effects are thought be to achieved by increases in GABA, an inhibitory neurotransmitter, and dopamine, a stimulating neurotransmitter, as well as by changes in serotonin levels.
7. Ginkgo biloba improves blood flow to the brain, increases the amount of neural transmission, and increases the number of receptor sites for neural transmission.

Recreating the Self Recreates the World

Awakening to our full human potential begins by eliminating the negative stress in our lives, detoxifying our brains, and overcoming the addictions that block the flow of our energy. By breaking the shackles that bind us, we release a power akin to a supernova. A brain that is irrigated with living foods, supernutrients, and a nurturing environment becomes alive to the world and its breathtaking possibilities. The premise and promise of the twenty-first-century mind is to transform our lives and manifest our inner genius. If ever there was a time to tap into the wellspring of creativity and vitality that resides within each of us, that time is now.

About the Author

Alessandro Tamborrino is a health and nutrition writer, medical copywriter, musician, and was a raw food chef at Hippocrates Health Institute. Early on in his career, he wrote satire for a national humor magazine. His writing has been featured on Gary Null's "Natural Living" radio program, and his work was commissioned by psychologist Armand DeMille for the WBAI radio program "The Positive Mind." At present, he is working on a communication program for mass media. Visit his Web site at http://www.VitaCreativa.com.

11

Love Your Body, Forgive Your Self

Laura Turner, MS, CHHP

This may sound a bit odd coming from me, but I believe that regardless of what you eat, how many times each week you exercise, or what particular diet you decide to try, if you do not have your inner life in order, it will be difficult to be at peace with yourself and your body.

In discussing ways to love your body, therefore, it is important to look at ways we can have peace with ourselves. Moreover, in this article, we will discuss an idea you may not have considered: forgiveness.

The Past Is the Past—Let It Go

The most important process we can undertake for our health and well-being is to make a conscious effort not to leave negative energy embedded in the past. In an effort to move into present time and be at one with our own bodies, it becomes essential to let go of all the hurts and struggles that have led us to this moment. There is only one road to this state of oneness, however: the act of letting go.

As it turns out, I'm not the only one who stands by the belief system of releasing the past in an effort to improve the health of our minds as well as our bodies and spirits. Caroline Myss, in her healing lecture series "Why People Don't Heal," makes the claim that forgiveness is the number one way to move forward in health. And she can back it up. She has used the healing process of letting go to transform people from near death to glowing health. With this in mind, then, ask yourself, Is there anyone or anything from my past that prevents me from moving forward? Said differently, is there something in your past that's holding you back?

Learn to Forgive Others—The Process

This brings us to the next step in our progress of releasing the past: learning to forgive others. Keep in mind that most often, others say and do things as a result of how they are feeling about themselves. In most cases, whether they are aware of it or not, unhealthy individuals inflict their wounds on us to salve their own pain. This can no longer affect us if we make a full effort to do as Don Miguel Ruiz says in his book *The Four Agreements* and "not take things personally." When we do take things personally, we really could gather up a lifetime of emotional baggage.

As it pertains to body image and self-esteem, however, is there anyone you need to forgive? Has someone knowingly or unknowingly inflicted a negative body view onto you? Here's my personal example: when I was in high school, I had a friend who was popular, pretty, and blonde. As an introvert and troubled youth, I took everything most personally. Imagine my emotional baggage when any time I would so much as mention my interest in a particular boy, she'd make sure to go out of her way to get his interest.

Needless to say, our friendship wasn't long term. And later, I learned that she was living in an unstable home. Yet when I was younger, her actions just plain hurt my feelings and gave me a negative self-image. Now I realize that my insecurities at the time were my wounds to heal, and once I'd forgiven her and not taken her actions personally, I could move forward without holding on to past insecurity.

Learn to Live in the Present—An Exercise

When we can learn to let go of the past and live fully in the present, we are also growing. After all, how could we grow if we have negative energy lodged in the past? Moreover, there are many other active ways to learn to live in the present. Begin the process by taking a current inventory of your body. I like to do this by using my journal (you do have a journal, don't you?).

Here's how it works:

- Take a scan of your body. First, take body part by body part, and make a note of what you are happy about. Ask yourself, What do I love about me? At first, this may seem awkward, but I cannot stress the importance of taking time to spend time with yourself and learning to know you.
- After you've noted all the positive aspects of yourself, make note of those parts you'd like to change. Keep in mind your boundaries—are these changes within your control? If so, make notes to yourself as to how you may go about making a change for the better. If changes are out of your control, take time every day to consciously send love to those parts of your body. Whenever possible, tell your mind that you accept your body and yourself for who you are, right now.

- When you've finished, take a look at your list. What can you do right now that would make you love a part of yourself? Consider this your permission slip: today, take time to do something good for yourself. Better yet, walk to the phone right now and make an appointment. My favorite self-love activities? Here are a couple suggestions. Ladies: a manicure or pedicure? Gentlemen: a massage?

Today, take time to focus on all your positive qualities. Make an effort to forgive the past and move into the present moment. Prepare to grow. Remember that exercise and proper nutrition are not always enough to achieve good health. You must be healthy on the inside first, and the first step toward emotional health is a positive self-image and mastering the art of forgiveness.

About the Author

Laura M. Turner is an author and certified holistic health practitioner through the Association of Drugless Practitioners. She publishes the "New Body News and Wellness Letter" (http://www.new-body-news.com) and is dedicated to inspiring and empowering others to live in the ways of health and wellness. You can heal yourself! Let Laura show you how with her latest book, *Spiritual Fitness: The 7 Steps to Living Well.*

PART TWO

Diet & Nutrition

Tell me what you eat,
and I will tell you what you are.

-- Jean Anthelme Brillat-Savarin

12

Going Organic: Why the Big Fuss?

Alia Almoayed, BSc, MA, Dip BCNH, mBANT

Someone once said, "I don't believe that paying extra for organic food will benefit anybody but those who sell it."

There are a lot of people out there who are opposed to buying or eating organic food. I do not know why, but it is possible that the main reason is that it is hard to change; the status quo is always easier to maintain.

When it comes to health in general, and organic food in particular, there is a lack of information. Consumers are bombarded with mixed media messages about what is better for them, and they do not know what they should do. Also, the size of the organic industry is relatively small; organic farmers and companies are still not big enough to compete with their nonorganic commercial counterparts.

Furthermore, organic laws are not standardized worldwide and do not even exist in some countries, which makes it hard for organic producers to thrive. As a result, organic food is not easily accessible and often has the image of being for so-called health nerds.

So what do you need to know about organic food? *Going organic* can have a tremendous effect on your health. Knowing about organic food and its effects on your body is the first step toward making your own choices about your health and well-being.

What Is Organic?

The definition of organic food differs depending on whom you ask. Most Western countries, Canada being the first in 1999, have established national organic standards that make the definition clearer.

In the United States, for example, organic food is defined as food that is produced by farmers who emphasize the use of renewable resources and the conservation of soil and water to enhance environmental quality for future generations. Organic meat, poultry, eggs, and dairy products come from animals that are given no antibiotics or growth hormones. Organic food is produced without using most conventional pesticides, petroleum-based fertilizers, or sewage sludge-based fertilizers, bio-engineering, or ionizing radiation. Before a product can be labeled "organic," a government-approved certifier inspects the farm where the food is grown to make sure the farmer is following all the rules necessary to meet organic standards. Companies that handle or process organic food before it gets to the local supermarket or restaurant must be certified too.[1]

Organic farmers also use methods such as crop rotation, recycling wastes to return nutrients to the land, effective pest management of encouraging beneficial predators and micro-organisms, and providing attentive care for farm animals.

After reading the definition of organic food, you start to realize that nonorganic food can have strange things. If "sewage sludge-based fertilizers" are not allowed on organic farms, are they used in ordinary farms? Sewage sludge! And that's not all: nonorganic food is treated and sprayed with a cocktail of pesticides, fertilizers, and chemicals that the average person is not aware of. And these chemicals are used even more abundantly in countries where the laws are not as defined.

Is Organic Food Better for Us?

Yes. In short, organic food is free of chemicals. Chemicals are toxic to the body. The more toxins we have in our bodies, the more prone to disease and illness we are. To get rid of toxins, our body uses all the essential nutrients, and we end up with very little to stay healthy.

People react differently to toxins, just like they do to medicines or foods. The effect of toxins will depend on the levels of toxins in the food, the period of exposure, and the health of the person receiving them. For example, a lot of cancers often occur at an older age because certain individuals have had a lifetime of toxin exposure that the body can no longer handle.

Some other effects of chemicals and toxins in our bodies include hormonal problems, infertility, asthma, eczema, allergies, headaches, and brain-related disorders such as mood swings, depression, autism, and attention-deficit/hyperactivity disorder.

Is organic food more nutritious? The nutrient content of the plant is determined mostly by heredity, but also by the mineral content of the soil. And because organic soil is exposed to crop rotation and many fewer chemicals, it is very likely that the products are more nutrient-dense.

Does organic food taste better? I think so, but I am biased. So try it for yourself and decide. To me, for example, the difference in taste between an organic and nonorganic apple is huge. A child once asked me, "Does organic food taste like

---

[1] Uncle Matt's Organic, "The Organic Advantage," http://www.unclematts.com/organicadvantage.html (accessed March 26, 2007).

fresh flowers?" I do not know because I have never eaten a flower, but I sure would like to think so.

Do organic fruits and vegetables look better? Probably not. Fruits and vegetables are not supposed to look perfect. If you buy a tomato, for example, and it looks perfect, then you take it home and it sits in your fridge for over a week, still looking perfect, then it's probably modified and sprayed. Natural fruits and vegetables have a shorter shelf life, and it is very normal to find them with some bruises and odd shapes.

What Can You Do?

- Do not stop eating fruits and vegetables for fear of pesticides and chemicals. The benefits of fruits and vegetables outweigh the possible risks of chemicals.
- Wash fruits and vegetables very well before consumption. Washing with water is not enough. Wash fruits and vegetables in a tub of water with added sea salt, vinegar, or baking soda to remove all the spray residues. You can also buy a small brush to scrub them with.
- Start your own vegetable garden in your backyard. This is very simple and economical, and as organic as you make it.
- Encourage local vegetable vendors by buying their produce if it is not sprayed.
- Find out which farms have organic milk and organic or free-range chicken and eggs, and buy from them.
- Buy organic food if you have access to it. Although organic products are marginally more expensive, you are not just paying for a more "natural" version, you are also paying for the organic farming and handling that went into it. With more people buying organic products over time, prices will go down.
- Buy organic food for babies and children. Children's bodies react very readily to chemicals, just as they thrive on natural foods.
- Get more information on how to get organic food by asking your local supermarket for their organic products or visiting a health food store.

Organic Food Myths

- Organic food has no pesticides at all. FALSE: Organic farmers are allowed to use various specific chemicals (not including cytotoxic chemicals that are carbon-based).
- Organic farmers use no antibiotics. FALSE: On organic farms, antibiotics would not be permitted as growth stimulants but would only be permitted to counter infections.
- All organic products are better for us than nonorganic products. FALSE: I saw a fruit jam at the supermarket that was labeled "organic." However, when I read

the ingredients, I found that the first ingredient was organic sugar. Although the product was organic and all the ingredients in it were organic, that jam had more sugar than it did fruit! Shop smart.

About the Author

Alia Almoayed, BSc, MA, Dip BCNH, mBANT, is a nutritional therapist running a busy nutrition consulting office in the Kingdom of Bahrain, serving the whole Middle East region. She writes regular health articles for several media publications, holds lectures and seminars about health and nutrition, and runs various weight loss projects. She is also the author *of I Want Healthy Kids,* a nutrition and lifestyle guide on how to raise healthy kids. For more information, to get regular email health tips, or to receive Alia's free report entitled *5 Secrets Your Doctor Won't Tell You About Your Health,* visit http://www.AliaAlmoayed.com.

13

Living Foods: The Next Evolutionary Step

Gabriel Cousens, MD, MD (H), DD

The power of live foods for healing is being more and more supported by traditional research. On the basis of recent journal articles, a calorie-restricted diet and upgraded gene expression (which come automatically with live foods) have become keys to understanding the clinical effectiveness of live foods.

The essence of understanding living foods is "if it isn't broken, don't fix it." Living foods, or raw foods, are those that have not been cooked, processed, "pesticided" or "herbicided," microwaved, irradiated, or genetically engineered. They represent an unbroken wholeness that is the original creation and nutritional gift of the divine. The understanding that the food we eat is an energetic whole greater than the sum of the parts reflects a quantum physics view of nutrition.

Research by Dr. Brekhman of the former Soviet Union illustrates a foundational truth about the power of live foods. When he gave whole, live foods to animals, their endurance was two to three times greater than if he gave them the same caloric value of food after it had been cooked. Brekhman's results can be explained, however, if we understand the effect of cooking on the whole food. Cooking not only destroys the ecological balance of the food, it makes 50 percent of the protein unavailable, destroys 60 to 70 percent of the vitamins, up to 96 percent of the B12, and 100 percent of phytonutrients such as gibberellins, anthrocyans, polyphenols, nobelitin, and tangeretin, which boost the immune system and other bodily functions. Cooking foods also disrupts the bioelectrical structure, the bioelectricity transfer power, and the bioluminescence. All these factors are important for building and maintaining our life force energy and health.

The famous European physician Dr. Bircher-Brenner, who started the first modern live food clinic in 1897, felt that eating raw foods was a way of restoring the diseased body and the mind's ability to heal itself. Many healers have gotten fantastic results using living foods with their clients: Dr. Gerson, who healed Dr. Albert Schweitzer of diabetes and Schweitzer's wife of tuberculosis, healed hundreds of documented cancer cases with live foods and published a book about it in 1958 called *A Cancer Therapy: Results of Fifty Cases*; Dr. Szekeley saw over 133,000 clients at his live food clinic in Mexico over a thirty-year period from 1940 to 1970 with impressive results; Ann Wigmore has success at her clinics; and the next generation, including the Tree of Life Rejuvenation Center (www.treeoflife.nu), has made the next step by using live foods not only for healing of physical disease, but for repairing mental and emotional imbalances and as a way to actively enhance spiritual life.

Cooking destroys enzymes in live foods. Enzyme reserves seem to be connected to life force, health, and longevity. There are natural enzymes in raw food that minimize the enzymes that need to be secreted by the body for digestion. The body's enzymes can then be converted and used for the process of detoxification, repair, and overall healing.

People have been eating live foods for thousands of years. Ancient cultures primarily ate live foods; for example, the inner circle Essenes, who were reported to be on live foods, seem to have had an extended life span of approximately 120 years and enjoyed a higher quality of health, vitality, and joy. In summary, live foods have the highest amount of bioactive food nutrients, phytonutrients, bioelectrical energy, biologically active water, and electrons and the most energized and organized subtle organizing energy fields.

The foods that we eat, or don't eat, communicate with our genes—for better or for worse. What we put into our bodies does not change the genotype, which is the physical structure of the genes, but the foods we eat do change the way the message in the genes is expressed in the phenotype. In other words, the genetic messages of our genes can be either turned off or turned on by the nature of our diets and lifestyles. What we eat and how we live directly affects our optimal phenotypic expression. An important corollary to this is that genes do not give rise to disease, but disease arises when lifestyle and diet alter the gene expression in a way that creates disease.

What we eat affects how we think and feel because it affects the genes that regulate how we think and feel. Well-documented journal research, for example, shows that alcohol decreases the healthy expression and production of endorphins, GABA, dopamine, noradrenaline, acetylcholine receptor sites, and various other central nervous system agents. In other words, not only what we eat, but how we live and the stresses we create, directly affect gene expression. The significance of this is that through proper living, diet, fasting, lifestyle, exercise, and emotional, mental, and spiritual development, we have the opportunity to activate our youthing genes.

Diets that are high in fruits and vegetables are very high in phytonutrients, which include a variety of antioxidants, carotenes, vitamin E, vitamin C, phenolic compounds, and terpenoids that specifically turn on not only anticancer genes, but antiaging genes and anti-inflammation genes.

In the author's experience, there are three main dietary practices that greatly increase the youthing process: undereating (calorie restriction), veganism, and live food nutrition (a natural form of calorie restriction) and spiritual fasting. Dr. Stephen

R. Spindler, professor of biochemistry at the University of California, Riverside, did research with calorie restriction using gene technology. His results give some deep insight into why live foods are such a powerful healing and rejuvenating dietary approach. He studied the expression of eleven thousand genes in the livers of young normally fed and calorie-restricted mice. He found a 400 percent increase in the activation of antiaging with a 40 percent calorie restriction. He found that there was a fourfold increase with short-term caloric restriction and a 2.5-fold increase with long-term caloric restriction in the activation of antiaging. He was able to reproduce this 95 percent of the time. Dr. Spindler's research is perhaps the first to show that caloric restriction could actually turn on the youthing genes and literally reverse the aging process. The research showed that calorie restriction seemed to quickly decrease the amount of inflammation and stress, even in older animals, and suggests not only an increase in antiaging gene activity, but also in anticancer, antistress, and anti-inflamation. These four points directly apply to the healing and rejuvenating effects of live foods.

Calorie restriction happens naturally and safely with a live food diet. According to the Max Planck Institute, when we cook foods, we lose 50 percent of protein, 70–80 percent of vitamins and minerals, and 95 percent or more of phytonutrients. By simple mathematics, we only need to eat 50 percent of the calories on a live food diet versus a cooked diet. Therefore a live food diet is a natural form of calorie restriction that turns on the antiaging, anticancer, and anti-inflamation genes. This is a powerful insight and scientific explanation for the youthing and health effects of a properly eaten live food diet that the author has observed in thousands of patients since 1983.

There are many levels to understanding the healing and rejuvenating power of live foods, but the simplest way to understand raw foods is "if it isn't broken, don't fix it."

About the Author

Gabriel Cousens, MD, MD (H), DD, diplomat of the American Board of Holistic Medicine, diplomat in Ayurveda, is the founder and director of the Tree of Life Foundation and the Tree of Life Rejuvenation Center in Patagonia, Arizona. Gabriel is the leading medical authority in the world on live food nutrition and uses the modalities of nutrition, naturopathy, Ayurveda, homeopathy, psychiatry, and family therapy blended with spiritual awareness in the healing of body, mind, and spirit. He is a best-selling author of many books, including *Spiritual Nutrition, Conscious Eating, Rainbow Green Live-Food Cuisine, Sevenfold Peace,* and *Depression-Free for Life.* He facilitates the spiritual, nutritional, and lifestyle support teleseminars, "Alive with Gabriel." His next book, *There Is a Cure for Diabetes: The Tree of Life 21-Day Program* is due to be released on January 8, 2008.

14

Know Your Good Fats

Ira Edwards

Are you weary of hearing about those bad, bad fats? "Don't eat that junk. It'll make you fat." Many writers can't resist the words *artery clogging* when they mention saturated fat.

I won't distinguish between fats and fatty acids or other complications, but there are distinctions that will help you make sense of the prattle. I promise that what you learn here will be useful, and different from what you have been taught.

Saturated fats are part of all fat products but make up more than half in meat and milk. A saturated fat in coconut oil is medium-chain triglyceride. *Saturated*, chemically, means that there are no double bonds. Double bonds are the places in a molecule where hydrogen can be added artificially. Palmitic and stearic acids are saturated.

Monounsaturated means that there is one double bond. Olive oil, avocado, and canola have a goodly portion of monounsaturated molecules. Oleic acid is monounsaturated.

Polyunsaturated means that there are two (sometimes more) double bonds. These are the common vegetable oils—corn, soy, and cottonseed—which have too much omega-6 oil. *Omega* refers to the placement of double bonds in the molecule.

Superunsaturated fats, the omega-3 oils, have three, four, five, or more double bonds. Most writers lump these with the polyunsaturated, but they are very different in effect. Food labels, to be useful, should list them separately.

Hydrogenated fats are unsaturated fats that have been treated with hot, high-pressure hydrogen to fill some of the double bonds. One result of this is *trans-fats*.

Saturated fats may not be so bad after all. Eskimos who live on blubber don't get plugged arteries, and in the South Seas, coconut oil users do fine. Most meat products have mono- and polyunsaturated fractions. Saturated fats increase both HDL and LDL, which may be a good thing. Remember, HDL is good. Very good. Don't trash saturated fats.

Monounsaturated fats are universally endorsed. Olive oil is credited for the good health of southern Europeans. Olive oil helps people of the island of Crete to be some of the world's healthiest people, which may also be due to a lot of purslane in their fare. Purslane is a common garden weed that happens to be rather good in salads and contains some omega-3 fat.

The Best Fat

Omega-3 fats are vital but very scarce in modern fare. When deficient, beware of developing heart disease, mental problems, and a multitude of chronic conditions. Plant sources provide linolenic acid (note that *n*). Flaxseed is a rich source of linolenic acid, and bits of this healthful fat are found in most plant sources. More vital DHA and EPA fats (with long chemical names) are found in animal sources, mainly cold-water fish and wild or grass-fed animals. These are necessary for healthy cell membranes. In commonly available foods, you won't get nearly as much DHA and EPA as you need. Salmon, cod, shad, herring, and a few other fatty cold-water fish are good. Sardines may be best of all. Unless you live in Alaska, it's hard to get a healthful amount of DHA and EPA. Eat fish, but also buy fish oil capsules or cod liver oil.

Now, Will the Real Bad Fats Please Stand Up?

Polyunsaturated fats, the omega-6 vegetable fats, are necessary nutrition in moderate amounts. An abundant type is linoleic (without the *n*). They are usually listed with good fats. *No!* They are in great excess in our modern fare, and they are inflammatory. Nearly all of our boxed and bagged snack foods have these fats, made even worse by hydrogenation. (Nuts have omega-6 oil but are very good nutrition anyway. Borage and primrose oils have a good form of omega-6.)

Trans-fats are the demons of this decade. No. Small amounts of natural trans-fat may be healthful. The problem is hydrogenation. Hydrogenation (partial hydrogenation) eliminates natural unsaturated fats and produces a variety of fats, including trans-fats, which the human body may have never before encountered. Food labels, to be useful, should list hydrogenated fat, not trans-fats, and the appropriate level is zero.

Cholesterol?

Much that you hear about cholesterol is wrong. Cholesterol is not a fat chemically, but it is often regarded as a bad fat. Wrong. Cholesterol, because of total insolubility, gives body cells stability in a water environment. It is also necessary for vitamin D and hormone production. High cholesterol may be due to a shortage of these products, as the body tries to compensate.

We were told not to eat egg yolks because of cholesterol. Wrong. It is unlikely that anyone was ever harmed from eating eggs. We were told that there is good cholesterol (HDL) and bad cholesterol (LDL). These are not cholesterol, but protein-cholesterol combinations needed for carrying insoluble cholesterol in the blood. HDL is indeed good, but LDL has minimal significance.

Taking drugs to lower cholesterol is the wrong treatment for the wrong condition. I have to say this, though it is contrary to almost all medical literature: low cholesterol may be more of a problem than high. The total cholesterol figure, which combines blood fat, LDL, and HDL, is useless and detracts attention from real risk factors, which are low HDL, high blood fat (triglycerides), and chronic inflammation. Homocysteine level is one of several indicators of inflammation. Cholesterol particle size matters, too, which is not so easily tested.

Is High Fat the Problem?

You have heard of the French paradox and places around the world where people eat high fat but don't get much heart disease. The explanation may be that they get many more plant-based antioxidants. They also get much more vitamin D than we do.

The problem with fats, mostly, is not that fats are bad. The larger problem is that they, along with sugar and starches, take the place of more vital nutrition. A person who fills up with meat, beans, and grain products will get very little omega-3 fat and little vital nutrition from low-starch vegetables. It is not necessary to avoid meat. It is necessary to get a good spectrum of nutrients, including a spectrum of different kinds of fat. Do you look for foods labeled "low fat"? Don't be fooled. These are often overpriced because they are presented as healthful. They leave you deprived of good fats. But first, eat your veggies.

Not Enough Veggies!

Protein is necessary, and high protein fare is good. Eat eggs: the white for protein and the yolk for wonderful nutrients. However, protein, fat, sugar, starch, beans, eggs, nuts, and whole grains must not take the place of spinach, celery, and onions. The onion and lettuce on your Big Mac barely count. However difficult the changes, you can be happy and healthy with lots of broccoli, asparagus, chard, beets, carrots, tomatoes, squash, cabbage, and berries. Include fruit, of course, but by all means, eat your veggies!

What You Should Remember

Healthful fare includes a spectrum of many nutrients, but with balance. Along with plentiful vegetables and some fruit, include a little saturated fat, more monounsaturated fat, much less vegetable oil than usual, and however you can do it, get EPA and DHA. While we are bombarded with messages about what is healthy and what is not, and as we gaze on endless aisles of packaged foods claiming to be low in fat, it is most important to remember that balance is key. Knowing the right combination of fats to consume is vital to your health.

About the Author

After forty years of adding to a good education in biochemistry, physiology, medicine, and other sciences, I thought I had learned nutrition. I was wrong. I found truth in nutrition so elusive that this study became an obsession that led to writing a book, *Honest Nutrition*. I'm still learning, still finding truth elusive, and still obsessed. For a description of *Honest Nutrition*, go to http://www.trafford.com/06-1866.

15

How Much Does Your Food Cost?

Marie Galdi, HHC, AADP

How much does your food cost? Have you ever given it much thought? Does your food budget dictate what you can and cannot consume? Do the weekly newspaper coupons, along with the sale end caps in your local grocery store, choose for you? Why are other people dictating to you what's going to be on your dinner table tonight? While you are pondering your thoughts on the rationale behind your food consumption, have you ever stopped and asked why, as a nation, we are the richest, yet we are the sickest?

The alarming rates of diabetes, coronary heart disease, and obesity plaguing our society suggest that something is terribly wrong! Moreover, we have the richest sources of natural whole foods available to us, but we often only consider processed and refined foods.

We expect a lot from our bodies; we want them to work like well-oiled machines. So how we invest our money in ourselves now will dictate what kinds of insurance premiums we have for our future health.

Ultimately, how we feed our bodies with food will show up physically in our energy levels and through our larger waistlines. It's also apparent that unhealthy processed food choices affect us mentally by clouding our thoughts and zapping our brain power. Consequently, diets comprised of refined foods are nutrient-poor and are causing many Americans to be highly mineral deficient. Over time, these deficiencies can lead to a plethora of degenerative diseases. Your food choice now ultimately determines the cost to you later.

What is the determining factor you use to purchase your food? Do you base your decision on economic principles coupled with quick preparation time? The food you choose could then be a frozen box of batter-dipped chicken breasts, a box of macaroni and cheese, and some frozen peas thrown on the side for good measure. Your purchasing power may be based on the perception that eating healthy may come at a higher price tag. The trade-off would be labor intensive and time consuming, albeit resulting in better-quality and fresher-tasting food. You may have come to the conclusion that you will have to pay more to get the desirable qualities. I disagree! You could still have an inexpensive and time-saving meal by choosing fresh, natural chicken breast seasoned with fresh herbs and tastefully grilled. To accompany the chicken, a wild rice pilaf with added fresh, sautéed vegetables would have fed you graciously for dinner and probably afforded you leftovers for the next day's lunch.

Optimally, the way we need to feed ourselves to sustain energy, vitality, and better health must come from whole foods. What is a whole food diet? Whole foods are basic foods in their most natural and original, plant-based states. The closer you are eating to the earth's soil, the more nutrient dense a food source will be. Such plant source groups and examples are fresh fruits (apples, oranges, grapes, peaches), vegetables (dark, leafy green vegetables, such as kale and collards, broccoli, cabbage, carrots, and sweet potato), whole grains (whole wheat berries, brown rice, buckwheat, and quinoa), and legumes (beans, lentils, and peas), nuts and seeds (almonds, pecans, sunflower and sesame seeds), just to name a few. The key here is to select a variety of fresh, seasonal foods whenever possible.

Does animal protein have its place in your whole food diet? Meat, poultry, and fish, along with dairy products, are not typically considered whole foods because they are not derived from a plant source. However, I believe they have their place on your plate. Consider them a condiment rather than a main dish when consuming them. Make sure you are choosing fresh, organic, or natural meat and poultry and freshwater or wild caught fish whenever possible.

I often hear the assumption that eating healthy costs more and that whole foods are hard to locate in the local grocery. I disagree! Whole grains and fresh, natural foods have arrived at many commercial supermarkets. They are tangible even in bulk portions, making them, pound for pound, less expensive. You optimally only buy what you need. You are not paying for advertising and pricey prepackaged foods sold in specific units. Most often, you need to purchase more quantity to account for the smaller packaging. This is an added expense. Bulk food gives you a plethora of options when choosing a whole grain source. Prepackaged foods are often loaded with enhancements to keep the food looking better, tasting better, and lasting longer. I personally don't want to consume a food that has a longer shelf life than my conceivable future!

I believe our bodies are rare entities. It is our given birthright to be as healthy as we choose. By consuming the purest, whole foods available, we are doing our bodies a great service. We are rewarded by the abundant energy, vitality, and healthy moods we can emulate to others. That's priceless!

You will be enlightened by the outcome when you begin to embrace the opportunity to replace refined foods with varieties of whole foods. Like a painter creating a fresh idea on canvas, you have your palette of choice colors to begin your original piece of art. Don't shy away from the brilliant colors as you seek new choices in the produce isle of your local market.

If you can grow your own fresh berries, herbs, lettuce, collards, and so on, your food costs will be reduced significantly. If you are unable to produce your own seasonal fresh foods, become a member of community-supported agriculture in your area. Signing up to purchase a share of farm fresh produce promotes a nutritious array for your personal culinary palette. You will also be supporting the dynamics of the farming community. As I began trying many foods for the first time, I recognized that quality, freshness, and taste were other key factors. I am no longer selecting foods just because they are on sale. Furthermore, I am very aware that I vote with my fork each time I eat. Remember, a *diet* is just another four-letter word. A *lifestyle* feeds us forever.

Five Nourishing Tips for Promoting a Whole Food Lifestyle

1. Replace white rice and plain pasta with whole grain brown rice and pasta. To transition from white flour products, use a half portion of whole grain flour, such as buckwheat, in a recipe.
2. Keep healthy snacks on hand. Select nuts (almonds and walnuts), nut butters, humus, or fresh-cut fruits and vegetables.
3. Select fats derived from plant sources over animal fat (avocado, olive and canola oil).
4. Drink plenty of water—especially during the cold winter months as we lose moisture through our breath.
5. Find a source of creative movement you can do daily (dance, walk in nature, buy a yoga tape for home use, take a swim, or ride your bike).

About the Author

Marie Galdi, BA, HHC, AADP, is the founder and director of Alternative Health Visions. She counsels others in living a life that promotes balance and wellness so that they can be at an optimal level of health for everyday living. Her journey began over seventeen years ago, when she found that the chronic use of medication was not the answer for what she and her family were ailing from. Delving further, her education and personal experience brought her to an understanding that certain foods can make us well or make us sick. In a new workshop series, Marie focuses on inspiring us to revisit our sacred space in the kitchen and begin again, nourishing ourselves with traditional whole foods. For more information about Alternative Health Visions, please visit our Web site at http://www.alternativehealthvisions.com.

16

All Aboard!
Riding Nature's Cycles to Better Health

Rafael Jerman, LMT, NCTMB

Optimum health and vitality are what most people strive to achieve and yet seldom do. If our bodies are, as we read so many times, perfect organisms, then how can sickness and disease possibly affect us? Contrary to what you might read in most entertainment magazines, a perfect body is not measured on a scale or in clothing size. Perfection of the human body, though inherent in all of us, is simply a raw potential for perfection.

Manifesting this potential requires daily replenishment of critical resources necessary for continuous cellular regeneration and constant maintenance to prevent a buildup of negative mental and physical stress.

Optimum health is dependent on several components, none of which should be omitted if health is truly what we desire. Unfortunately, our food today is sorely lacking the essential nutrient content of, say, a couple decades ago. According to agricultural experts, there are many reasons for this, such as soil quality, fertilizers, crop rotation, maturity at harvest time, and so on. Charles Bembrook, PhD, who has conducted a fifteen-year study on the nutritive value of organically produced foods, explains that nonorganic methods that include soluble nitrogen fertilizers produce higher yields because with their use, plants and vegetables absorb more water. While the fruits these plants produce are larger, they tend to suffer in nutritional quality due to the nutrient dilution.

If we closely examine what passes for food these days, it becomes quite clear that the average commercial nourishment sources are laden with more of the things that are *not* conducive to the replenishment of spent nutrients and less of the things that are. The widespread use of antibiotics, hormones, and other substances on cattle and poultry farms increases the production of milk, beef, eggs, and so on. The effects of these practices have yet to be proven safe for human consumption. The labels on most of today's supermarket products list a number of preservatives, food coloring, artificial flavoring, and taste enhancers. Avoid foods that contain the word *hydrogenated*: this process creates a known carcinogen and shows no signs of being removed from our food supply anytime soon.

We further compound this nutrient deficit by failing to incorporate an adequate physical, mental, and spiritual maintenance program, which is essential for optimum health, vitality, and longevity, and in not doing so, we unknowingly accelerate our bodies' overall deterioration. Something as important as the key to our survival deserves more than just a casual commitment.

We are a nation teetering on the edge of chronic obesity. Many people tend to have misconceptions as to why they may have accumulated this excess fat and usually try to counter it by subscribing to every fad diet, pill, or gadget that comes along, and when that fails to work, as is generally the case, they resort back to eating infrequently, eating the wrong foods, or not eating at all. There is a general consensus among dietary experts that advocates increasing the frequency, diversity, and quality of our food intake and drastically diminishing the portion size of each meal. Failure by most to adapt to this concept is one reason for this excess accumulation of fat that plagues our society today.

Obesity is a product of many years of miscommunication with our bodies and the contradictory information we unknowingly send it. Though there are certainly more complex causes to explain such a condition, the root cause will always be one of imbalance somewhere along the line.

The body is designed to forgo unnecessary tasks, and fat storage becomes redundant when a steady stream of high-quality nutrition is frequently being supplied. Cooperating with your body's natural cycle is the surest way to attain optimum health, so the most important thing to do is to choose your foods carefully, then introduce them in relatively small and balanced portions during the time when your body is most prepared to accept and digest them. There are three eight-hour cycles, and each is designed for specific tasks. The first cycle is the elimination cycle, which begins at 4:00 a.m. and continues until 12:00 noon. Your body will discard all unwanted material, such as toxins and waste, in various forms. During this phase, it is highly recommended that you consume only fruit, fruit juice, or vegetable juice. These foods enhance this detoxifying stage without taxing your digestive system.

Next comes the appropriation cycle, which runs from 12:00 noon until 8:00 p.m. This is the time to eat frequent, small, and balanced portions since the body is most active and can easily break down foods. These mini meals should consist of alkalizing (neutralize acid) foods such as green leafy vegetables and salads of various colors and tastes such as green salads, cucumber, zucchini, to name a few. Our bodies also require pungent tastes, not just sweet and salty ones. It is further suggested that we eat healthy fats such as those found in avocados, olive oil, and flaxseed oil. Alkaline and healthy fats should represent 70 percent of each portion.

The remaining 30 percent should consist of acid-forming foods such as meat, dairy, breads, etc. Applying this 70-30 rule will help you make better food choices and improve your energy level and overall health. Highly processed foods, such as smoked meats, fried foods, white flower, sugar, bread, and sodas, should be eliminated as food choices altogether.

This 8:00 p.m. cutoff period for food consumption is critical as the next phase is the assimilation cycle, which begins at 8:00 p.m. and continues until 4:00 a.m. Now, the extraction of nutrients from the foods you consumed during the previous phase begins. No eating whatsoever should take place during this time. If the food consumption up until that point has been adequate, any feeling of hunger will most probably be of a psychological nature rather than a physiological need, and a cup of hot tea or room-temperature filtered water will probably quell the sensation of hunger; your body will also adjust in time.

We can greatly accelerate our metabolism by adding exercise to our health plan, and this can include a game of golf or tennis or simply going for a brisk walk. If you opt for a more complete training program, check with professionals, and let them tailor an exercise program to best meet your needs and personal goals. Your mental outlook is also important—take time out each day to contemplate all that is good in your life.

Finally, these cycles can be modified to fit any lifestyle. If you work the swing or late shift, you simply move the cycles so that when you wake up, you begin cycle 1. If you are taking any medications, please check with your care provider first before starting any new diet or exercise regimen.

Today, we know enough about the human body to understand that *when* you eat is equally as important as *what* you eat. Armed with this knowledge, let us give this most marvelous of organic machines the opportunity to reach its perfection potential and experience total health, vitality, and longevity. Let us strive to reach our inherent perfection in the absence of sickness, disease, and overall imbalance.

About the Author

Rafael Jerman, LMT, NCTMB, is president of Like Night & Day Inc. and has established a reputation as a knowledgeable and caring professional in his field. His unique blend of several modalities, such as Shiatsu, neuromuscular, Myofascial Release, and Swedish techniques, have made him a consummate body worker and has earned him high praise among his peers. In addition to massage, he is also one of only 120 certified Cranial Release Technique practitioners in the country. Rafael has his own exclusive Sansage rejuvenation treatment line and has written articles for periodicals in both English and Spanish. He is a frequently invited guest on local radio and television programs in Miami. Visit his Web site at http://www.likenightanddaybody.com.

17

Stevia: A Better Alternative to Sugar and Artificial Sweeteners

Lisa Jobs, MJ

Most medical experts would agree that one of the best ways to improve your health is to reduce your sugar intake. Doing this can help decrease your chances of getting diabetes and being overweight or obese—both epidemics in this country with adults and children alike. Consider these facts:

* Since 1985, childhood diabetes has increased tenfold. The Centers for Disease Control predict that if this trend continues, one out of every three children born beginning in 2000 will develop diabetes in his lifetime.
* About two thirds of U.S. adults are overweight or obese, while up to 30 percent of children are overweight, compared to 4 percent in 1982. In the past twenty-five years, obesity in children has more than doubled, affecting at least 15 percent of school-aged children![2]
* The average American ingests over 150 pounds of sugar annually! That represents a whopping thirty five-pound bags of sugar each year! In reality, much of this sugar is in the form of high fructose corn syrup prevalent in foods because it's much cheaper than sucrose, common table sugar.

While some might think that artificial sweeteners are the best solution to curb our love affair with sugar, others disagree. Artificial sweeteners do eliminate the high calories and carbohydrates associated with sugar; however, many believe that these alternatives are unsafe and are actually worse than sugar. So is there yet another alternative available?

If there were an all-natural sweetening ingredient that's been used safely for over thirty years in other parts of the world for food applications and diabetes management with no ill effects, would you be interested? Well, such a substance does exist, and it's called stevia.

The use of stevia, an all-natural alternative to sugar and artificial sweeteners, is gaining increasing popularity worldwide. *Stevia rebaudiana*, its botanical name, is derived from a plant in the chrysanthemum family grown primarily in South America and Asia.

---

[2] "Report: Obesity Will Reverse Life Expectancy Gains," http://www.cnn.com/2005/HEALTH/diet.fitness/03/16/obesity.longevity.ap.

The plant's intense sweetening qualities are derived from a complex molecule called stevioside that is a glycoside made of glucose, sophorose, and steviol. This, and a number of other related compounds, is what makes stevia up to three hundred times sweeter than sugar and noncaloric. These glycosides do not get absorbed into the body; rather, they simply pass through, leaving no calories. The Japanese have used stevia in food applications from soft drinks to soy sauce since the 1970s, and recent reports indicate that stevia commands up to an incredible 50 percent share of Japan's commercial sweetener market. Moreover, countries like Brazil use stevia for the treatment of diabetes.[3]

The advantages to stevia are numerous, so the following are the most frequently cited. In its pure form, it's noncaloric and doesn't affect glucose levels, an advantage for diabetics and hypoglycemics. Also, it has no carbohydrates or fat, so it's great for dieters, especially those watching carb intake. Unlike artificial sweeteners, high-quality stevia has little aftertaste when measured properly. It has no known side effects like some chemical sweeteners and has been safely consumed around the world for decades. Actually, stevia's original medicinal uses date back centuries ago to the Paraguan Indians, who mixed the herb in teas for its healing properties. Since stevia is sugar-free, candida sufferers can use it. Health-conscious consumers take advantage of stevia to avoid sugar and help prevent diabetes and obesity. The Web site http://www.ncbi.nlm.nih.gov, under the direction of the National Institutes of Health, the National Library of Medicine, and the National Center of Biotechnology Information, offers abstracts from stevia studies which indicate that it may also aid in lowering blood pressure, controlling the development of plaque and cavities, and regulating glucose levels.

The average consumer may not have heard about stevia until recently because of its current Food and Drug Administration (FDA) approval as a dietary supplement, not as a sweetener or food additive. Numerous studies worldwide tout its overall safety and health benefits. As of this writing, twelve countries, including Japan, Paraguay, and Brazil, have approved stevia as a sweetener and/or food additive. The FDA approved the use of stevia only as a dietary supplement since 1995. This means that stevia companies must maintain a fairly low profile, thereby limiting its distribution and marketing potential. For instance, health food stores and natural grocers must place stevia in the supplements section, not with the natural sweeteners, for fear of the FDA mandate. The stores cannot promote the sweetening qualities of stevia, even though that's why it is purchased.

Interestingly enough, the most exciting recent news about stevia came in May 2007, when Coca-Cola and Cargill announced their partnership to develop food and beverage products using "rebiana," a derivative of stevia. In addition, Coca-Cola has filed 24 patent applications related to using, formulating and processing high potency sweeteners, including "rebiana." In an effort to build support for a petition requesting

---

[3] David Richard, *Stevia Rebaudiana: Nature's Sweet Secret* (Bloomingdale, IL: Vital Health Publishing, 1996).

FDA permission to use "rebiana" as a food additive in the USA, Cargill is conducting clinical trials using the sweetener. Although the newly developed products will be sold in other countries initially, their hope is to eventually sell them in the USA once "rebiana" is FDA approved[4]. While the possibility of enjoying commercial food products using stevia is very encouraging, keep in mind that it may take years before it becomes reality in the USA.

Stevia can be used as a healthy substitute in most sugar applications, including baking and cooking, since it is heat stable. The average conversion rate of sugar to stevia is one cup of sugar per one teaspoonful of pure stevia extract. Clearly very little stevia is needed to replace sugar. When used in beverages, stevia dissolves quickly and easily and, depending on your taste preference, only a pinch is needed. The real challenge to using stevia effectively is knowing what ingredients to use in a recipe to make up for the volume and consistency lost with the elimination of sugar, especially in baked goods. That's why it's a good idea to find stevia cookbooks with proven recipes when you're starting out. You can also find some free recipes online. Finally, stevia is not appropriate in recipes that require sugar caramelizing or browning such as meringues.

Stevia is available in many forms, including liquid, teas, plants/leaves, pure white and green powdered extract, and powdered blends with different fillers. In baking, the pure extract is used primarily, and in some cases, the liquid variety is used. Stevia can be purchased at health food stores, natural grocers, food coops, and online. Currently, a big push is under way to expand distribution into grocery stores, vitamin shops, and drugstores.

Since there are a number of factors that can influence your stevia purchase experience, the following guidelines provide some good advice:

- You often do get what you pay for; don't buy based solely on price—taste and quality matter.
- A higher percentage of stevioside doesn't necessarily make the stevia better; you can find excellent tasting pure stevia extract powder with key plant concentrations of even 80 percent.
- If you purchase the green powder for its slightly higher health benefits, it will usually have more aftertaste than the white powder.
- The product's country of origin doesn't matter; it's farming, manufacturing, and processing experience and techniques do.
- At this time, stevia production is not standardized, so taste and strength do differ depending on brand.
- Use a minimal amount; it can be overwhelming if you add too much initially, so add more later if needed.

---

[4] http://www.usatoday.com/money/industries/food/2007-05-31-cokecargill_N.htm.

The widespread use of sugar and artificial sweeteners is at dangerous levels. The negative side effects and controversial studies regarding their proposed safety suggest that another alternative is desirable and necessary. Stevia may be a welcome option for those who want to ingest more natural ingredients with no known side effects, no calories, no carbs, no fat, no effect on glucose levels, and no sugar or artificial sweeteners. Stevia may also be advantageous in the prevention and treatment of diabetes, obesity, and other health conditions. Check with your doctor before including stevia in your diet. If he or she doesn't recommend it, politely ask why to see if the reason is satisfactory to you.

About the Author

Lisa Jobs, BA, MJ, is the author of *Sensational Stevia Desserts* and president of Healthy Lifestyle Publishing LLC. As a former co-owner of @Stevia LLC for ten years, Lisa created two stevia products. During that time, she also developed hundreds of dessert recipes, the best of which are showcased in her book. Lisa is often interviewed about stevia on radio and television. She is currently working on another book project. For more information about stevia, free recipes, or to order her book, visit http://www.steviadessert.com, http://www.healthylifestylepublishing.com, or call toll-free (888) 8STEVIA (878-3842).

18

Chocolate! Chocolate! Chocolate!

Carol (Coco) Klingsmith, RN, CES

It's everywhere. Is this media frenzy funded by Hershey's or Mars? Or could it be true? There is a type of chocolate that really is good for you! The headlines read, dark chocolate increases energy and reduces chronic fatigue; a natural way to enhance mood and mental clarity; reduces the risk of heart attack and supports normal blood pressure and cholesterol levels; can chocolate really replace aspirin as a blood thinner?; chocolate for shiny hair and smooth skin (I am so confused—I thought chocolate caused pimples!); what does the future hold in store—betty ford treatment centers for chocolate addiction?

Personally, I knew all along that chocolate was good for you. After all, it is a vegetable, isn't it?

Chocolate contains antioxidant compounds called flavanols. According to data from the U.S. Department of Agriculture and the *Journal of the American Chemical Society*, dark chocolate is the food richest in antioxidants. Antioxidants are measured by oxygen radical absorbance capacity (ORAC). Dark chocolate has 13,120 ORAC units per 100 grams. Prunes, raisins, and blueberries contain 2,400–5,770 ORAC units.

If the above information is true, why do we feel so guilty when we eat chocolate? Part of the problem may stem from the commercialization of chocolate. The "Food of the Gods" has become adulterated with refined sugar, wax, lard, hormone-treated dairy, and other cheap fillers.

Conventional cocoa plantations use a huge amount of pesticides. In addition to the ecological damage caused, these pesticides can be retained in the fat of foods. And since chocolate contains high quantities of cocoa butter, it can retain and store pesticides applied to the plant.

These are very good arguments for avoiding chocolate, but let's go back and visit the ancient civilizations of the Incan, Mayan, and Aztec peoples. When chocolate was first discovered, health and nutrition were common sense. Historians recount that a chocolate drink produced a happy sense of euphoria, a warm-all-over sensation (oh, my childhood cup of cocoa!). They didn't know whether to call it a food or a medicine. They eventually called it *Theobroma Cacao*, which translates as "Food of the Gods." Only the royal family was allowed to drink it. Montezuma reportedly drank it with his royal court and concubines for enhanced energy and virility.

When Cortez sailed to the New World, he was greeted and treated as a god. He was given many gifts, chief of which was the ceremonial *Theobroma Cacao* drink. He and his men quickly recognized the value of this treasure and took it back to Spain.

For the present, I will let science and Hershey's and Mars continue their fight to prove the health benefits of chocolate. But I will not wait for the results of these studies. Instead, I will continue incorporating an ounce of quality dark chocolate into my day and into those of my weight loss–seeking clients because, personally, I think of chocolate as a SuperFood: a food that provides health benefits far beyond its recognized nutritional value. SuperFoods help embrace health, instead of fighting disease. When you increase your SuperFood consumption, the inevitable result is a more nutrient-dense, lower-calorie, health-promoting diet. I believe SuperFoods make creating health fun and pleasurable. And shouldn't eating be pleasurable? It used to be.

I offer Coco's Chocolate Clues for Healthy Living:

- Choose organic ingredients.
- It should taste like pleasure feels.
- Don't chew chocolate or swallow it right down. Savor and enjoy it—let it melt in your mouth.
- There is some debate about the percent of cacao and claims that it needs to be 70 percent or higher. I do believe it should be at least 60 percent cacao, but for some people, the higher cacao content tastes bitter.
- Most important to me is the list of ingredients. I like to see as few listed on the label as possible. The ingredients should come from Mother Nature, rather than a laboratory. Note the difference in the ingredients of the following two chocolate bars.
  - o Dark Chocolate Bar A: organic dark chocolate, organic raw cane sugar, organic chocolate liquor, organic cocoa butter, soy lecithin (used as an emulsifier), organic vanilla (65 percent cacao)
  - o Dark Chocolate Bar B (name brand bar): sugar, chocolate, cocoa (processed with alkali, milk fat, lactose), soy lecithin, PGPR (emulsifier), artificial flavor, milk (50 percent cacao)
- If you choose to use chocolate as your only SuperFood, know that you will probably gain weight. Chocolate is about 50 percent fat. Although I use chocolate as a part of a healthy weight loss program, I recommend a portion size that yields fifty to one hundred calories. I find that that portion of healthy chocolate provides satisfaction and pleasure and helps decrease carbohydrate cravings.

Coco's recipe for improving health includes an ounce of healthy dark chocolate added to ten to fifteen SuperFoods every day. Other SuperFoods include apples, almonds, avocados, beans, berries, broccoli, cinnamon, extra virgin olive oil, garlic, wild salmon, oats, flaxseed, brown rice, sweet potatoes, and quinoa. What makes these foods super? As mentioned earlier, a SuperFood offers health benefits far beyond its nutritional value. Quinoa, for example, is a high-energy protein, rich in minerals—including calcium. It eases digestion. Quinoa is gluten-free, which makes it great for those with wheat intolerances. There are many SuperFoods, each with their own health benefits, so go for variety. In addition to SuperFoods, drink adequate amounts of pure water and engage in thirty minutes of daily exercise, preferably outside. Stir and watch as your hair shines, your skin glows, and you come alive with newfound health.

About the Author

Carol Klingsmith, RN, CES, is a nurse and health coach. She is also a clinical exercise specialist and lifestyle and weight management consultant with the American Council on Exercise. She lives in Missouri and has an international coaching practice. Her focus is on prevention and treatment of health issues through education and natural sources. She may be reached at cklingsmith@gmail.com. For information on 24 Karat Chocolate™ and other whole food products, go to http://www.carolswellness.com.

19

Protect Your Cells with Antioxidants

Julie Merrick, ND

Good health starts at the cellular level. For the body to be healthy, cells must be healthy, and to be healthy, cells need nourishment and protection. Nourishment is provided by nutrients, and protection is dependent on a variety of factors such as your immune system, the nutrients that make up your cell membranes, and very importantly, *antioxidants*.

To understand the significance of antioxidants, you must understand oxidative stress. Every day, during normal metabolism, your body produces molecules known as free radicals. These molecules are unstable: they have an unpaired electron that causes them to take electrons from other molecules, disrupting their structure. This is the process of oxidation.

In a state of optimal health, the body's oxidative processes don't cause ill health, but in some situations, such as illness, inflammation, stress, intense exercise, nutritional deficiencies, and smoking, the oxidative processes in the body overwhelm the body's ability to deal with them, and oxidative stress results. This may cause damage to cells and increase the likelihood of cellular dysfunction and premature aging. This is where antioxidants come in.

What Do Antioxidants Do?

Antioxidants, as their name implies, are against oxidation. They help prevent free radicals from disrupting cells by allowing free radicals to oxidize *them*. In a way, the antioxidant is sacrificing itself to protect other cells. They defend against oxidative stress and help maintain cellular structure and integrity. A cell that is protected will last longer and function effectively.

Where Do Antioxidants Come From?

Antioxidants are found in various foods, especially fresh fruits, vegetables, and other plants. The color variation of plant foods depends on their constituents, including the antioxidants that are present. For example, the orange color of carrots is due to carotenoids such as beta-carotene, an antioxidant that is converted to vitamin A in the body. Other antioxidants include vitamin C and bioflavonoids, vitamin E, selenium, lipoic acid, and coenzyme Q_{10}. Some antioxidants protect the water-soluble parts of cells, and some protect the fat-soluble parts of cells. To defend against oxidative stress, both parts of the cell need to be protected. That is why it is important to have a good supply of various antioxidants by eating a wide variety of foods.

What Can I Eat to Increase My Intake of Antioxidant-Rich Foods?

- Brightly colored vegetables such as carrots, peppers, spinach, and broccoli
- Citrus fruits, pineapple, grapes, and strawberries
- Berries such as raspberries, blueberries, and blackberries
- Almonds, cashews, and brazil nuts
- Egg yolks, oysters, and tuna
- Alfalfa and garlic

Should I Take a Supplement As Well?

Although it is preferable to eat a varied and healthy diet high in antioxidants, it is becoming more difficult to get everything we need for optimal health from food alone. This is due to such things as green harvesting, which doesn't allow plant foods to naturally ripen on the vine and fully develop their nutritional value. Also, storage for long periods of time may cause a loss of some nutrients, and processing often removes important nutrients and antioxidants. During processing, some nutrients are added back into the food synthetically, but this is not usually as good as the real thing because it is often the naturally occurring complex or combination of nutrients in a plant that is responsible for its beneficial effect, rather than a particular nutrient on its own. In addition, some cooking methods, such as boiling and frying, can cause a loss of nutrients and antioxidants, further adding to the depletion caused by modern farming practices.

Your first step should always be to improve your diet as much as possible, and the addition of an effective antioxidant supplement may also prove worthwhile in maximizing your cellular protection and improving overall health.

How Do I Choose an Antioxidant Supplement?

Choose an antioxidant supplement that has clinical research supporting its effectiveness, rather than just picking one up off the shelf. It is best to take a supplement that is natural and that contains a combination of plant ingredients, rather than separate antioxidant nutrients added together in a formula. The plant's constituents work synergistically and are usually more effective when used whole.

Many antioxidants are tested for effectiveness via the oxygen radical absorption capacity (ORAC) method, which is an in vitro testing procedure.[5] The supplement is then given an ORAC value: the higher the value, the more effective the supplement. This method only measures the antioxidant potential of *water-soluble* molecules, however, so the sORAC method, which tests the antioxidants in *serum* (a component of blood), is a more accurate predictor of how a supplement will work in the body. This is because it also tests fat-soluble molecules, and your cells are made up of both fat- and water-soluble parts, which both need protection.

Look for a supplement that has a high ORAC, or preferably sORAC value, and make sure you check whether the value is per gram of supplement. For example, sometimes an antioxidant supplement will claim to have a high ORAC value, but the fine print says that it is per twenty grams. Divide the value by twenty, and you may in fact have a low ORAC value!

How Else Can I Protect My Cells?

In addition to an optimal intake of antioxidants, other ways to protect your cells and maximize their health are getting adequate sleep, not smoking, balancing intense exercise with periods of rest, learning to deal with and prevent stress, getting enough anti-inflammatory nutrients like essential fatty acids from fish, and achieving and maintaining a healthy body composition.

Your cells are designed to protect you, but make sure you also protect them! Start increasing your antioxidant intake, and notice the difference in your health and well-being.

About the Author

Julie Merrick is a naturopath with a health science degree in complementary medicine. She is the owner of Intrahealth Naturopathic Clinic in the Blue Mountains of Australia (http://www.intrahealthclinic.com), where she helps patients with a variety of health challenges to take control of their health with nutrition and natural medicine. Julie is also a certified practitioner of Hemaview™ live blood screening and is the author of the e-book *Stop Stress! And Get Your Life Back!* She has developed a Web site (http://www.proactivenaturalhealth.com) dedicated to educating people about natural health and encouraging people to take a proactive approach to their health care.

---

[5] S. McAnalley, C. M. Koepke, L. Le, E. Vennum, and B. McAnalley, "In Vitro Methods for Testing Antioxidant Potential: A Review," *Glycoscience and Nutrition* 4 (2003): 1–9.

20

What Is in Our Foods?

Kathryn Morrow, DD, MS

Never, no never does nature say one thing and wisdom another.
—Johann Christolph

The influence of nutrition exceeded that of any other health measure,
including medical intervention.
—Thomas McKeown

We all will agree that our health is the most important aspect of our success in all areas of our lives. Food is the dynamic force in all that we are. We are seeing proof of this in our country every day. Unfortunately, what we are seeing is mostly the result of poor choices. Most people do not realize that it is the food we consume every day that results in how we feel, look, and think. The health of the general public is declining, and health care costs are escalating to an all time high; the time has come for alternative health education and guidance specifically in what I call "holistic nutrition."

Isn't time we went back to how Mother Nature intended us to eat? Isn't it time to view food in its whole, true form? Foods need to be viewed not only as calories, proteins, fats, or carbohydrates, but with the understanding that food interacts on many different levels. Food interacts on a physical body level and on an emotional mind level as well. Healthy, whole food helps us look and feel healthy, helps us think clearly, and helps our state of mind, fending off depression, insomnia, and emotional issues.

Obesity is the number one health concern, affecting one out of three adults. Every twenty-five seconds, someone suffers a heart attack. Diabetes is the third leading cause of death in the United States. We are seeing an epidemic of type 2 diabetes in children that was unheard of a generation ago. We are seeing an increase of autoimmune diseases in younger and younger people. We are seeing more and more people with low IQs and, even more startling, less and less people with high IQs. Some are calling this the dumbing down of society. Is this intentional or just a result of a science experiments gone wrong? Could our food be playing a major role in this?

It is not only what we eat, but how the food is produced that may cause harm to our health. Information on what is healthy and what is not is sometimes overwhelming. At times, even if you are able to understand the ingredient list of the food you are choosing, some ingredients are not even listed on the product since the food industry does not have to list ingredients if they are less than 5 percent, and they don't have to list things that were used during the manufacturing of the product. They only have to list the ingredients that are in the final product. For example, an additive used in manufacturing ice cream is diethyglycol, which is a cheap chemical used as an emulsifier instead of eggs and is the same chemical used in antifreeze and paint remover.

What Is Genetic Engineering?

Genetic engineering is a revolutionary new technology still in its early experimental stages of development. This technology has the power to break down fundamental genetic barriers—not only between species, but between animals and plants. By randomly inserting together the genes of nonrelated species—utilizing viruses, antibiotic-resistant genes, and bacteria as vectors, markers, and promoters—and permanently altering their genetic codes, genetically altered organisms are created that pass these genetic changes onto their offspring through heredity. *Genetically engineered* (GE), *genetically modified* (GM), and *transformed* are all terms that relate to a wide range of agricultural, industrial, and medical products in which genetic codes have been altered using recombinant DNA techniques. Genetic engineers intend to confer on the genetically engineered organism new, desirable characteristics not found in the original, unmodified organism. By genetically modifying crops, often, the goal is to eliminate the use of pesticides and make farming more productive and affordable. And while many experts believe that GM foods may someday help prevent illnesses such as cancer and osteoporosis, critics claim that GM foods could cause health problems (allergic or toxic reactions) and damage the environment.

The use of GE crops increases the pesticidal pollution of food and water supplies. Most research done is to enable plants to handle more pesticides. Since the green revolution, the use of pesticides has increased, and yet the crops destroyed by insects have doubled. The Food and Drug Administration (FDA) has had to classify genetically grown corn and potatoes, which have been engineered to produce toxins that kill insects, as insecticides instead of vegetables.

Presently, certified organic foods are the best bet for the anti-GM consumer. However, even with the best intentions, companies attempting to exclude GM ingredients from their products have found contamination from GM crops. An organic company recently had to recall a batch of organic tortilla chips after tests showed that they contained GM maize. The company believes that cross-pollination of crops was to blame. A supermarket chain tried to ban GM ingredients from its own brand products but had to write its suppliers acknowledging that some GM contamination is unavoidable because of cross-pollination of crops. Meanwhile, organic farming is under threat from the biotech companies. In the United States, lawyers from the biotech companies are trying to force the government to require that GM crops be declared organic. Some U.S. states have succumbed to Monsanto's pressure and banned GM-free labels on food. Monsanto has successfully sued dairy farmers who labeled dairy products as free from Monsanto's genetically engineered bovine growth hormone.

How Do I Find Non-GM Foods?

It might help to look at the produce stickers, those little stickers on fruits and vegetables. They contain different PLU codes depending on whether the fruit was conventionally grown, organically grown, or genetically engineered. The PLU code for conventionally grown fruit consists of four numbers, organically grown fruits have five numbers prefaced by the number 9, and GM fruits have five numbers prefaced by the number 8.

Many people believe when they enter a health food store that everything in the store is healthy, but that is not the case. There's a lot about the natural foods industry that is dishonest, and it seems like the larger the companies get, the more dishonest they become. The small companies still offer genuinely natural foods without all the additives, preservatives, and taste enhancers, but once they become large and successful or get purchased by a larger food company, it seems like all the formulas suddenly change, and it's just another "natural" brand of junk food. This is why we always have to read the ingredient list, even on products we trust. This is where we find most of our answers, but as I stated before, not all.

Conclusion

When we consume whole, real food, our bodies respond in health. Authentic farming is how all food is produced by the growers who sell it. Fresh fruits and vegetables are sold within a 50- to 150-mile radius, making all food at its highest nutritional quality. The soils are naturally nourished, and cover crops are included along with crop rotation. Pest control is treated as an imbalance, where the problem is addressed, not the symptoms; healthy crops have no pest problems. Eating organic and authentic foods is a powerful way to protect our health, our children's health, and the health of our planet.

We have the power to refuse to consume what is detrimental to our health and to the planet. Since there is very little control by the U.S. government, the responsibility lies with us. Let us put our money where our mouths are. Buy organic whenever possible. We have the power to restore the world to one that is aligned with the healing harmony of the way nature has intended us to eat.

About the Author

Kathryn Morrow has a doctorate of divinity in holistic and spiritual health through the American Institute of Holistic Theology and a master's in holistic nutrition through Clayton College. She is an integrated health care professional, educator, counselor, professional speaker, author of the book *The Color of Nutrition*, a talk radio show host, a Reiki master and intuitive counselor, and a lecturer at local colleges. Her motivational and inspirational talks and private consults assist people to better understand nutrition and how healthy food enables a healthy body, mind, and spirit. Contact her at (727) 596-0783, by e-mail at Kmorrow3@tampabay.rr.com, or at http://www.kathrynmorrow.net.

21

Nutrition Strategies to Turbo-Charge Your Metabolism

Scott Tousignant, BHK, CFC

This article is not about a new miracle pill that melts the fat off your body. The best strategy of fat loss is to *earn it*. Forget about any shortcuts and quick fixes—they do more damage than good.

The first step in earning a lean and tight body is to consume five to six small meals per day. It is something so simple, yet many of us choose to ignore it. This alone is enough to kick-start your metabolism.

- You should eat every two and one half to three hours. Each meal should be small and leave you feeling satisfied but not full. If you are not quite hungry three hours after you've consumed your meal, it's a sign that you ate too much. Basically, take what you would eat during your three meals each day and spread it out over six meals.

To get the most out of each meal and turn up your metabolic furnace, it's best to combine a lean protein, a complex carbohydrate, vegetables, and essential fatty acids with each meal. I am a firm believer in this food combination.

Eating carbohydrates alone will result in quick digestion and an insulin spike. Protein takes longer to digest and requires your body to burn more calories during the digestion process (thermic effect of food). Consuming proteins with your carbohydrates will cause the digestion of the carbohydrates to take longer, and you will stay satisfied longer as well.

The serving size of each meal is based on each individual's needs and should be evaluated on a weekly basis by measuring your weight and body fat percentage. Modify your portions so that the result is one or two pounds of fat loss each week.

If you are losing more than two pounds each week, I suggest that you increase your caloric intake slightly. If you lose too much weight in a short period of time, chances are you are sacrificing some muscle mass and reducing your metabolism in the process.

This is a very common problem with the typical low-calorie diet, where there is a significant reduction in calories and holding them there at that low level. During the beginning stages of the diet, you may lose a significant amount of weight, but then you notice that your results start to decrease, until eventually, you are no longer losing weight, even though you are still following the strict diet.

At this point, you figure that you probably hit a plateau, and you decrease your calories a little bit more so that you can lose those last ten pounds. The plateau that you have experienced is due to your body's defense mechanism—it is on red alert and screaming, "I'm starving!"

So what does your body do?

It releases more fat-storing hormones and enzymes into the bloodstream and decreases the fat-burning hormones and enzymes. Why? The answer is that your body is simply trying to protect itself, so it stores whatever it can as fat to prepare for this famine that you are putting yourself through. The end result is a decrease in your metabolism. So what can you do to prevent this from happening?

- Use "calorie cycling." To lose weight, you definitely need a caloric deficit, meaning that you need to burn more calories than you are taking in. You should never drastically reduce your calories. Aim for a 15 to 20 percent reduction in calories.

Other diets fail because they maintain this deficit for an extended period of time. With calorie cycling, you follow this deficit for three days, and on the fourth day, you go back to your maintenance caloric intake, which is the amount of calories that you could eat without gaining or losing any weight. You then repeat the cycle.

What this strategy does is just when your body starts to think that it better make some changes to lower your metabolism and store up some fat, you trick it by slightly increasing your calories. This also gives you a boost in energy and does not leave you feeling deprived.

- The second strategy improves on calorie cycling and is called "carbohydrate cycling." If you reduce your calories by 15 percent, the reduction would come entirely from carbohydrates. Follow the three days of reduced carbohydrates, and on the forth day, increase your carbohydrate intake back to normal. This is not your typical low-carb diet. A 15 percent decrease is not an absurd amount, and you get to bring it back to normal on the fourth day, which will replenish your glycogen stores in your muscles to give you more energy and strength to get through your workouts.
- The third strategy is called "calorie tapering." In a five- to six-meal-per-day plan, you consume more calories in your first few meals of the day and reduce the amount of calories in each meal as the day goes on. For example, at breakfast, mid morning, and lunch, you may consume four hundred calories at each meal. Then for the next two meals, you consume three hundred calories and, finally, two hundred calories at your last meal.

To improve this strategy, you should consume your starchy carbohydrates, such as oatmeal, sweet potatoes, and brown rice, in the earlier meals, and for the remaining two or three meals, consume fibrous carbohydrates such as vegetables. The reason for this is that the starchy carbohydrates are more calorie-dense, meaning that a small portion of them would equal the same amount of calories as a large portion of vegetables. By consuming the starchy carbs in the morning, it will provide you with the right amount of fuel to get you through your day.

It's not realistic to maintain a perfect nutrition plan for an extended period of time. There are several diet plans that allow a cheat day. I find that most people go way overboard on their cheat days. If you are serious about your nutrition program, you should limit yourself to one or two cheat meals per week. This would depend on how many meals you consume each day. If you are eating five to six meals each day, then two cheat meals per week is great. Make sure that the rest of your day is perfect.

This is not a quick fix weight loss strategy. Incorporating nutrition-packed, whole, natural foods into small, frequent meals is not rocket science, but it definitely works. It will take some planning to prepare meals ahead of time, but the results will be worth it. Best of all, this is a program that you can follow for life. Eating frequent meals will leave you satisfied, and the temptation to binge will be reduced.

Nutrition is a very large piece of the puzzle in your battle for fat loss and should be taken seriously. To truly ignite your metabolic furnace, it is absolutely necessary to include weight training, cardio, and the most important piece of the puzzle, which is developing a powerful mind-set. Your body will only go as far as your mind will take it.

About the Author

Scott Tousignant, BHK, CFC, is a certified personal fitness trainer, motivational coach, author of *The Fit Chic* and *The Fit Bastard,* and creator of Unstoppable Fat Loss. For a limited time Scott is granting you Private Access to one full month of fat burning and body sculpting workouts. Women claim your gift at http://www.FitChicFatLoss.com. Men claim your gift at http://www.AskTheFitBastard.com while this special offer lasts.

22

The Secret to Healthy Weight Loss and Unlimited Energy

Thomas Von Ohlen, MS, NC

For many years, I have seen the equation diet + exercise = weight loss. Let me explain the problem with this equation. Can you imagine trying to sit on a three-legged stool that had one leg missing? Missing one third of the parts will cause you to fall short of your intended outcome every time. Let me fill in the missing part of the weight loss equation: diet + exercise + *metabolism* = weight loss. You see, tens of millions of Americans have dieted and exercised for years with intense dedication and still not gotten the results they were searching for. Without taking into account your metabolic function, you can never properly assess your weight control needs!

So what exactly is your metabolism? Metabolism is the sum of the processes by which your body changes phytochemicals from food into the energy needed to move, breathe, think, and, essentially, live. When you eat food, your metabolism converts the phytochemicals in the food into other chemicals your body needs such as vitamins, minerals, amino acids, glucose, and water. You may wonder why some people have a fast metabolism while others are slow, or why some who once had a fast metabolism now have a slow one. Well, three main systems in your body help regulate your metabolism. They are the liver, thyroid gland, and most importantly, your adrenal glands.

Each of your two adrenal glands is located above each kidney and does numerous things for your body. They first and foremost regulate over forty hormones, or chemical messengers, which play a crucial role in your metabolism! The same glands also initiate the immune response, regulate blood pressure and blood sugar levels, and produce much of the digestive juices you use in breaking down your foods. The two reasons that our adrenal glands are weakened have to do with input and output. First, we will discuss adrenal output.

What you may not know is that every day, you experience physical, mental, and chemical stress, which affects your body chemistry on a cellular level, and it is the cells in the adrenal glands that take the brunt of these stresses. Over years of stress, the adrenals become fatigued and can no longer regulate all the constituents of a healthy metabolism properly. Sometimes the adrenals, in a weakened state, are referred to as "insufficient," and as the progression of adrenal breakdown continues, it leads to so-called adrenal burnout, as described by the late Dr. Paul Eck, who researched adrenal function and tissue analysis for decades. In either stage, a person may exhibit symptoms such as weight gain, chronic infection, allergies, high blood pressure, high and low blood sugar levels, PMS, depression, and anxiety.

When your adrenals are fatigued, you look for an outside stimulant to jump-start them. Increased intake of caffeine may be an indicator of coping with adrenal weakness. Unfortunately, caffeine is also a chemical stressor. While the average cup of coffee contains 100–150 milligrams of caffeine, just 250 milligrams of caffeine has been shown to cause insomnia, headaches, nervousness, and even stomach ulcers. Other diseases associated with different levels of caffeine intake are miscarriages, bladder cancer, breast cancer, ovarian cysts, and prostate cancer. The reason caffeine has been linked to such disorders is that when the adrenals are synthetically stimulated over and over, they make mistakes and send hormones to the wrong places in our bodies, which leads to cellular imbalance.

Other substances that push the adrenals are sugar, enriched and bleached flours, nicotine, alcohol, diet pills, and sometimes even excessive exercise. We need to rest and feed our adrenals after years of stress, but instead, we push them chemically, like whipping a dying horse.

There are other dietary intake factors that slow your metabolism as well. The intake of dairy products affects your hormone levels and immune system. When dairy products are pasteurized, the high heat destroys the enzyme phosphatase, which is necessary for the absorption of calcium. Also, the addition of hormones and antibiotics to the dairy cows will cause more biochemical imbalance and toxicity. Red meat from cows also slows our metabolism due to the same chemical processing as well as the high fat and protein, which take a great deal of digestive enzymes to break down. Remember, when the adrenals are insufficient, it will negatively affect digestive enzyme production as well. Hydrogenated fats are found in almost all packaged foods today, and they will most definitely slow down your metabolism since the body was never intended to break these man-made fats down.

Regarding the input to the adrenal glands, this is where a large problem remains. You can cut out all the chemical stimulants and dietary intake of metabolism killers, but what are you doing to rebuild your already weakened adrenal glands? I have often given my patients the analogy of the body and a bank account. Let's say that for years, you made withdrawals from your bank account until there was almost no money left in it. You realize you better stop taking money out or you won't be able to pay your bills. Even if you stop making withdrawals for many years, the interest on the little amount left in your account will not build the account back up to where it once was. To restore your finances in that account, you need to make deposits.

This means that we need to put back the proper nutrients into our human bank accounts.

On top of all the toxic chemicals that are allowed into your food sources, a big problem is that there are very small amounts of nutrients in your food at all! According to *Earth Summit Report, 1992*, 85 percent of the nutrients in North America's soil have been depleted! That statistic is from fifteen years ago, and things have certainly not gotten any better on our commercial farms. Since your metabolism relies heavily on proper nutrients, which are no longer found in adequate amounts in our soil, you need to supply your body with an alternate nutrient source.

Following are some tips to strengthen your adrenals and have a superior metabolic rate:

- Make sure you are getting proper amounts of sleep. The body needs to shut down at night to repair from the damage of the day.
- Try to purchase your meats, fruits, vegetables, and grains from organic sources whenever possible, and always drink plenty of purified water!
- The addition of whole food vitamin and mineral supplements is always a good idea to ensure you are getting the nutrients you need to keep your metabolism working the way it was designed to.
- If your body is already showing signs of adrenal insufficiency or burnout, you should consult a health care professional about an adrenal gland supplement.
- Do not let yourself get into stressful situations, and if you find yourself in one, resolve it as quickly as possible to lessen the amount of stress to the adrenals.

Once you heal your adrenal glands and maintain them at peak performance, your new energy level will amaze you. Now apply this knowledge daily, and watch the results!

About the Author

Thomas Von Ohlen, MS, NC, is a clinical nutritionist and developer of Plasma Pro software for doctors. After suffering for many years as a child and young adult with his own health ailments, he dedicated all his time to finding the truth about health. Today, he continues that same dedication to helping others who are sick and tired of being sick and tired. In his fifteen years in private practice, he has helped thousands of people from all over the world achieve their health goals through education and specific product recommendations. His *free* newsletter and full report on *weight loss* is available at http://www.healyourbodynow.com.

23

The Secret Link between Nutrition and Behavior: Addressing Intolerance to Food and Your Mood

Rose Forbes, HHP, CNC

If you find yourself feeling unwell and can't figure out why, you may be suffering from a food intolerance. Unexplained fatigue and tiredness as well as brain fogginess, which make it difficult to concentrate or remember, can be linked to eating a food that doesn't agree with your body.

Food Allergies

When you hear the term *food allergy*, you may think of a severe reaction to a food or environmental hazard that results in a rash, hives, breathing difficulties (anaphylactic shock), or loss of consciousness. If you know someone with a peanut allergy, for example, you know that he cannot come into contact with the offending allergen by smell, touch, or taste. A simple definition for *allergy* is a condition in which the body has an exaggerated response to a substance like a food or drug. A blood test can often diagnose a true allergy.

What Is Food Intolerance?

Food intolerances may not have the obvious physical symptoms of an allergy. However, they can have a profound impact on health. The definition of food intolerance is a reaction to a specific food or food ingredient.

Major Symptoms of Food Intolerance

Symptoms of food intolerance include the following:

* mood swings
* irritability

- impatience
- anxiety
- depression
- sleep disorders
- headaches
- skin rash
- diarrhea
- bed-wetting
- asthma
- eczema
- infertility
- weight gain or loss.

The top food intolerances that people experience include dairy (75 percent of people), yeast (33 percent), wheat and gluten (15 percent), and sugar (35 percent).[6] Other relevant intolerances are monosodium glutamate (MSG), soy, corn, eggs, artificial colors, artificial flavors, and artificial sweeteners, including aspartame, saccharine, and sucralose.

Food Intolerance–Related Disorders

Food intolerance can affect different systems of our bodies, including the following:

- gastrointestinal (stomach and intestines)
- respiratory (lungs and breathing)
- skin (rashes, hives, etc.)
- neurological (pain, memory, and mood)
- muscle and bone
- reproductive (genital and fertility issues)
- immune (ability to fight infection).

Since reactions may take two to three days to present themselves, linking the food to a food intolerance illness is often difficult. Physicians are not usually knowledgeable enough about food intolerances to make a diagnosis or suggest a remedy.

---

[6] See http://www.zipworld.com.au/~ataraxy/Salicylates_list.html and the Food Intolerance Support Group at http://foodintol.com.

Determining the Link

Here are some ideas of how each food intolerance may be linked to specific symptoms.

Dairy
A dairy intolerance may result in intestinal imbalance, digestive problems, diarrhea, skin rash, gas, bloating, nausea, and cramps. After age two, many humans develop an inability to digest lactose due to an enzyme deficiency as our bodies produce less lactase. Some may find relief by taking a lactose enzyme tablet before eating dairy products to aid in the digestion of lactose. Read labels carefully to identify processed foods containing whey, lactose, milk, butter, cheese, yogurt, or curds.

Yeast
Candida albicans, or yeast, is normally present in the body. When the beneficial bacteria balance is compromised by antibiotics, excessive intake of sweets and refined carbohydrates, or immune issues, Candida can grow unchecked. Symptoms include mood swings, fatigue, memory loss, headache, and cravings for sweets.

Wheat and Gluten
Wheat and gluten intolerance may result in gastrointestinal and digestive problems such as skin rash, diarrhea, bloating, and gas.

Sugar
Sugar should be considered to include all refined carbohydrates (which convert to sugar), including table sugar, sweets, breads, pastas, and so on. Primary symptoms include irritable bowel syndrome, gas, bloating, and weight gain. The enzymes lactase, maltase, and isomaltase are needed to break down the disaccharides; when one or more is inadequate, the result is carbohydrate or sugar intolerance.

ADD and Autism

Many of our precious children as well as adults are being routinely diagnosed with autism spectrum disorders, including attention-deficit disorder (ADD), attention-deficit/hyperactivity disorder (ADHD), Asperger's syndrome, sensory issues, and autism.[7] Although mood-altering drugs like Ritalin and Aderal have a place for

---

[7] Doris Rapp, "Is This Your Child?" (http://www.drrapp.com).

some, many can avoid these drugs by changing their diets to remove known and unknown allergens and food intolerances. Likely foods that may be culprits include wheat, dairy, and artificial colors and flavors. Dr. Feingold, a pioneer in the autism field as an allergist and pediatrician, believed that food additives and salicylate-containing foods, aspirin, medications, or skin care products may be the culprit.[8] Some foods with high concentrations of salicylates include dried fruits, berries, and citrus products. Behaviors that teachers, physicians, or therapists commonly label as ADD/ADHD can often be stopped, or at least reduced, by following a restricted diet.

Dietary Changes Are the Key to Success

If you believe you may have a food intolerance, you are probably right. Fortunately, a change in diet is the only remedy you should require. After eating an offending food, you may know that you are experiencing a reaction. In other cases, you may need to embark on a rotation or elimination diet,[9] which will help you cycle through different food groups to pinpoint where your intolerance lies. Many of these intolerances include similar symptoms, so it may be necessary to use a rotation diet to determine the exact food that is causing you problems. A basic rotation diet will allow a limited number of whole foods (healthy carbohydrates, fats, and proteins) usually on a four-day cycle. Dairy, wheat, gluten, eggs, sugar, yeast, coffee, alcohol, dried fruits, soda, and other common contributors to food allergies are eliminated. Followers must choose from a list of acceptable foods. For example, day 1 includes a selection of lamb, beef, clams, tomato, and spinach, to name a few. On day 2, chicken, celery, tuna, cherries, and peaches are among the options. Days 3 and day 4 also come with their own lists of foods.

Once you have discovered which foods are not agreeing with you, eliminating them will be the ultimate test. This will generally take thirty to ninety days of experimentation. In many cases, you will be able to add back small quantities of the offending food and may be able to tolerate it again after your body readjusts and balances itself. In other cases, you may need to keep the food out of your diet for a longer time before you can tolerate it well. It is getting easier to maintain a diet without dairy, wheat, or gluten with plenty of tasty and inexpensive options becoming available. It will take much more vigilance on your part to stay away from

---

[8] See http://www.feingold.org.

[9] See http://www.cfids.org/about-cfids/elimination-diet.asp, http://curezone.com/diet, http://www.askdrsears.com/html/4/T041200.asp.

foods that contain sugar, yeast, and MSG (which often masquerade on food labels as "natural flavors") as they are commonly added to almost all processed foods.

The final solution? Eat a diet of fresh, whole foods that are as close to nature as possible. This means unprocessed and mostly raw vegetables, fruits, nuts, and seeds. Avoid factory-farmed meats and animal products that may contain hormones, antibiotics, pesticides and harmful bacteria. Choose organic meat and produce whenever possible, and avoid processed foods that come in a box, can, jar, or bag with added chemicals, artificial colors and flavors, sweeteners, and other unknown and unnatural ingredients.

Making these changes will go a long way to improve your outlook on life, increase your energy level, and give your body the fuel it needs to stay well. Good health and wellness to you!

About the Author

Rose Forbes, HHP, CNC, is a board-certified holistic health practitioner and nutrition consultant practicing in Asheville, North Carolina, at the Nutrition Makeover Wellness Center. She founded the Brevard, Florida, chapter of Families for Natural Living and has been active in La Leche League and Attachment Parenting. She organized several vaccination education conferences and developed an expertise in the link between nutrition/food and behavior. She has merged her passion for cooking and nutrition as the owner of Green Mountain Bed and Breakfast, an organic and green B&B offering health and cleansing retreats. For more information, please visit Rose's Web sites: http://www.nutritionmakeover.net and http://www.greenmountainbb.com.

24

Seven Emotional Blocks to "Eating Right"

Tricia Greaves

If you're like me, you'd sooner write a nutrition book than follow one! If you've read at least one nutrition or diet book in your lifetime (or perhaps dozens), then you know what to eat. You may even have it down to a science: a cup of this, four ounces of that, two tablespoons of this, and so on. Yet when you are hungry and really want to eat, you're sitting down on the couch with a bag or box, not your measuring cup. When you have that "gotta eat" glaze, all intellectual reasoning and knowledge leaves the room: it's time to eat!

The truth is that eating right isn't as much about knowing what to eat as it is about wanting to eat it! I could have written a book on nutrition by age eighteen, but did it matter? My weight problem (fifty extra pounds!) wasn't caused by lack of nutritional know-how, it was caused by uncontrollable emotional eating. My eating was as bottomless as my emotional hunger.

We know what overeating does *to* us, so let's take a closer look at what overeating does *for* us. We don't overeat simply because we love food (if only it were that simple!). We overeat and snack on unhealthy foods out of emotional impulse. Freedom comes when we identify what emotional function overeating is playing and take action to fill our needs in healthier ways.

In the following paragraphs, I discuss the seven emotional blocks to eating.

1. The Stress Effect

The number one cause of compulsive eating is stress. When our energy is low from overactivity and burnout, we use excess food to power us through. Eating relaxes us—temporarily.

Often, our stress is self-created; we subconsciously seek validation from our professional, social, and family obligations. Are you aiming to please at the expense of your own health?

Action: Adopt a meditation or yoga practice and embrace the silence; allow peace to be your new craving, instead of approval and food. For "easy-to-do" meditation, visit http://MeditationYouCanDo.com.

2. The Great Escape

Overeating dulls our emotions. The more we eat, the further away our troubles seem to be. Eating starch and sugar causes a secretion of serotonin in our systems, creating a feeling of euphoria and a numbing of our senses. The caveat is that the further we escape in food, the harder life becomes; our problems pile up, and our ability to cope diminishes.

Action: Overeating solves nothing. Ask for help from a friend, coach, counselor, or family member to face difficult issues. The sooner you face them, the sooner you'll solve them.

3. Self-Protection Plan

Studies prove that there is a very strong link between obesity and experiences of early childhood sexual abuse. The fact is that when our bodies are violated in any way, it is natural to want to protect ourselves from further harm. Maintaining a large (or underweight) body can also be an unconscious attempt to shut down our sexuality and keep our own sexual impulses in check. We not only construct a physical prison with the intention of keeping others out, but also to trap ourselves in.

Action: Begin exploring your relationship with your body and your sexuality. Join a supportive dance or exercise group and seek assistance from friends, a coach, or a counselor.

4. Buried Alive!

We use food as a pillow to muffle our inner voices. We all have that still, small voice (God, Spirit, Holy Spirit, conscience, intuition) inside, directing and protecting us. When we listen to it, our lives are relatively smooth and orderly. When we deny it and act from our ego mind, we create chaos. We often bury this voice to avoid the responsibility of following its guidance.

Action: Affirm daily: "I welcome, embrace, and eagerly follow my inner voice, for this brings me energy, protection, and unlimited good!"

5. Self-Sabotage Solution

Gaining weight and living in a body we cannot stand erodes our self-esteem and self-confidence. We often have a deep-seated belief that we are bad and subconsciously take perverse pleasure in our food lashings. We easily feel guilt for things we have thought, said, and done, and instead of addressing these issues directly, we seek to deliver our own punishment by overeating and suffering the consequences.

Action: Start today to forgive yourself for all that you perceive you've done wrong. Next, become diligent about amending any hurts you cause, even slight ones. When you say or do something that offends or if you make a mistake, apologize and move on.

6. Self-Care Crisis

Emotional eaters take better care of others than themselves. But if you don't take care of yourself, no one else will or can. Eating right is about self-care, not self-control. If you don't make self-respecting choices in your life, you won't be able to make self-respecting choices when it's time to eat.

Action: Spend the evening fixing and savoring a fresh, organic meal at home. Relax, and enjoy the experience!

7. Decrease the Deficit

Most compulsive eaters are compulsive doers. We pride ourselves in our near-superhuman strength and endurance. How do we do it? We overeat. At the end of a hard day, we refuel with a binge, telling ourselves that after all we've accomplished, we deserve it. The fact is that we create a deficit when we try to do more than our bodies and minds can reasonably do in a day. If we have to compensate for all do we by overeating, we are doing too much.

Action: Identify one activity a week you can cancel or pass to someone else. Everything will get done without your being there to do it.

Conclusion

As you can see, there are many reasons why we don't follow a proper eating plan. If you want real answers, look within. Chances are it's not because you have the wrong diet, running shoes, or exercise equipment. The food you crave is filling an emotional need that must be addressed and healed for you to have lasting success. Since the inner mechanisms that cause overeating also cause other chaos in our lives, when you identify and heal these mechanisms, your entire life improves, not just the number on the scale. It's only when you change your life that you can truly change your waistline!

About the Author

Tricia Greaves is a speaker, author, and private coach helping emotional eaters move beyond diets to lasting change. Register *now* for your companion *free* report "Is Your Emotional Debt Making You Hungry?"at http://www.healyourhunger.com. Tricia is also the founder of Be Totally Free!, a nonprofit organization for overcoming emotional eating, eating disorders, and various addictions. For more information, visit http://www.betotallyfree.com.

25

EveryBody Is Unique

Suzanne Monroe

Consider the fact that no one fingerprint is alike. It's amazing to think that no one in the entire world will ever share your same fingerprint. Your fingerprint is your identification, your unique marking, your signature. Just as your fingerprint is one of a kind, so is the rest of you. No one thinks exactly like you, no one talks exactly like you, and no one is you! Even if you have an identical twin, you are still an individual with an inimitable soul, body, and mind. This one and only you holds the answers to your perfect health.

When it comes to your health and eating, it's easy to forget that you are a unique being. In your quest for the perfect, flawless body, you assume that the latest fad diet advertised on the newsstand must be the way to a better-looking you. Twisted notions come to mind such as, "If it worked for my friend Jane, then it will work for me!" and "If my coworker can lose ten pounds fast by eating nothing but cottage cheese, so can I!" But when the peanut butter and celery diet fails, you are left wondering what went wrong. So you jump on the next diet roller coaster that barrels into the public eye. Stop! Don't blame yourself. There is an answer.

The truth is that there is no one right diet that will work for everyone. Despite all the dietary information available today—Vegan Is Victorious, Macrobiotic Is Marvelous, Low Carb Conquers, Raw Food Rules—you remain utterly confused. You are left with only one tool. That tool is your body's own wisdom. Yes, the answer to what and how to eat lies within you, not on the cover of your favorite magazine.

It's fascinating to think of everything you learn in your life. You learn to wake up on time and arrive at school before the bell rings. You learn either to get good grades or fail. You learn to operate bikes, automobiles, computers, and more. But when it comes to your own health, you may never take the time to learn how to operate your own system. It's your body's wisdom that will tell you when you are hungry, what you should eat, and for how long you should sleep. You just need to learn to listen to what your body is saying to you.

You may be wondering, "Why can't I hear any of this then?" Well, your body speaks to you every day. It whispers to you quietly, though, and if you're not listening, you may miss it. Somewhere deep inside, as you are craving that hot fudge sundae, your body is talking to you. Perhaps it's really saying that you are scared, lonely, tired, depressed, happy, angry, or sad and that what it really needs is some physical touch or a listening ear. But the hot fudge sundae is easy; it will work to cover up your feelings . . . until the next craving.

So how can you begin to listen to your body's inner wisdom to achieve your perfect health? Do you want to reach your ideal weight, feel comfortable in your own skin, or increase your energy? There are four steps to getting in touch with the inner wisdom of your body that will send you on the path to a healthier you.

1. Slow Down

Consider that the world is not as fast paced as you think it is. By changing your belief about the world, your view of it will change. Begin to picture your world as slower and calmer. When you begin to experience stillness throughout your day, your body will thank you. Take a few moments to meditate during your daily routine. Most people avoid stopping to reflect because they are fearful of what they might discover within themselves. When you step out of your daily routine and take even just a moment for peace, you quiet the endless chatter in your head and allow your body's wisdom to speak up. Pick two times during the day to stop what you are doing, breathe, reflect, and give thanks for your incredible body that breathes, sleeps, and operates each day.

2. Chew Your Food

If such a simple step sounds insignificant, think again! If you come to the table in a rush, your body will remain in the stressful state of the fight or flight response. Imagine your body as it tries to digest food, thinking that it is going to fight a war. It's impossible! Your body will choose to store the food for later. (Huh! . . . So that's how all of those extra pounds got packed on!) Chewing your food allows your digestive juices to do their job by helping you properly assimilate food and absorb nutrients. And also, chewing your food and experiencing the taste, texture, and smell of each bite will lead to a more enjoyable experience. You can be eating the best food money can buy, but if you are disconnected from the process of experiencing your food, you will never be truly satisfied. When you relate with your food in this way, you will be less likely to go looking for something else in the pantry an hour later.

3. Eat and Listen

Now this is not your everyday food journal. Keep a log of what you eat every day and how you feel two hours after eating it. Are you still hungry? Are you too full? Are you satisfied? Is your stomach settled? What are you craving? By listing not only what you are eating but also how it makes you feel, you will begin making a connection to what you eat and how it affects your digestion, your energy level, and your mood. You are learning to turn on your inner radar so that you can listen to what your body is telling you. Most importantly, you will create the mind-body connection that is often missing in today's dining experience.

4. Honor Your Body

Start by making your health and your body a priority. Try a new exercise routine, go for a brisk walk, or participate in a yoga class. When you take time for your health and well-being, you send positive messages to your body such as, "I honor you and my health. I am in touch with you so that you can be in touch with me." Begin to talk to your body as the home of your soul. Eliminate the negative messages that you subconsciously send to your physical body. Try this exercise: begin by standing in front of the mirror naked. Stand there for five minutes and notice what you love about your body. Then state it out loud. Repeat this several times a week until you feel connected to both your physical and emotional self. When you concentrate on the beauty that you have, you will by law attract more beauty.

When you slow down, chew your food, eat and listen, and honor your body, you will reconnect with that inner voice that tells you each day all you need to know about what to eat, when to eat, and how much to eat. There is no one, single miracle diet that will tell you what your own body needs to be happy, fulfilled, and healthy. You are your own guide for healthy eating and living.

About the Author

Suzanne Monroe is an accomplished holistic health and nutrition counselor trained in holistic health counseling, Eastern and Western nutrition theories, the use of nutrition as therapy, and wellness lifestyle coaching. She is the founder of Intelligent Health Group, LLC, a health and wellness company that offers organizational wellness programs, one-on-one nutritional counseling in person or via phone, grocery store seminars, and healthy cooking classes. To sign up for her free e-newsletter or weekly recipe subscription, visit www.intelligenthealthgroup.com, http://www.milwaukeehealthcoach.com, or
http://www.online-nutrition-counseling.com.

26

Why You Can't Lose Weight

Dr. Dan Pompa, DC

Part I—The Hormone Connection

It is time to bring the science of weight loss out of the Dark Ages and apply a new understanding of hormones and their impact on metabolism.

In 1995, a hormone called leptin was discovered. This hormone is the one that tells your brain to burn fat for energy. If your brain is not receiving the correct message from this hormone, then your body will not be able to burn fat for energy. What does this mean? Simply put, you will not lose weight, regardless of what you eat or how much you exercise. Drug companies scrambled to develop a synthetic form of leptin in an attempt to be the first to have the solution to obesity. They figured that if leptin tells the brain to burn fat, then overweight individuals must be leptin-deficient, right? Wrong! They soon realized that obese and overweight people had elevated leptin. Why? It is analogous to type II diabetes. A diabetic has plenty of insulin, but his cells just can't use it. This is due to the overconsumption of processed grains and sugars as well as to toxicity. The constant sugar elevation causes the body to release more and more insulin. Because insulin is constantly elevated along with sugar (glucose), the cells' receptors for insulin become burned out. In other words, the cells cannot hear what insulin is saying—a.k.a. insulin resistance.

The same thing is happening with leptin. Leptin is produced by your fat cells to tell your brain that there is too much fat, and therefore the command is to burn it. Just like with insulin, if this system is challenged enough, it will eventually break down. The increase in leptin will eventually cause your brain not to hear the signal to burn fat. The receptors in your brain (hypothalamus) burn out—a.k.a. leptin resistance.

Once this hormone mechanism fails, it will become nearly impossible to lose weight—a.k.a. weight loss resistance.

However, there is hope The Healing Diet. A diet that eliminates everything that turns to sugar and that is high in good fats will allow insulin and leptin receptors to heal and therefore reset the hormonal mechanisms. This means a diet that has no sugar and grains because grains turn to sugar within four seconds of entering the mouth. Once an individual's insulin and leptin receptors have been burned out and they are in a state of insulin or leptin resistance, even whole, healthy grains such as oatmeal or whole wheat products will not be tolerated. The receptors will only regenerate if we control the elevation of sugar (glucose). Therefore fruit is not allowed on this diet, unless it is berries and used sparingly. Protein must be kept in moderation, averaging between fifteen and twenty-five grams per meal, depending on body size and activity. Protein can turn to sugar and therefore must be limited. Last, an increase in healthy fats helps control glucose and insulin and heal their receptors. The increase in healthy fats will also restore depleted hormones. As you can see, this is not a low-carb or high-protein diet. I would more accurately describe it as a high-fat, moderate-protein, and moderate-carbohydrate diet due to the increase in vegetables.

Who Needs The Healing Diet?

Besides someone who simply cannot lose weight despite diet or exercise, there are five additional factors to determine who needs this diet. Any one of the five qualifies you.

1. *Triglycerides/cholesterol.* If your body cannot hear the hormone leptin, it is unable to burn fat for energy, and therefore circulating blood fat in the form of triglycerides or cholesterol will eventually be elevated.
2. *High blood pressure.* High blood pressure is caused by a narrowing and/or hardening of the arteries initiated by oxidation of cholesterol and inflammation within the arterial wall. By eliminating glucose (sugar), you are controlling hormones such as insulin and leptin, which reduces inflammation and therefore blood pressure.
3. *Elevated glucose, leptin, or insulin.*
4. *Genetics.* Some individuals, depending on their ancestral origins, do better on certain diets than others. This is why some people do well with low-carb diets and others do better with high-carb diets. Because there is not a simple test to take for this factor, the only advice I can give you is if you are someone who has tried other diets and failed, have a family history of heart disease, diabetes, and/or obesity, then this diet is probably for you.
5. *Neurotoxicity.* Neurotoxins cause systemic inflammation affecting hormones, especially those dealing with weight loss. Neurotoxins such as heavy metals (mercury, lead, etc.) and biotoxins (mold, lyme, etc.) enter the body and, in the genetically susceptible, attach to fat and nerve cells. Neurotoxic individuals will not lose weight, regardless of diet (even this diet) or exercise, unless this issue is addressed; therefore this subject will be discussed further in Part II.

Part II—The Toxicity Factor

After addressing the hormones leptin and insulin with diet, only one problem potentially remains. According to Dr. Richie C. Shoemaker, "one-third of all leptin-resistance comes from the chronic biotoxic illnesses that are now spreading rapidly across America."[1] When we add in general toxicity from heavy metals, food, and our environment, the problem is epidemic. Dr. Shoemaker is the utmost respected authority on biotoxic illnesses and believes that 98 percent of those who are significantly overweight are leptin-resistant, most of which he feels is due to toxicity.

If The Healing Diet is the correct diet for you based on the five factors, the weight will come off with ease. If not, toxicity must be considered and is likely the cause of your uncontrollable cravings, diet failures, and inability to lose weight.

When toxins enter your body, they have an affinity for fat cells due to the fact that they are fat-soluble. When the toxins attach to the outer cell membrane, which is made of a lipid bilayer (two layers of fat), they cause the cell to continually release leptin. When leptin is continuously elevated, just like insulin in type II diabetes, the receptors burn out, and the message is not heard. Remember, leptin is the hormone that tells the brain to burn fat for energy; therefore weight gain that does not respond to exercise or diet is inevitably due to leptin resistance. The toxins also cause the unregulated release of chemicals, called cytokines, that damage leptin receptors in the brain (hypothalamus). Once the receptors to leptin have been damaged, weight loss resistance is only the first of many problems. Your body makes an extremely important hormone called melanocyte stimulating hormone (MSH). MSH is produced in the hypothalamus by leptin and is at the top of the hormone chain and therefore controls numerous body functions: immune system, inflammation, skin and mucus membrane defenses, endorphin and melatonin production. If your brain cannot hear leptin due to toxicity, you will eventually become MSH-deficient[2].

What Does This Mean?

It means that every immune and hormone response in your body will be altered. Practically speaking, you feel horrible and cannot figure out why. You find yourself on medications, chasing symptoms on a never-ending downward spiral—the pitfall of modern medicine. The key to twenty-first-century medicine is understanding how toxins affect this hormonal cascade, causing inflammation that leads to so many

---

[1] Ritchie C. Shoemaker, *Mold Warriors: Fighting America's Hidden Health Threat* (Baltimore: Gateway Press, 2005), 482.
[2] Ibid, 91-99.

new-millennium diseases such as depression, diabetes, cancer, heart disease, chronic fatigue, and fibromyalgia, just to name a few.

The solution lies in proper detoxification. This does not mean some simple colon cleanse or liver detoxification program. These neurotoxins must be chelated (detoxed) very specifically, depending on the toxin; therefore proper testing is also very important. This being the case, working alongside a doctor experienced in this kind of toxicity is of paramount importance because this is your health, and there are so many fad detoxification programs on the market today. True detoxification must occur at the cellular level.

In conclusion, the majority of Americans cannot lose weight, despite diet and excessive exercise. The amount of processed grains and sugars and the onslaught of toxicity are causing major hormonal problems, which lead to uncontrollable cravings, the inability to burn fat for energy, a decrease in metabolism, muscle wasting, and eventually, a new-millennium disease.

Following The Healing Diet and ridding your body of toxins properly will reset your entire hormonal system and bring your body back into balance. You will finally have success, even if you have had many failures in the past, because you will be getting to the cause of why you can't lose weight.

About the Author

Dr. Pompa received his bachelor of science degree from the University of Pittsburgh. He earned his doctor of chiropractic degree at Life University in Marietta, Georgia, in 1995, where he graduated second in his class. Today, he is internationally known for his expertise in neurotoxic illness, nutrition, and structural correction chiropractic care. As a sought-after doctor and educator for the treatment of such neurotoxic-mediated illnesses as autism, chronic fatigue syndrome, and fibromyalgia, his teaching is transforming lives around the world. His philosophy of using natural solutions with the latest research in these misunderstood conditions have brought healing to the seemingly incurable and are being replicated by other physicians he teaches across the nation.

For doctors trained in the protocols discussed in this article, visit these pages: http://www.pompahealthsolutions.com and http://maximizedliving.com/Programs/Chiropractors/currentCNP.aspx.

PART THREE

Energy Healing
& Other Unique Techniques

Energy and persistence alter all things.

-- Benjamin Franklin

27

Bowen: The Key to Optimal Health and Pain Elimination

Raymond Augustyniak, PhD

Bowen is a multidimensional healing system that alleviates human pain and suffering. It was discovered and developed by the late Tom Bowen of Geelong, Australia. It is a natural health care solution that safely and gently awakens and revives the self-healing mechanisms of the body by applying the minimal amount of treatment to generate the greatest positive response. It rapidly restores a state of optimal health and healing in the body without the need for medication or surgery. Simply put, Bowen is the best-kept secret in health care today!

Bowen works by using a particular series of "activations," a type of gentle soft tissue manipulation, over precise points on the body. The practitioner uses a specific series of activations to address the body in very particular ways to elicit specific responses. The activations that are used are determined by what area of the body needs to be released or what specific health issue needs to be addressed. The practitioner *only* performs activations that are in agreement with the body's specific needs and what it can process and use that day. Each individual activation utilizes the central and autonomic nervous systems to send direct signals that stimulate the entire body to awaken, reenergize, and revive core healing mechanisms and initiate cellular level changes. Ideal organ and system functioning, optimal health, and elimination of pain are the result in nearly every case.

Bowen is consistently effective in eliminating pain and addressing a very long list of conditions and ailments ranging from tension to severe muscular and joint pain, fibromyalgia, carpal tunnel syndrome, plantar fasciatis, acid reflux, depression, stress, asthma, TMJ, allergies, respiratory problems, PMS, and erectile dysfunction to name just a few. Its consistency in addressing all kinds of pain and mild to severe health-related issues with a high level of success is unrivaled.

The benefits of Bowen are numerous, including elimination of tension and anxiety, improved breathing, restful sleep, calm children, increased energy, greater stamina, improved mental clarity and focus, rapid recovery from surgery, and rehabilitation from injury.

People commonly resolve 50–60 percent of their long list of ailments within the first seven days after just one treatment. With Bowen, the body will continue to heal and change for three to five days after a treatment *as though it received a treatment every day*. Between treatments, the body will continue to peel off layers of signs, conditions, disorders, and dysfunctions until core issues are addressed. In most cases, once a core issue is addressed, it clears itself from the body, and the results are almost immediate and long lasting.

In nearly 90 percent of all cases, people are restored back to optimal health within an initial set of only three to five treatments. Each treatment is generally spaced five to ten days apart, with seven days between treatments being optimal for most people. After the initial set of treatments, maintenance is performed on an as needed basis, similar to a tune-up for a car. Urgent, nonemergency care can be performed immediately after an injury or trauma to quickly initiate the healing processes and to get the body out of shock. Athletes who sustain an ankle sprain or neck, shoulder, or muscle strain, for example, can rapidly return to competition in as little as two to five minutes at 80–100 percent. Another case, an asthma attack, can be stopped in as little as ten to twenty seconds using a very specific, yet simple, set of activations.

Bowen is very gentle in its approach. Anyone, ranging from newborn infants through aging adults, with *any* condition can receive treatment without any potential health risk or risk of harm or injury. Athletes use Bowen to provide a very rapid, all-natural, exceptional, and superior competitive edge.

A treatment can take as long as sixty minutes to complete or, in some cases, as little as ten minutes, depending on what the body needs and can optimally receive *and* use that day. One of the key elements to Bowen is that each successive treatment builds *and compounds* on the last one. This directly influences and accelerates healing on much deeper levels, greatly improving overall health and well-being as multiple layers of ill health and dysfunction are removed.

Bowen is very unique in its approach to the body and clearly exceptional. It is unlike any other bodywork or physical treatment method. During a treatment, the practitioner performs just a few activations at precisely located points on the body and then walks away for a few minutes. The practitioner returns, activates a few more points, and then leaves again, continuing in this manner throughout the course of the treatment. The waiting times placed in between a series of activations are an integral part of the treatment. They allow the body time to take in the signals that were given, while also allowing it time to respond and make much needed adjustments or changes. This process of only slightly activating the body before leaving it to respond and change also protects the body from overstimulation as overstimulation quickly causes the body to become defensive. The waiting time also gives the practitioner time to observe and identify any changes the body has made in direct response to the work that was performed. The responses, or, in some cases, a nonresponse, give the practitioner solid clues to the true current state of the body on deep levels, and they show the direction it is heading and also give subtle hints for the practitioner to follow. These hints communicate to the practitioner what the body wants or needs next. This unique and proactive relationship between the response of the body and the practitioner has a direct correlation to the extraordinary, very predictable, and lasting results Bowen achieves.

Bowen is simple, straightforward, and deliberate. It works *with* the body and what it presently needs, causing the body to stimulate healing from the inside out, in the reverse order that issues came. It also allows the body to heal what *it* knows is most important first as it aligns with and draws on its own optimal health and healing blueprint once again. The body does the work, not the practitioner. Bowen just simply opens pathways that have been dormant. Once the pathways are opened, neural-chemical changes instantaneously radiate throughout the entire body at lightning speed, setting off numerous chains of events that directly and powerfully impact every system, organ, and muscle in the body to varying degrees. The results of the overall impact on the body produce monumental shifts that can actually be felt during a typical Bowen treatment.

Characteristically, many of these shifts are experienced as a form of heat or heating up, vibration, a slight tingling sensation, body shifting, and/or slight involuntary muscle movements as the body begins to open and communicate with itself again. People often report that they can actually *feel* their bodies calm down, rebalance, and let go as the stress, tension, and pain simply disappear. Many also report that their minds calm down, and mind chatter vanishes, allowing them to feel a deep sense of peaceful well-being and restfulness that has been long overdue.

When the body is at rest, it begins to participate actively in resetting its own healing mechanisms, causing a myriad of acute and chronic health issues simply to resolve themselves on their own, without the need for any other outside effort or interference. Health issues that are commonly resolved include those on physiological, mental, emotional, and energetic levels. Healing on these levels transforms the entire body from a dis-eased or ill-at-ease state to a near-effortless or at-ease state of functioning and balance.

The focus of the practitioner is to concentrate initially on addressing the body as a whole, getting it to relax, open, and quickly let go of whatever it can, and *then* individually tailor the remainder of the treatment for the needs of the individual. Each consecutive treatment is tailored on the day of and during treatment to address very specific areas or conditions that are yet present in the body to achieve optimum results *as soon as possible*. As a treatment series progresses, it becomes more specific, and the length of treatment may shorten because the entire focus of the treatment will turn to more specific areas of the body that haven't yet responded, with the sole purpose of focusing the body's resources directly to a nonresponsive area or two.

Bowen simply addresses the entire body by activating key receptors that remind the body to function at its most efficient and vibrant state at all times. If the body *can* heal, it *will* heal with Bowen.

Many physicians and health care professionals around the world who have seen or experienced the superior and consistent results that Bowen produces are convinced of its profound effectiveness in addressing a long list of difficult-to-treat pain and health-related issues.

Dr. Robert Jay Rowen, MD, has written that Bowen is "the gentlest, most effective pain therapy *ever!*"

About the Author

Raymond Augustyniak, PhD, became involved with Bowen after it saved his life 14 years ago. He is the founder of the Bowen Healing System™ Centers and the Natural Healthcare Institute™ in California and regularly lectures and teaches classes both nationally and internationally. He is an author of the book *Awaken the Doctor Within!*, which explains Bowen in detail. His book also includes case studies, testimonies, a chapter on Bowen for animals, discoveries, and other theories about Bowen. His book includes over one full page of conditions that he has witnessed Bowen commonly address specifically for men, women, infants, children and teens, and athletes. More information can be found at http://www.bowenhealingsystem.com.

28

G-Jo Acupressure:
Safer, Faster, and More Effective
Than Most Drugs or Surgery

Michael Blate

Centuries ago, even ordinary families had something most people lack today: ways to relieve suffering and heal themselves without doctors, drugs, or surgery. Instead, when they fell ill, they used nature's medicines: herbs, food, and other such remedies. Perhaps surprisingly, there are actually *many* simple self-health techniques that take only minutes to learn and moments to apply yet can bring dependable relief from most common aches and ailments.

One of the safest and most effective of these is called G-Jo Acupressure—a kind of acupuncture, but without the needles. Here tiny spots, or *acupoints*, on the body are triggered in a deep, goading massage for a few seconds when a person is suffering from headache, back pain, or another common complaint. In most cases, relief follows instantly. Though ancient, G-Jo (pronounced GEE-joh) is so powerful and effective that people have continued using this safe, reliable technique in spite of modern (and often dangerous) drugs and surgery.

There are nearly two hundred G-Jo Acupressure points on the body. When you notice a pain or discomfort—say, a headache—simply reach for the appropriate G-Jo acupoint, trigger it in the special G-Jo way for a few seconds, then find and trigger the same point on the opposite side of the body. By the time you've finished, the headache should be gone. If it isn't, just reach for the next headache control point—there are more than twenty of them—and repeat the process. Nearly always, at least one of them will bring immediate relief.

Try it for yourself right now. To actually relieve that headache, begin by finding G-Jo acupoint number thirteen. Place your right hand so that the palm faces the floor. Now put your fingers out straight, side by side, and squeeze your thumb tightly against your index or pointer finger. You should see a small, fleshy mound pop up on the back of the right hand between the thumb and index finger.

Next, place the tip—not the pad or fleshy part—of the left thumb (or if you have a long thumb nail, the bent knuckle of the left index finger or even the eraser tip of a pencil) on top of that mound. Keeping the left thumb tip in place, relax the right hand and begin pressing deeply in the webbed or fleshy area that is formed between the thumb and pointer finger. Press around deeply until you feel a tender "ouch" point. This will feel like a toothache or pinched nerve when you contact it.

The more the acupoint hurts, the better it is likely to be for your headache (or other health problem since this broad-acting G-Jo point has many healing uses). Once you locate the spot, do step two of this very easy three-step process: trigger the point deeply, in a digging or goading kind of fingertip massage. Make it hurt a little. Do this for fifteen or twenty seconds on the right hand. Then stop and do step three: duplicate the find-and-trigger technique on the back of the left hand for another fifteen or twenty seconds. That's all it takes. By now, your headache should be gone.

G-Jo Acupressure works the same way for hundreds of other health problems and disorders. However, there are usually one or two best points that not only bring prompt relief, but actually stimulate the body's own self-healing mechanisms as well. Compare this to most conventional medicines, which may mask or block pain but do little to heal and restore health.

G-Jo is used symptomatically (not preventively), that is, only when symptoms manifest themselves or are suffered as a result of injury. The same good points are then triggered again as soon as the target symptom returns. The goal is to gain increasing spans of relief time, time between the return of symptoms and necessary restimulation of the best acupressure points.

Normally, you'd only need to trigger a good acupoint several times a day in the beginning, then less as time passed. In an emergency—say, to control the pain and bleeding from a cut or similar injury—you might have to stimulate the same G-Jo acupoint as often as two or three dozen times the first day or two, but, again, less as the healing process continued.

There are several types of acupressure, but G-Jo is the most easily learned form. Once you master the procedure, all you need is knowledge of where these two hundred control points are located and each of their many uses. This is what the G-Jo Institute teaches. Some acupoints are found on the hands or arms, others on the feet, legs, or body. And each G-Jo acupoint can have dozens of uses. G-Jo point number thirteen, for example, can relieve or heal some fifty health problems. Best of all, once you possess this knowledge, it is yours for life. Then you and your loved ones have become essentially health self-reliant.

Along with G-Jo point number thirteen, there are at least five other basic acupoints that everyone should know. These control large portions of the body. While not always the best G-Jo points for a specific symptom, one or another of them can usually bring quick relief from most minor or emergency—though not necessarily chronic—symptoms we are likely to encounter in our lives. Three of these points are found on the hands and arms, three on the feet and legs.

Basic training in this simple yet powerful healing method is free and takes only minutes to accomplish. But even mastering G-Jo Acupressure is remarkably fast, easy, and inexpensive. Remember, this method has been successfully used by ordinary families for many generations and for nearly every common health problem, so simplicity and ease of use are its key.

Of course, self-help can have its limits. Before using G-Jo—or any other self-health technique—first check with your doctor or other health care professional if you are a pregnant woman, especially beyond your third month of pregnancy; a chronic heart patient, especially one who wears a pacemaker or similar energy-regulating device; or if you take regular or daily medication for serious health problems.

About the Author

Author, lecturer, and media personality Michael has been sharing G-Jo Acupressure and other self-health techniques since the early 1970s. He has appeared on nearly two thousand radio and TV talk shows as a tireless promoter of health self-sufficiency. He is a cofounder of the G-Jo Institute, one of the world's largest natural health educational organizations. All the G-Jo acupoints, and the more than 250 health problems you can self-treat, are revealed in the Master of G-Jo Acupressure Home-Study Certification Program from the G-Jo Institute. You can contact the G-Jo Institute by e-mail at office@g-jo.com, by phone at 828-863-4660, by post at P.O. Box 1460, Columbus, NC 28722-1460, or at http://www.g-jo.com.

29

Feel Alive!
Thrive with the Cross Crawl

Gwenn Bonnell

Do you ever feel uncoordinated and out of balance? Or do you find it hard to focus and comprehend new information? Are simple tasks, such as reading, writing, and listening, overwhelming? Is it impossible to lose weight? Are you unable to heal? Have you lost your motivation?

What's going on? Any sort of traumatic stress, or a continual level of stress, stops the body's energies from "crossing over."

Just as the left side of the brain sends information to the right side of the body, and vice versa, our energies are meant to cross over at the neck as well. Normally, our entire system contains these crossovers. Our DNA is built on this pattern. We thrive when these crossing patterns are fluent in our physical system and energetic body.

The good news is that walking is the natural motion that reinforces this crossing pattern. Unfortunately, often, when we walk, we inhibit the natural crossover by carrying a handbag, a suitcase, a briefcase, or a child. Even holding a dog's leash sends the body's energies off balance.

We are not born with these crossing patterns. As we grow, crawling, walking, and running stimulate the receptive as well as the expressive hemispheres of the brain. These crossover patterns improve coordination, breathing, spatial awareness, hearing, vision, and overall health.

Dr. George Goodheart Jr. developed applied kinesiology, the study of how muscle movements influence health, for use by medical professionals. Robert Frost explains in *Applied Kinesiology* how Dr. Thie simplified the program for use by laypersons in his *Touch for Health* manual.[1] The *cross crawl* is one of these easy-to-learn techniques that does a lot of good. Even if done incorrectly, it is not harmful.

---

[1] Robert Frost, *Applied Kinesiology: A Training Manual and Reference Book of Basic Principles and Practices* (Berkeley, CA: North Atlantic Books, 2002).

A branch of applied kinesiology, educational kinesiology is the study of using body movement to empower learners of all ages. *Brain Gym*,[2] by Paul and Gail Dennison, explains how the cross crawl exercise reinforces the natural crossover of energy between the brain's left and right hemispheres, making learning easier. The cross crawl is also a great exercise whenever you feel lethargic and unmotivated.

Cherise, who was living HIV for twelve years, was feeling sluggish and showing signs of attention deficit disorder. Although she was eating mostly fruit, she was fifty pounds overweight. Cherise's body language reflected her increased energy level immediately on doing the cross crawl. Cherise reinforced her crossing energies with daily walks, lost thirty pounds in three months, regained her appetite and concentration, and slept more soundly.

If you don't have time for a daily walk, take a minute to cross crawl, and help maintain your health.

The Cross Crawl

1. Stand in place and perform the natural walking motion of lifting the *opposite* arm and leg together while breathing deeply. This involves lifting your right arm and left leg simultaneously. As you lower them, lift your left arm and right leg.
2. If you are not able to walk or stand, you can sit and move the opposite arm and leg together, reaching to touch the opposite knee or ankle with your hand or elbow. For infirmed people, this can be done while lying on a bed. You can have someone else move your legs and arms for you.
3. As you repeat the motion, exaggerate the lift of your leg and the swing of your arm. Even more effective is tapping the opposite knee with your hand or elbow. The important motion is to cross the midline of your body.
4. Continue this exaggerated march for at least a minute, breathing deeply in through your nose and out through your mouth.

For best results, perform the cross crawl at least once daily. The positive effects could include

- improved focus and concentration
- boosted metabolism and overall energy
- greater coordination and balance
- enhanced breathing and stamina
- better hearing and vision.

---

[2] Paul E. Dennison and Gail E. Dennison, *Brain Gym: Teacher's Edition Revised* (Ventura, CA: Edu-Kinesthetics, 1994).

There is a reason why most diet and exercise programs emphasize walking as a simple way to lose weight. Walking, especially power walking, not only burns calories, but more importantly, emulates the cross crawl motion, therefore boosting metabolism and overall energy levels.

Some people, however, will not feel immediate positive effects from walking or the cross crawl exercise; in fact, walking will actually weaken them.

Experiencing stress knocks our energies into a homolateral pattern. This means that our energies move straight up and down the body instead of crossing at the neck. Normally, we compensate, and as the trauma passes, our energies begin to cross once again. However, when we are under continual stress or experience a major trauma, this homolateral pattern becomes embedded in our system.

When our energies are no longer able to crossover, we feel slow and sluggish. Our physical body only gets about half the energy it needs; we are in survival mode. What little energy we have is used for breathing, digesting, and eliminating. Our metabolism slows.

We lack the energy needed to think clearly, to learn, to create, to concentrate, to be enthusiastic or passionate. As all our physical processes slow down, we feel less alive, and we might feel depressed. Our immune systems become hypervigilant, yet we may be chronically ill and unable to heal for unknown reasons. Donna Eden, in *Energy Medicine*, says, "You cannot get well if your energies are homolateral."[3]

Henry's father had passed unexpectedly a month before, and instead of his natural energetic, aggressive business persona, he slipped into an apathetic attitude. Losing all motivation, he stopped making phone calls, which was lethal for his home-based business. After a few minutes doing the homolateral correction, he was back to his positive self, and he continues to expand his business!

If the cross crawl is difficult for you, if you feel uncoordinated lifting your opposite arm and leg together, or if it exhausts you, then your energies are probably running straight up and down instead of crossing. Use the homolateral correction to gently instill the crossover pattern.

Homolateral Correction

1. Stand in place, and perform the walking motion. But this time, lift the *same side* arm and leg, first on one side of the body, then on the other side, to a count of twelve. Keep yourself comfortable. If it's easier to do this while sitting or lying down, that's OK. If you are ill or weak, another person can lift your arms and legs for you. *Do not*

---

[3] Donna Eden with David Feinstein, *Energy Medicine* (New York: Tarcher/Putnam, 1998), 233.

strain as this will send your energies back into homolateral. It's important to breathe deeply and rest when you get tired.

2. Next, perform the cross crawl motion: lift the *opposite* arm and leg to a count of twelve (each side).
3. This is one set. Repeat this two more times for a total of three sets.
4. Finish with an additional twelve cross crawls.

Perform this routine at least twice a day for ten to thirty days. Even though you'll probably feel immediate benefits, it may take a month or so for the crossover pattern to stabilize.

Once the crossover pattern becomes established, keep doing the cross crawl on a daily basis to maintain long-term benefits. Be aware: this is often a life-changing experience!

About the Author

Gwenn Bonnell is an internationally renowned author, teacher, and trainer, sharing Emotional Freedom Techniques (EFT) and energy medicine with the south Florida community since 1999. Gwenn's manuals include *Tap Away Those Extra Pounds with EFT* and *The Foundational Energy Psychology Training Manual*. Her audio programs include *Tap Your Troubles Away (An EFT Tutorial)*, *Remove Your Blocks to Success with EFT*, *Personal Peace*, and *Chakrativity*. For more information, visit http://www.tapintoheaven.com or call (954) 370-1552.

30

EFT:
The Universal Healing Tool That Modern Medicine Has Missed

Gary Craig

New Discovery Takes Chinese Medicine to a New Level

Thousands of years ago, physicians in China mapped the body's electrical system. They charted fourteen energy paths, or meridians, and documented how stimulating specific points along those paths released energy blocks, restored the normal flow of Chi, or healing energy, and improved health.

Acupuncture, in which very thin needles are inserted at precise locations, is one way to achieve this result. Acupressure, in which massage or pressure stimulates the same points, is another.

But until recently, no one realized that tapping on key acupuncture points while focusing on a specific problem could eliminate or significantly reduce physical, mental, or emotional symptoms.

That's why Emotional Freedom Techniques (EFT) is such an exciting discovery.

EFT's underlying premise is that the true cause of every negative thought and most physical symptoms is an energy block along one or more of the body's meridians. The combination of tapping and mental focus releases both the energy block and the problem it causes. No matter what they worry about, people of all ages, including small children, can change their minds from stressed to relaxed and improve their health and happiness, usually in less time than it takes to read this chapter.

Versatile and Widely Accepted

At first I didn't realize how versatile EFT would become or how dramatically it transforms physical as well as emotional symptoms. Then the reports began to arrive. Whenever someone asked whether EFT works on a particular condition, such as allergies, high blood pressure, colds and flu, indigestion, arthritis, asthma, insomnia, sprains, or anything else, my answer was always the same: try it, and let me know what happens.

Soon, thousands of people with no special training were sharing their results. They had tapped and lost weight, stopped smoking, recovered in minutes from muscle sprains, chased migraine headaches away, stopped pain, and recovered from all types of illness or injury.

Many medical doctors and licensed health care practitioners have adopted EFT and use it routinely. Their patients often recover without the drugs or surgery they were scheduled to receive, or they heal faster, or chronic conditions that persisted for years suddenly improve or disappear.

Physical therapists working with athletes report that sports performance improves whenever EFT is part of the treatment. Many amateur and professional athletes use EFT to increase their stamina and coordination and to prevent injury. In fact, quite a few have used EFT to significantly improve their performance in everything from golf, baseball, bowling, soccer, or gymnastics to running a marathon.

Medicine's Major Miss

What excites me most about EFT is its application to physical health and wellness. I'm convinced more than ever that modern medicine has walked right by a major contributor to chronic and acute diseases. Our unresolved angers, fears, and traumas show up in our physical bodies and manifest as rheumatoid arthritis, cancer, multiple sclerosis, Parkinson's disease, and hundreds of other illnesses.

Just about everyone knows this intuitively. Whenever Los Angeles physician Eric Robins, MD, shows patients how to do EFT, he explains that past traumas can be stored in muscles and organs in the body and that releasing past events and all the emotions they generate may alleviate physical symptoms. Dr. Robins reports that most patients grasp this concept at once, and as soon as they tap away their anger, frustration, or unhappy memories, their symptoms improve.

Psychologists have always known that there are powerful connections between mind and body, but conventional talk therapy seldom cures anything, and neither do psychoactive drugs.

But balancing the body's energy can help cure everything, and it's as simple as tapping on your head and torso while focusing on the problem. As Dr. Robins explains, this simple procedure releases or neutralizes the illness's underlying cause, and as soon as that happens, the illness itself disappears.

Ever since I discovered how simple and effective EFT can be, I've been a man on a mission. So far, 350,000 people have downloaded my free EFT manual (it gives all the basics), my free online newsletter goes to several hundred thousand subscribers, and more than thirty books have been written about EFT. To help spread the word, those who purchase my inexpensive instructional DVDs have my written permission to make one hundred copies of each disc to share with others. Thousands of EFT practitioners around the world teach classes and work with clients. These practitioners include nurses, doctors, chiropractors, acupuncturists, massage therapists, physical therapists, nutritionists, clinical psychologists, licensed social workers, and counselors of every description.

No technique or procedure works for everyone, but by all accounts, approximately 80 percent of those who try EFT for a specific problem experience significant results. That's a stunning statistic.

In Most Cases, Try EFT First

EFT has come a long way in ten years, but it's not even a blip on conventional medicine's radar. When it is noticed, it's often relegated to the "support therapy" category, something to be used later, after conventional treatments. I hope that will soon change. Unless there is a medical emergency that requires immediate attention, EFT should be the *first* treatment that doctors offer. This, in my observation, will dramatically reduce the need for drugs, surgery, or radiation. Even in emergencies, such as accidents or injuries, EFT can be extremely helpful, for it helps people think clearly while reducing pain and discomfort. In all situations, it speeds recovery and healing.

To satisfy my curiosity about EFT's effectiveness in the treatment of serious diseases, over the last two years, I traveled to different cities giving three-day seminars, in which I worked onstage with actual patients. As a result, I know more than ever that EFT is a truly universal healing tool. The same basic approach that treats diabetes, chronic fatigue syndrome, and multiple chemical sensitivities works as well for eyesight, muscular dystrophy, rheumatoid arthritis, asthma, allergies, pulled hamstring muscles, high blood pressure, and heart disease. And when it comes to fears, phobias, and anxiety, EFT is in a class by itself.

EFT is so new that it's still evolving. I encourage practitioners and newbies alike to experiment—to try it on everything. It's so versatile that you can use it on yourself, others, and animals. Some have even used it on plants, cars, and computers. It makes sense that if your energy is balanced, everything inside you and everything around you benefits.

I hope that everyone who reads this will be curious enough to try EFT. It's easy to learn, easy to do, and can literally save your life.

About the Author

EFT was introduced in 1995 by Gary Craig, a Stanford engineer in lifelong pursuit of personal well-being. He recognized at a young age that the quality of his thoughts were mirrored in the quality of his life and has been intensely interested in personal improvement ever since. He has been self-taught in this field, seeking only those procedures that, in his opinion, produced results. EFT is his latest finding, but he also has high regard for NLP, in which he is a certified master practitioner. He is an ordained minister through the Universal Church of God in southern California, which is nondenominational and embraces all religions. He is a dedicated student of A Course in Miracles and approaches his work with a decidedly spiritual perspective. However, there is no specific spiritual teaching connected to EFT or its practitioners. You can learn more at the EFT Web site: http://www.emofree.com.

31

Anti-Aging Acupuncture: Why Many People Think It's the Next Best Thing to the Fountain of Youth

Dr. Bruce Eichelberger, OMD

Thousands of years ago, physicians in China mapped the body's electrical system. They charted fourteen energy paths, or meridians, and documented how stimulating specific points along those paths released energy blocks, restored the normal flow of Chi, or healing energy, and improved health.

For better or worse, people respond to you based on how you look. If you look old and tired, people treat you differently than if you look young and energetic. This affects everything from your likelihood of getting a job or promotion to the quality of your relationships and even your self-confidence.

In the quest to look younger, there are many modern options available. For example, some people take the medical approach of surgery, injections, or topical creams. Of course, such approaches focus entirely on outward appearance, without taking into account how the inner health of the person contributes to his looks.

To Truly Look Your Best, You Must Also *Feel* Your Best on the Inside

Simply stated, the health of your internal organs reflects in your face. In Oriental medicine, an entire branch of practice uses someone's facial appearance as part of assessing his underlying health. For example, you can easily see the effect of internal organ health on the faces of longtime smokers—they tend to have a gray, ashen appearance.

Because there is such a strong relationship between inner health and outer beauty, looking and feeling younger have long been goals in Asian culture. In fact, many of the old texts from the Orient mention the quest for the "elixir of immortality." They were constantly looking for ways to live long, healthy lives. And they found some very interesting approaches in their quest.

Very specialized techniques evolved over thousands of years to achieve a longer, more youthful life. Various herbal preparations, individual self-care techniques, and specific acupuncture procedures developed and were tested extensively. The ancient emperors were particularly interested in learning ways to keep themselves going and constantly sought out experts who knew how to achieve this.

This body of knowledge eventually became what we now know as Anti-Aging Acupuncture. Through the use of specific herbal formulas, self-care techniques, and the stimulation of specific acupuncture points, people live longer, more energetic lives. In addition, those who adopt these techniques look and feel younger.

How You Can Benefit

I'd like to share with you several self-care techniques that you can use to help yourself enjoy the benefits of this ancient knowledge. But before I do, you should know something about what improvements these techniques can bring.

Related to appearance, people experience the following:

- improvement in fine lines and a diminishing of deeper wrinkles
- improved facial muscle tone and a firmer jawline
- moisturized, softer, and more even skin tone
- increased metabolism, resulting in reduced puffiness
- reduction or elimination of rosacea and acne.

These are fairly impressive benefits. Because they are based on also supporting underlying health, additional improvements happen:

- reduction in mild anxiety and/or depression
- reduction in hot flashes and the discomfort and embarrassment they can cause
- increased energy and stronger immunity, a crucial factor as we age
- better sleep, making every other part of life better
- improved digestion and elimination.

Not bad for something that also helps you look your best.

Specific Steps to Take

Obviously, you wouldn't practice acupuncture on yourself (or anyone else) without specialized training. And since the specific antiaging herbal formula best for

119

you depends on your underlying health situation, I won't confuse the issue here by talking about the wide array of possible herbs you might use.

I can, however, share with you some of the very specific self-care techniques that will improve your overall sense of well-being and energy. Like any exercises, these are best practiced regularly, ideally every day. You get the most benefit from regular practice over time.

1. *Stimulating the Leg Three Miles points.* Just below your kneecap and slightly to the outside of your shin bone, you can find a point traditionally called "Leg Three Miles." The story goes that in the old days, people took long walks through the mountains, and when they got tired, they'd rub this point for a few minutes. This gave them more energy, enough so that they could walk three more miles.

These points exist on both legs and are easy to find. Simply slide your fingers lightly down your shin bone from your knee until you reach the bottom of the bump at the top front of the shin bone. The point is about one finger width toward the outside of your leg at this level. When you press on the area, you may notice a slight deep ache.

Ideally, sit down to do this technique. Stimulate the point by tapping on it twenty-one times on each side. Use your thumb and first two fingers together, and tap with the tips.

2. *Stimulating the Sea of Blood points.* Just above your kneecap and slightly to the inside is another longevity point. This one is called the "Sea of Blood." This name refers to the effect of this point on invigorating blood flow.

Locate the point about two finger widths above the inside top of the kneecap. There will be a slight indentation at this spot on your leg.

As with Leg Three Miles, sit down to do this technique. Stimulate the point by tapping it twenty-one times on each leg. Use your thumb and first two fingers together, and tap with the tips.

3. *Slow walk.* In our everyday lives, we all tend to rush around too much. This creates tension and stress, both of which speed the aging process. This exercise is an excellent way to help you slow down and get regrouped.

As the name implies, walk, but very slowly. Take time to feel the shift in weight as you put all your weight on one leg. Then lift your other leg and slowly place it in front of you and then back down on the ground. At this point, shift your weight toward the front leg until all weight is on it. Then lift the back leg and slowly bring it forward in front.

Walk this way for at least three to five minutes, breathing deeply and allowing yourself to relax your shoulders, neck, and arms.

4. *Stirring the Sea of Energy.* Locate the point called "Sea of Energy" by placing your palm just below your navel. The point is located about one third of the way down between your navel and your pubic bone.

With your right palm touching your abdomen, make twenty-one clockwise circles over this point. You can do this standing, seated, or lying down. Again, focus on breathing deeply, and relax your shoulders and neck.

5. *Brushing the face.* Rub your hands together briskly for a few seconds. Then very gently brush your palms across your forehead with a very light touch. Start from the center of your forehead, and move toward the sides.

Then rub your hands together again. This time, very gently brush your palms across your cheeks, starting below your eyes and moving outward toward your ears and jaw. Again, use a very light touch.

Finally, rub your hands together one more time. Place your palms on your temples and hold for fifteen to twenty seconds.

As simple as these exercises sound, practicing them every day can bring you profound improvement in your health and sense of well-being. Try them for yourself!

About the Author

Dr. Bruce Eichelberger practices Oriental medicine, specializing in Anti-Aging Acupuncture™. Anti-Aging Acupuncture helps you look and feel five to fifteen years younger, regardless of your age. By supporting healthy balance in the organs and systems of the body as well as increasing vital energy and circulation, you naturally look better and have more energy. Anti-Aging Acupuncture combines individualized acupuncture, herbal medicine, nutritional support, and self-care techniques to rejuvenate you inside and out. Get your free copy of the downloadable report "37 Proven Stress Busters" by going to http://www.RenoAlternativeMedicine.com.

32

An Introduction to Energy Healing

David Herron

Energy healing is a practice that promotes positive change. It involves an exchange of subtle energy that enables change toward greater peace, harmony, health, and vibrancy. Energy healing is practiced in many forms; some are modern, while some are drawn from ancient practices reaching back to the earliest human history.

All forms of energy healing involve the use or manipulation of subtle energies. These energies are known under various names such as animal magnetism, bioenergy, biomagnetism, Chi, prana, and so on. This subtle energy is said to be intertwined into everything in the universe, and some claim that the material world is created from the subtle energies. The human aura is one depiction of the subtle energies. The halos drawn in paintings of holy people may be a depiction of the subtle energies. Master Yoda's lecture to Luke Skywalker about the Force, despite it being in a movie, was a decent explanation of these subtle energies.

In energy healing practice, the healer takes some sort of action with the intent to affect the subtle energy of the client. Change in one's subtle energy tend to positively affect physical or emotional well-being in a process related to the mind-body phenomenon. There may be a transmission of energy into the client, an extraction of energy from the client, a clearing of stuck or blocked energy, disentangling or repair of energy structures, discovery or extraction of subtle energy objects, and much more. The movie *Karate Kid* contained a depiction of transmission of energy to cause healing, and the movie *The Green Mile* contained a depiction of energy extraction.

The better known energy healing practices include acupuncture, Brennan healing science, core energetics, EMDR, EFT, healing touch, Jin Shin Jyutsu, pranic healing, Reiki, quantum touch, Shiatsu, therapeutic touch, Qigong, and yoga.

Characteristics of the subtle energies show up in normal daily conversation. Take the phrase *quit yanking my chain*. This is related to an energetic structure called a "cord." Many energy healers recognize that human relationships create relationship cords. These cords carry subtle parts of the relationship using subtle energy exchanges that occur, usually, without conscious awareness. Ideally, cords are connected between the core essence of each person. Often they are not, and cords can be used in harmful ways. One way is a tugging on the cord, perhaps with the intent by one person to control the partner, leading to that *yanking my chain* phrase or other similar phrases. Another phrase is the *heart connection* and the way broken relationships can feel like tugs, yanks, or rips in the heart.

Another phrase in normal daily conversation is a *sinking feeling in the pit of the stomach*. The third chakra, one of the structures in the human aura, is located in the solar plexus. When someone is worried or anxious, often the third chakra becomes twisted or tied up in knots. This, like other energetic disturbances, can feel like a physical sensation. One wonders how many people who think they have ulcers really have a twisted third chakra?

Another phrase in normal daily conversation is when one throws *verbal darts* at another. Many energy healers find astral objects embedded in their clients, and often they are attached to people via a verbal dart. Astral objects take many forms, such as spears, arrows, really almost any sort of object you can imagine. Astral objects may represent oaths or curses. A common treatment is to remove these objects via extraction, or the healer may transmute the object into pure essence.

You may be wondering, how does energy healing help someone? There are various explanations, depending on who you ask. One general principle is that a healthy person has freely flowing energy through his or her subtle bodies. A healthy flow of energies promotes physical or emotional health. The human energy field (aura) is made of both subtle energetic structures and a flow of subtle energy through those structures. In Chinese medicine, these are the acupuncture meridians. In Chinese medicine, they discuss several types of Chi, and imbalances of Chi can describe almost every illness. The word *chakra* comes from Hindu mysticism. The chakras are a part of a system of energy channels called *nadis*, which carry an energy called *prana*. These two systems probably describe the same energetic structures.

The energy channels can be blocked or tangled in several ways, impeding the flow of energy. Energy healing can release stuck energy or can repair and disentangle these channels. Either promotes a return to healthy flow of the subtle energies.

In any traumatic event, we generally experience only a portion of the event. This leaves the rest of the event hanging around as energetic residue that can feel like the heavy burden some people are said to carry. Most forms of energy healing can help one release such residue, which can truly feel like the lifting of a heavy weight from the body.

Some practices, especially Brennan healing science, have techniques to directly structure the chakras, organs, or other parts of the human energy field. The organs in the human body are seen to have related structures in the etheric body, and when an organ is diseased, often the etheric body will be tangled in the vicinity of the organ. Restructuring the energetic structure of the organ often positively improves the organ itself. Similarly, restructuring chakras or other parts of the aura often positively improves the person's well-being.

Wilhelm Reich, the developer of Reichian psychology, was one of Freud's students. Reich's branch of psychology has developed into a wide range of therapies known as body psychology. He identified an energy he called "orgone," widely recognized to be Chi, and ways that people held armoring that impeded the free flow of emotions and/or this orgone energy. His work inspired bioenergetics, core energetics, Brennan healing science, biodynamics, Hakomi, and other therapies. Often, the patient is asked to get into various postures, which help him release the stuck energies, thus helping him return to a free flow of life force. The word *Reiki* comes from the Chinese symbols *rei* and *ki* and is translated as "universal life force energy." Reiki teachers say that Reiki energy is intelligent and knows where to go within the client and what to do to promote healing. The Reiki practitioner is asked to simply open himself to the flow of Reiki for the highest good of the client.

Prayer and laying on of hands is a religiously oriented form of energy healing. Most energy healers recognize that they are interacting with the divine, and they may recognize the presence of divine beings, or they may utilize prayer in their healing practices. The various energy healing practices draw from the whole gamut of spiritual practices from around the world, testifying to the core divine presence in all spiritual practices.

Energy healing is often a gentle practice performed through touch, though it may also be sent over long distances. The recipient may experience heat or cold, tingles, memories, emotions, or divine presences of relatives or ancestors, or the recipient may experience nothing. Recipients frequently fall asleep during the session, waking up at the end.

About the Author

David Herron is an energy healer, trained in Brennan healing science, Reiki, and several other forms of energy healing. David is also a blogger and lives in Silicon Valley. You may find lots more information about energy healing at http://energy-healing.info.

Copyright © 2007, David Herron

33

Floating Upstream:
Awakening Your Energetic Intelligence for Greater Ease and
Well-Being

Laura Maciuika, EdD

How much energy do you have by the end of the day? Do you usually feel vital, alive, ready to interact warmly with family or friends? Or do you feel stressed, weary, ready to eat and just watch TV?

If you feel low energy after a typical day, you're not alone. It's common in our hurried society for people to feel worn out by day's end. Yet many people push through weariness because of multiple worries and demands. They can end up feeling stressed, rushed, and worn out all at the same time. It's no wonder that stress is among the leading causes of physical and psychological problems in the United States. Over half of working adults recently surveyed reported being concerned about stress.[1] Chronic stress can negatively affect our physical and emotional health,[2] contributing to anxiety, depression, obesity, hypertension,[3] heart trouble,[4] and general weakening of our immune system.[5]

Keeping our energy strong and reducing stress can involve nutrition, exercise, and so on; those important topics are covered elsewhere in this book. Here I want to consider

---

[1] Z. Stambor, "Stressed Out Nation," *Monitor on Psychology* 37 (2006): 28.

[2] L. Winerman, "Reducing Stress Helps Both Brain and Body," *Monitor on Psychology* 37 (2006): 18; G. E. Miller, S. Cohen, and A. K. Ritchey, "Chronic Psychological Stress and the Regulation of Pro-inflammatory Cytokines: A Glucocorticoid-Resistance Model," *Health Psychology* 21 (2002): 531–41.

[3] Stambor, "Stressed Out."

[4] American Psychological Association Practice Directorate, "Stress and Emotion Can Negatively Affect Heart Health: APA Provides Tips for Mind/Body Health," news release, January 26, 2006, http://apahelpcenter.mediaroom.com/index.php?s=press_releases&item=22.

[5] S. C. Segerstrom and G. E. Miller, "Psychological Stress and the Human Immune System: A Meta-Analytic Study of 30 Years of Inquiry," *American Psychological Association Psychological Bulletin* 130 (2004): 601–30; Winerman, "Reducing Stress."

one way we consistently either build or drain our energy: through some of the decisions we make many times each day.

What kinds of decisions make such a difference? Usually not the smaller, external ones, like what you will wear today or what you will have for lunch. I'm referring to the subtle decisions we make. Our internal choices, our ingrained habits of thought and feeling, can be so automatic that we may not even notice we made a choice. Yet these decisions engage our energy and can either build up or deplete our life force.

One way we use our energy without noticing is through mental storytelling. Have you ever rehearsed an upcoming conversation or challenging situation? Many of us do this mental rehearsal. It can be helpful if used deliberately to build up our confidence and energy. But the kind of rehearsing we do without awareness is an energy drain. On and on our thoughts and feelings go. We often end up anxious, imagining worst case scenarios.

Along with future rehearsing, many of us do not easily let go of past upsets. Can you recall a recent difficult conversation? Once it was over, how many times did you play it over in your mind? Did your feelings get involved? Did you feel confusion or anger, frustration or helplessness?

We are prone to these replays. We review what he said, what she said, and if only I had said ... But as we vividly imagine our story, our bodies don't really know the difference between what's imagined and what's real. Our heart rate goes up, our breathing becomes shallower, and we use our energy to elaborate the experience, creating upsetting feelings and their biochemical reactions in our bodies.[6] The truth is, we choose to jump on those trains of thought and feeling. But many of us make this choice so quickly and automatically that we don't even notice we chose to jump and just get carried away. The good news is that we can learn to notice these choice points and redirect our internal focus and energy in more productive ways that leave us happier and stronger.

Imagine what life would be without such negative visualizations. You'd be in the present moment more—the only place we live anyway, and which many spiritual traditions teach is a doorway to inner peace. Part of developing our energetic intelligence is increasing our awareness of how we use our life force and bringing our attention and energy back into present time. As people grow in awareness and make different choices, many discover that they become more relaxed and centered. It's easier to be relaxed when we're not using so much energy to mull over past upsets or imagined, negative future events!

When we're not scattering our energies among past, present, and future, we have more energy available to nourish our entire system. We become more internally spacious and better able to respond instead of reacting, even in challenging situations. Our sense of

---

[6] C. B. Pert, *Molecules of Emotion: The Science behind Mind-Body Medicine* (New York: Touchstone, 1999).

humor returns. We become better able to float through the usual stream of stress more calmly—paradoxically, we become more productive, with greater ease and less striving.

Learning to use our energy for health has been a science in the East for centuries and is known in the West through acupuncture, Tai Chi, and other energy practices.[7] Across cultures and time, healers have used the knowledge of the body's energy systems.[8] Einstein was the first Western scientist to demonstrate that all matter is really energy. Currently, energy psychology is examining techniques that use the body's energy to heal emotional distress and wounding.[9] Some scientists in medicine and physics are predicting a major shift in focus from matter to energy as the basis for human healing and transformation.[10]

So what does this mean for you and your well-being? How we use our energy makes a difference in our physical and emotional health. Becoming attentive to our internal choices is one part of developing our energetic intelligence: our inherent ability to be aware of our energetic decisions and to learn how to use our energy more skillfully to be happier, healthier beings.

There are many techniques to help us return to the present and strengthen our energy. Becoming aware of our breath (which is always in present time), moments of silence, meditation, and energy exercises including Qigong are all helpful. Getting curious about our own energy use is an excellent starting place for awakening our energetic intelligence.

Try this simple exercise to gather your extra energy back at the end of the day: before you sleep, notice where you still have active energy about people or events from your day. Where are you still using energy through thoughts or feelings; where are you still having leftover reactions? Without jumping on any train of thought, just note a few places where your energy is still connected—maybe your job, your family, or the commute home. Then visualize a glowing energy ball in your heart area, like a bright ball of string or twine. Each strand of that twine is your life energy; some strands are still stretched out into your day. Imagine the ball beginning to turn within your heart, pulling back the energy strands of leftover feelings or thoughts about the day. Allow the ball of energy-twine to grow in your heart as all the strands gather back to your center. When it feels complete, allow the energy to glow brighter and gradually fill your entire body with soft warmth and relaxation.

---

[7] K. Serizawa, *Tsubo: Vital Points for Oriental Therapy*, 14th ed. (New York: Japan Publications, 1999); L. K. Chuen, *The Way of Energy: Mastering the Chinese Art of Internal Strength with Chi Kung Exercise* (New York: Simon and Schuster, 1991).

[8] R. L. Bruyere, *Wheels of Light* (New York: Fireside, 1994).

[9] F. Gallo, *Energy Psychology: Explorations at the Interface of Energy, Cognition, Behavior, and Health* (Boca Raton, FL: CRC Press, 1999); J. L. Oschman, *Energy Medicine: The Scientific Basis* (Edinburgh: Churchill Livingstone, 2000).

[10] N. Shealy and D. Church, *Soul Medicine* (Santa Rosa, CA: Elite Books, 2006); W. Tiller, *Science and Human Transformation: Subtle Energies, Intentionality and Consciousness* (Walnut Creek, CA: Pavior, 1997).

Try this exercise for a week. See what you notice about your sleep and dreams or your daytime energy levels and choices. Become aware of how your body feels when you have greater awareness of your energy, and notice your interactions with others.

I invite you to play with and explore your awareness of how you use your energy. Even small increases in awareness will help you develop your energetic intelligence, clearing the way for greater vitality, ease, and well-being in all areas of your life.

About the Author

Laura Maciuika, EdD, is a licensed psychologist in California and Massachusetts, and holds the advanced EFT Certificate of Completion. In her Integrative Psychotherapy practice in California, Dr. Maciuika includes energy psychology approaches, including Emotional Freedom Techniques (EFT), to reduce stress and anxiety, to heal old wounds and patterns, and to help people step into the freedom of their truest selves. Her work includes in-person and phone consultations and workshops on stress reduction, emotional freedom, and EFT. Dr. Maciuika is on the research committee of the Association of Comprehensive Energy Psychology and is working on a book on energetic intelligence. Visit her online at http://www.tapintofreedom.com.

34

Bursting with Health: Two Health-Improving Techniques

Deborah Miller, PhD

Would you describe yourself as bursting with vitality, energy, love, joy, enthusiasm, passion and excitement? Or would you describe yourself as tired, anxious, stressed, confused, worried, sad, depressed, angry, bitter, disappointed, frustrated, and overwhelmed? Most of us hold on to old hurts and traumas, and many add new hurts on top of the old. Yet everyone's had a moment that made him or her burst with energy, joy, delight, and enthusiasm. Remember one of those moments now and how your body felt. Even remembering it brings back the vibrant, tingly sensation in your body. Being in a positive emotional state helps us gain and maintain health, while a negative one leads to the opposite.

Want to release old traumas and burst with energy and vitality? Use the following techniques: (1) Emotional Freedom Techniques (EFT) and (2) the Law of Attraction.

Emotional Freedom Techniques

EFT is an extraordinary technique for eliminating emotional and physical problems by rebalancing the energy system of the body. Our bodies' energy system interacts with our thoughts, emotions, and physical bodies. Since our thoughts and emotions are energy, they in turn affect the energy system. Thus when our bodies' energy system is out of balance, it influences our overall health.

Imagine this energy system like a simple household electrical circuit. When you turn on a light switch, electrical current flows through a pathway provided by electrical cables that subsequently pass through a lightbulb, causing it to shine. You are similar. As long as your energy system is open and flowing, your light shines, whereas negative experiences or emotional traumas inhibit the energy system, and that is analogous to turning off a light switch.

EFT consists of tapping with the fingertips on strategic points on the face and body to stimulate the energy system while bringing to mind a specific problem—

whether an addiction, pain, or traumatic event—and stating affirmations about the topic. This process clears the short circuit from the body's energy system, thus restoring balance to the mind and body. This restoration of balance simply eliminates emotional problems and many resulting physical problems.

Can being healthy be as simple as unblocking your energy flow so that you feel better, emotionally and physically? EFT practitioners find that it has a great effect. Let's do a round of EFT on health so that you can get an idea of what it is all about.

Notice a tension in your body. Where is it? How intense is it on a scale of 0–10, where 10 represents maximum tension? Begin by tapping on the karate chop point, the fleshy part on the outside of one of your hands, with the fingers of your other hand. Then state out loud, "Even though I feel tension in my body, I love and accept myself. Even though I worry about my health, I love myself completely. Even though I don't know how to stop worrying about my health, I love myself."

Now use two or three fingers of either hand to tap on the following points while stating the accompanying affirmation out loud:

- *Eyebrow:* "I feel tension in my [name area of tension]."
- *Side of the eye:* "I hold stress there. It feels tight."
- *Under the eye:* "My body is tense."
- *Under the nose:* "I feel so anxious that I forget to breathe deeply. Then my cells don't get enough oxygen to function well."
- *Chin:* "I hold on to my fears and anxiety. It stops my energy from flowing."
- *Collar bone:* "I keep telling myself that I'm not healthy."
- *Under the arm:* "No wonder my body doesn't feel good. I keep telling it how poorly it functions."
- *Eyebrow:* "I breathe deeply. The stress leaves my body."
- *Side of the eye:* "I relax. The tension drops off."
- *Under the eye:* "I let go of my anxiety now. It is OK to do so. I choose to relax."
- *Under the nose:* "I choose to have a healthy body."
- *Chin:* "I let my energy flow. My body knows how to be healthy. I choose to get out of the way and let it do its job."
- *Collar bone:* "I feel so relieved to let go of this stress. My body relaxes. My body is healthy. My body is bursting with energy."
- *Under the arm:* "I can breathe deeply now, and that nourishes my body. My body thanks me for sending more life-giving oxygen. My body is bursting with energy and health."
- *Top of the head:* "I love myself completely and profoundly. I love my body and appreciate that it knows how to create and maintain perfect health."

Take a deep breath.

Did all or some of the tension release? Do you feel relaxed? This example shows how EFT shifts the body's energy system. Shifts may occur in one round of EFT, like what we just did, or after repeated rounds including different wording. Either way, EFT is a fabulous tool to move toward greater health.

The Law of Attraction

The Law of Attraction states that anything on which you focus your energy or attention is drawn to you. So how can you use the Law of Attraction to obtain better health? Become aware of your inner dialog to become aware of what you attract into your life. What do you say to yourself? How often do you say something negative about your body and health? Something positive?

Let's change some negative statements to positive ones:

- I'm tired. → I feel refreshed when I take three deep breaths.
- My body aches. → I stretch to maintain flexibility.
- I feel old. → I have wonderful memories reminding me to enjoy each moment of my day. That keeps me young.

Which would you rather attract?

Why is it important to use the Law of Attraction? Changing your focus restructures the neural net within your brain by breaking old and creating new associations about being healthy. Think of your mind as a recorded tape. Essentially, you are erasing the unwanted and recording new information about being healthy.

Take a look at your inner dialog. Have fun creating a vibrant, healthy body by changing your inner dialog into something positive, uplifting, and joyous. That is using the Law of Attraction to create health.

Enjoy using EFT and the Law of Attraction to create the health you desire.

About the Author

Deborah Miller, PhD, is an EFT practitioner, SRT practitioner, Reiki master, and prosperity guide. She has facilitated EFT and instructed many on the Law of Attraction in person, on the radio, and in teleconference sessions. She is the author of What Have You Got to Be Thankful For?, a thirty-day gratitude journal. She has created EFT scripts and audios to help individuals with the EFT process. Deborah specializes in empowering individuals by helping them release their blocks and inhibitions, followed by instilling new beliefs that allow them to step into their own power. Find out more about Deborah at her Web sites http://www.findthelightwithin.com and http://www.youcanchangeyourlife.net.

35

The Buteyko Breathing Method: Physiochemical Rebalancing or Psychospiritual Practice?

Dorisse Neale

To meet everything and everyone through stillness instead of mental noise is the greatest gift you can offer to the universe.
—Eckhart Tolle

As contrary as the title may sound, the Buteyko breathing method is actually a very simple set of tools and techniques used to correct chronic patterns of hyperventilation, or overbreathing.

Buteyko breathing is modeled on the research and physiological findings of Ukrainian Dr. Konstantin Pavlovich Buteyko, who developed a system of breathing retraining in the late 1950s that has been used successfully in Russia, Australia, and internationally (New Zealand, Great Britain, Thailand, the United States, Canada, Europe) to treat thousands of individuals afflicted with chronic respiratory, nervous, cardiovascular, and immunological illnesses.

Chronic "hidden" hyperventilation is now being recognized as one of the underlying causes of all disease. Normal breathing, as measured in liters of airflow in and out of the lungs per minute, is approximately four to six liters. Chronic overbreathers can get up to fifteen to seventeen liters per minute on a regular basis; during an acute asthma attack, the airflow can increase up to twenty-four to twenty-six liters. At these rates, a vicious cycle is established that encourages contraction of the bronchi, inflammation of the airways, and a severely decreased efficiency of oxygen release into the bloodstream. Asthma and respiratory disorders are on the rise, and it is estimated that up to 90 percent of people in the Western world are afflicted with chronic hyperventilation syndrome.

The Buteyko breathing method seeks to break the cycle of hyperventilation by normalizing ventilation through a series of eucapnic (normal amounts of carbon dioxide) exercises aimed at increasing carbon dioxide (CO_2) levels.

There is a myth in our modern world that CO_2 is a waste gas; in truth, it is only a waste gas in excess, as it is in fact essential for the utilization and release of oxygen in the body. CO_2 is a natural bronchodilator, as it relaxes the smooth muscle of the airways as well as decreasing inflammation. Hyperventilation leads to a loss of CO_2, which affects pH and ultimately every system of the body. By increasing CO_2 levels, oxygenation and circulation are improved.

The most efficient means of regaining optimal CO_2 is by slowing the breathing rate and depth. Breathing in and out always through the nose will ensure a healthy maintenance of CO_2, as rapid exhaling through the mouth depletes CO_2 more rapidly than any other factor. CO_2 is retained via specialized cells in the paranasal sinus during exhalation. Consistent abdominal breathing will allow for optimal diaphragm movement up and down with each breath, no matter the size or depth. A classic Buteyko breath analogy is "less is more."

It is estimated that about 85 percent of the work of maintaining normal pH in the body is carried out by the respiratory system; the lungs regulate carbon dioxide, which is the primary acidic component of the blood. The kidneys respond via their regulation of bicarbonate, which is the alkaline component. These two organs, the lungs and the kidneys, work together to keep this delicate balance of internal equilibrium.

Stressors such as dehydration, nutritional deficiencies, overstimulation of our senses with constant noise, lights, temperature regulation, and illness all contribute to overbreathing since breathing is the place where our body automatically speeds up to compensate. Human beings have created an external "world out of balance," as reflected in planetary changes that are taking place. We have internalized this world out of balance by our increasingly frequent dysfunctional breathing patterns.

Learning to breathe properly and integrating eucapnic breathing exercises into one's life on a daily basis can result in a dramatic improvement in health and significantly reduce the amount of medication used for chronic conditions.

When (eucapnic) Buteyko exercises are practiced regularly and correctly,

- circulation and metabolic rate improve
- the immune system is strengthened
- high *and* low blood pressure begin to normalize
- rapid pulse begins to lower, including atrial fibrillation
- diabetic complications improve, and weight normalizes
- insomnia becomes a vague memory of the past
- energy and alertness, inner calm, mental clarity, and concentration are improved.

Often, conditions that are not the focus of attention also improve or become eradicated. These have included chronic fatigue, infertility, hormonal problems, thyroid conditions, erectile dysfunction, tinnitus, digestive complaints, constipation, menopausal conditions, cramps, migraines, headaches, autoimmune diseases, and tumor growth.

The exercises are easy to learn, even for children as young as five years old.

Remedial breathing, with eucapnic techniques as a foundation, encompasses the Wise Woman traditional model of healing, where common sense, plants, whole foods, compassionate listening, simple ritual, and living in synchronicity with Earth's natural rhythms support and nourish health and wholeness. The Wise Woman tradition is the world's oldest healing tradition. Its symbol is the spiral. Illness and injury are doorways of transformation. Each one of us is inherently whole, yet seeking greater wholeness; perfect, yet desiring greater perfection. Body, feeling, thought, and spirit are inseparable and intertwined—the embodiment of deep healing at the source, beginning with the breath.

The three primary facets of remedial breathing are

- optimal breathing
- eucapnic—Buteyko breathing exercises
- health and wellness—oriented lifestyle (breathing, nutrition, hydration, rest, exercise).

Using the Wise Woman tradition model, the first step in remedial breath training is noticing the following:

- Do you breath primarily through your nose or mouth?
- Does your belly move with your breathing?
- Are your inhalations and exhalations equal?
- Can you hear yourself breathe?
- Is your breathing irregular and interrupted throughout the day by sighs and yawns?
- Do you often feel as if it's hard to get a breath?
- How was your health and well-being as a child?

Nasal and abdominal breathing are the hallmarks of optimal breathing. Successful remedial breathwork practice depends on connection with the physical body. Put your hands on your body, and feel the movement of breath—stay connected. Eucapnic breathing brings us back home to the body.

Exercise: Go for a walk, and breathe only through your nose both during inhalation and exhalation. Use the comfortable rhythm of the breath to govern your pace. Count how many steps you take for one complete cycle of inhalations and exhalations. Speed up your pace until you feel the need to open your mouth to breathe; if you do so, you will bypass the body's own perfect breathing apparatus (the nose), and your body will switch over to anaerobic (lacking oxygen) metabolism. Instead, keep your mouth shut and slow down until nasal breathing is comfortable again—this will maintain a healthy aerobic (using oxygen) state. Then pick up your pace and repeat.

Breathing is the source of life energy, and breathing correctly is preventative medicine. The Buteyko breathing method offers us one of the greatest tools to retrain our breathing toward a goal of increased physiological health and well-being and repair of physiological damage already done. All it takes to master the method is patience, plenty of slow time, commitment, and a willingness to go beyond our comfort zones to experience our true selves, where no emotion, psychological trauma, or intellectual story exists. It gives us an opportunity to embrace fully the present as we quietly observe and slow our breathing and as we learn to embrace and enjoy the pauses between the breaths. Breathing efficiently is at the heart and foundation of wellness.

About the Author

Dorisse Neale, respiratory educator, registered nurse, mother, dancer, and herbalist, has been involved in the wellness movement for over thirty years. An early member of the Holistic Health Association and the American Holistic Nurse's Association, her experience ranges from critical care/emergency nursing to midwifery and home-based natural health care. Dorisse has traveled, lived, taught, and published internationally and has pioneered the Buteyko breathing method in North America. With graceful enthusiasm, Dorisse offers a new paradigm of health—wellness versus illness—inviting individuals to reclaim optimal health via the respiratory system through workshops and events for ages 5–105. She is the founder of BreathDance—Wellness Through Breathing, based in Asheville, North Carolina (http://www.breathdance.org).

36

Bioelectromagnetic Medicine

William Pawluk, MD, MSc, and Donna Ganza, ND

W e are only as healthy as our cells. Having healthy cells is not a passive process. We can help our cells become and stay healthier. Cells can be fine-tuned daily in only minutes using bioelectromagnetic medicine (BEM).

Bioelectromagnetic Medicine (BEM): What Is It and How Does It Work?

The earth and sun create magnetic fields, without which life would not be possible. Science teaches that everything is energy. Energy is always dynamic and therefore is almost always time varied, meaning that it has frequency and changes by the second or minute.

All energy is electromagnetic in nature. All atoms, chemicals, and cells produce electromagnetic fields (EMFs). Science has proven that our bodies actually project their own magnetic fields and that all seventy trillion cells in the body communicate via electromagnetic frequencies. Nothing happens in the body without an electromagnetic exchange. We are all familiar with the electrocardiogram and the electroencephalograph, which measure the electromagnetic activity of the heart and brain, respectively. When electromagnetic activity ceases, life ceases.

Electromagnetic energy controls chemistry, which in turn controls tissue. Whatever the initial cause, disruption of electromagnetic energy in cells causes impaired cell metabolism. This is the final common pathway of disease. If cells are not healthy, the body is not healthy, in whole or in part.

BEM is the use of EMFs to address the impaired chemistry and thus the function of cells, which in turn improves health. BEM delivers beneficial, health-enhancing EMFs and frequencies to the cells. Low-frequency EMFs of even the weakest strengths pass right through the body, penetrating every cell, tissue, organ, and bone without being absorbed or altered! As they pass through, they stimulate the electrical and chemical processes in the tissues. BEM fields are specifically designed to positively support cellular energy, resulting in better cellular health and function.

Electromagnetic Fields (EMFs):
The Good, the Bad, and the Ugly

"But aren't EMFs *bad* for you?" They can be. Evidence is mounting that a new form of pollution, electrosmog, is a very real threat because it is disruptive to cell metabolism. Man-made, unnatural EMFs come from electrical wiring and equipment, for example, power lines, communication towers, computers, TVs, and cell phones. Electrosmog EMFs are not designed with the body in mind. They can be a strong inducer of stress in the body and therefore drain our energy. Electrosmog is all around us and cannot be practically blocked. But we can take measures to decrease our exposure. And now, with BEM, we can purposely add beneficial balancing frequencies to the body.

The EMFs in BEM use specifically designed frequencies, applied in controlled ways, to have more natural and beneficial actions. They act in basic and fundamental ways in tissues, positively affecting many biologic and physiologic processes, for example, to

- reduce pain, inflammation, the effects of stress in and on the body, and platelet adhesion
- improve energy, circulation, blood and tissue oxygenation, sleep quality, blood pressure and cholesterol levels, vasodilatation, the uptake of nutrients, cellular detoxification, and the ability to regenerate cells
- stimulate the immune system and RNA and DNA
- accelerate repair of bone and soft tissue
- relax muscles.

Because of these effects in the body, daily use of EMFs supports healthy aging and may even slow aging. EMFs have been used extensively for decades in many conditions and medical disciplines, and results can be seen in animals as well as humans. The National Institutes of Health made BEM a priority for research. In fact, many BEM devices have already been approved by the Food and Drug Administration.

EMFs and Magnets: What's the Difference?

BEM utilizes time-varying, or frequency-based, EMFs to help a wide range of conditions, applied to either the whole body or parts of the body. EMFs may only be needed for short spans of exposure, while the effects last for many hours, setting in motion cellular and whole body changes to restore and maintain balance in metabolism and health. The body does not acclimate or get used to the healthy energy signals of time-varying EMFs, even if used for a long time.

Stationary (or static), non-time-varying magnets of somewhat fixed strengths are used in mattresses, bracelets, knee wraps, and the like. Most have very shallow penetration into the body, resulting in a very limited ability to affect deeper tissues, and they rarely cover all the cells of the body simultaneously. Also, they can be awkward to use. They are more likely to cause the body to acclimate to the field and no longer provide benefit.

Modern Problems Require Modern Solutions

The concept of healing is quite simple: get the bad stuff out (detoxification and elimination) and get the good stuff in (oxygenation, circulation, and nutrient assimilation). Therapeutic EMFs do both and, at the same time, stimulate repair of damaged cells and tissues.

Now, in the United States, there are BEM EMF systems available for daily in-home use that can help meet the needs listed above.

Scientists worldwide are interested in the benefits and applications of BEM. The use of BEM is supported by more than thirty years of research, with various devices developed by teams of international scientists. Medical researchers are even working in the world's space programs with therapeutic EMFs.

One whole body EMF system, the Quantron Resonance System, has been available in the United States for almost a decade and has been used in Europe by tens of thousands of people for a wide variety of problems without significant negative effects for over twenty years. It is now being used in National Institutes of Health–supported research at the University of Virginia on rheumatoid arthritis. Another system, the Magnopro, can improve tissue oxygen by a full 1 percent, among other benefits. These whole body systems have been used worldwide not only by health-conscious individuals for health improvement and maintenance, but also by world class and Olympic athletes for increased endurance, enhanced performance, and faster recovery. They are natural, safe, gentle, and effective. There are even devices designed for horses and pets!

Conclusion

Bioelectromagnetic medicine is a new frontier of medicine. For health and wellness, it can be an important answer to healthier cells and healthier bodies. It is now generally available, and without the need for consultation with or prescription by a physician. In any event, most physicians don't yet understand bioelectromagnetic medicine.

About the Authors

William Pawluk, MD, MSc is an integrative physician in Baltimore, international expert on magnetic therapies and author of www.drpawluk.com, an authoritative website on magnetic therapies.

Donna Ganza, ND, is a leading natural health consultant and speaker on how EMF can effect the body either to harm or to heal. For more information and product resources for health enhancing EMF devices, as well as products to protect against harmful EMF's, visit www.donnaganza.com.

37

Speleotherapy and Halotherapy for Healing Lungs and Skin

Isabella Samovsky

As we are increasingly exposed to pollutants in the air that we breathe and the water that we bathe in, it makes sense that respiratory and skin problems are on the rise. These health issues take the form of asthma, seasonal allergies, breathing difficulties, skin rashes, and countless other modern maladies.

Medical researchers are still discovering new ways in which humans are adversely affected by airborne and waterborne pollutants. Some people think that their primary exposure to the outside environment is through the food and drink they consume. But actually, your skin and lungs are your main interface to the outside world. In fact, your skin is your body's largest organ, and it plays a crucial role in regulating your body's temperature and keeping the outside, outside! Your lungs and skin can easily absorb toxins for which they were never intended.

What are the most effective and healthy ways to reduce or completely eliminate these ailments that afflict our lungs and skin? Conventional Western medicine typically turns to prescription drugs to try to cure the problems or mask the symptoms. But these unnatural chemicals often do more harm than good. Consequently, people interested in more natural solutions are getting terrific results from speleotherapy and halotherapy. Speleotherapy is essentially the treatment of respiratory diseases using the air found in underground caves. When people hear this for the first time, they usually wonder if we are kidding, or just plain crazy. But scientific studies have demonstrated that such air is typically bacteria-free and is rich in healthy ions and salt microns, which have been found quite effective in reducing asthma, allergies, and other breathing problems, in addition to soothing irritated skin and restoring ionic balance within the body.

Speleotherapy is most popular in former Soviet Bloc areas, such as east Germany, Romania, Armenia, and the Ukraine, for several reasons. Initially, eastern European health practitioners and medical clinics did not have the financial resources for purchasing expensive Western pharmaceuticals, and so they turned to more traditional and lower-cost methods, including speleotherapy. The mountainous regions of

Europe and Asia are well known for having the best mines for ancient salt as well as being the primary source for crystal salts. These natural crystals, formed countless millennia ago, are also handcrafted into beautiful lamps that give off healthy negative ions, which have unique healing properties.

References

There are numerous medical modalities used by speleotherapy practitioners. For example, at the world-renowned Ukrainian Allergologic Hospital (UAH) located in the foothills of the Ukrainian Carpathian Mountains, three major types of treatment are offered: the healthy microclimate deep in their salt mines, water from those salt mines, and brine and mud from a nearby salt lake. UAH utilizes speleotherapy to treat patients with bronchial asthma, psoriasis, neurodermitis, allergic dermatitis, postburn conditions, nervous system dysfunction, sex disorders, and chronic nonspecific lung diseases (CNLD). During more than thirty years, an estimated sixty thousand patients are reported to have been cured of their maladies.

As a result of people all over the world learning the benefits of speleotherapy, clinics outside of eastern Europe are simulating the deep cave microenvironments, offering halotherapy in specially constructed rooms, halochambers, whose surfaces are coated with medicinal salt. Natural ionization of the air is supplemented with a dry sodium chloride aerosol to maximize the health potential of the treatment while the patient is there. Halotherapy clinics have the advantage that they are more accessible to people living outside of eastern Europe. Yet patients only get exposure to the healthy ions while they are at the clinic, which might be for only a few days or weeks per year.

That is why the most cost-effective solution by far is to create your own mini halotherapy environment in your own home and/or office. Thus you derive the health benefits of this remarkable therapy any day you choose, without having to travel anywhere. With the right products, creating your own halotherapy environment in your home or office is simple.

Here are some ways you can get started in creating your own halotherapy environment. Many experts consider one device, the Salin device, to be the best air purifier/salinizer, partly because it is so effective at creating a halotherapy microenvironment, and also because it is quiet and well made. In fact, Canada considers the Salin device to be a Medical Device Class I, just as various clinical studies have demonstrated its value in alleviating respiratory diseases. The Salin device emits tiny microns of salt crystals into the air, almost like salt dust found in salt caves. The salt microcrystals are one to five micrometers in diameter and are able to penetrate deep into the lungs. Leave the machine on for at least eight to ten hours a day in the room you are in. Within hours, you will notice the air quality difference with it being easier to breathe, nasal passages opening, and decongestion clearing. Use the Salin device every day.

Using salt crystal lamps hand carved from the salt mines is another option. The beautiful crystalline structure of ancient salt deposits is a result of their constituent minerals drying under intense pressure, not unlike diamonds. But salt crystals are far more colorful, ranging from light shades of pink, yellow, and orange to the more intense hues of dark red, deep blue, and lavender. Not only do people find the light of natural salt lamps to be quite soothing, but the negative ions given off by the lamps are the wonderful ions we smell in the air after a thunderstorm. These ions have a refreshing and energizing effect, helping to purify the air and thereby benefit the people and pets breathing that air. Salt lamps are being used worldwide in holistic spas and medical treatment centers. The most common types of disorders treated are breathing problems such as asthma, emphysema, bronchitis, and various allergies. Place several salt lamps throughout your house to experience clean, healthful, energized air.

And when you are at work, on the road, or traveling out of state, keep enjoying the benefits of salty air halotherapy with the portable salt pipe, which is made of porcelain and whose daily use helps flush away impurities from the nasal passages as well as helping to heal and calm inflamed lungs and airways.

All three products are complementary to each other and can help create a mini halotherapy environment in your home or office. When you are ready, you can add a natural salt floor or salt box and even add salt tiles or salt rocks to your existing sauna to enhance the concentration of natural salt ions for an even greater health effect.

About the Author

Isabella Samovsky founded world-renowned Solay Wellness when she was just twenty-nine years old, after falling in love with a salt crystal lamp. As she tells it, she was instantly drawn to the lamp's striking beauty and energy as well as its strong health benefits. But Samovsky didn't stop there. After doing research, she learned how beneficial natural salt is and about its many uses as well as how it can be used to help people look and feel better. This prompted her to create Solay Wellness and eventually launch her own top-selling product line, which now includes Solay Simple, a line of 100 percent natural, nontoxic cleaners; Solay Gourmet, a natural food line that includes Solay Gourmet Granola and natural Himalayan salts for seasoning; Solay Smile, a natural tooth power; Solay Therapy Pillows for people and pets; and more. A reputable source for all of these items—and a place to learn more about halotherapy and its many benefits—is Solay Wellness Inc. at http://www.solaywellness.com, 8051 N. Ridgeway Avenue, Skokie, IL 60076, (312) 224-2710.

38

Relieve Stress Magically with Passive Qigong

Al Simon

What is Qigong?

Have you heard of Qigong? Many people haven't, but you may be surprised to learn that over eighty million people not only have heard of it, but actively practice it each day!

Originally from China, but now practiced the world over, Qigong helps its practitioners improve their health and fitness, aid in healing and recovery of illness, develop energy and vitality, and gain a better sense of connection to themselves and the world around them.

The term *Qigong* (pronounced chee-GUNG) literally means "energy practice." It refers to a family of practices for health, fitness, energy development, and stress relief. Qigong includes yoga-like movement exercises, standing and sitting meditations, massage, therapeutic healing techniques, and other health- and energy-building practices.

One of the areas where Qigong excels is in relieving mental tension, stress, and simple anxiety. These mental problems have been shown to cause disease. In addition, stress increases the time it takes for us to heal from even non-stress-related illness. Even if it doesn't cause problems in and of itself, certain types of mental tension and stress can prevent us from physically, mentally, and emotionally feeling our best.

To help us clear ourselves of accumulated stress, tension, and simple anxiety, Qigong includes a number of physically passive techniques, that is, techniques that involve no body movement and are more like meditation. These passive techniques use the intention of the mind, rather than movement of the body, to clear ourselves of stress and have us looking and feeling great.

Mental Clarity Qigong

I'd like to teach you two simple passive Qigong practices. The first is called "mental clarity Qigong."

143

Mental clarity Qigong uses vocalization—the making of sounds. These vocalizations may at first seem a bit silly, but they work almost magically to relieve mental tension, stress, and anxiety.

You can use these exercises any time you need to release mental tension. They are also particularly valuable when you need clarity and focus such as when learning new skills or information. You can practice these three exercises before any learning situation to help increase mental clarity.

I prefer to do them while lying down, but they can be done in any position— sitting, standing, or lying. However, you will need some privacy to do these exercises as you will be making vocal sounds to help you clear your mind.

1. Lie comfortably on your back with your head supported by a pillow or mat. You may also wish to place a pillow underneath your knees to take pressure off your lower back. Allow your arms to lie comfortably at your sides.
2. Once you've made yourself comfortable, do each of these exercises in turn, spending at least two minutes or longer on each one.
3. *Sighing.* Begin inhaling using deep abdominal breaths, expanding your stomach (not your chest) on each inhalation. Then exhale through your mouth, creating a long, audible sigh. Sigh out loud during the entire exhalation using an "ah" sound. Practice sighing for at least two minutes before moving on to the next step.
4. *Chattering.* After two minutes of sighing, continue to inhale with abdominal breathing. But now, on the exhalation, make chattering noises using your lips and tongue. For example, make sounds like "babababababa" or "tatatatatata" or "dadadadadada," or any mixture of these sounds. Chatter out loud for at least two minutes before moving on to the next step.
5. *Making faces.* After two minutes of chattering, forget about your breathing. Instead, spend some time making faces. For example, roll your eyes, squish up your face, stretch your face out, stick out your tongue, stick out your jaw, or wrinkle your forehead. Try to move, squish, and stretch every muscle in your face and forehead as much as possible. Make faces for at least two minutes.

After you've completed sighing, chattering, and making faces, relax quietly for a minute or so, noticing any sensations in your body or mind. Do not dwell on any sensation, but merely observe and note it, then move on to look for other sensations.

Falling Water Qigong

The second passive Qigong practice is called "falling water Qigong."

Falling water Qigong uses visualization, and visualization is a great way to help relieve tension and stress as well as reinvigorate yourself.

Falling water Qigong is great for relieving stress, focusing concentration, and releasing tension in both mind and body. It can also be used at bedtime as a safe and effective way to fall asleep. We've even had a Qigong student use it to stop migraine headaches when she first felt them coming on!

While the instructions below are for lying down, falling water visualization can also be done in any position—sitting, standing, or lying.

1. Lie comfortably on your back with your head supported by a pillow or mat. You may also wish to place a pillow underneath your knees to take pressure off your lower back. Allow your arms to lie comfortably at your sides.
2. Begin imaging or visualizing your body full of water, from the top of your head to the bottom of your feet. Really feel yourself completely full of water. Stay with this image for a few moments.
3. Once you have that image in mind, imagine four small drain holes opening in your body. Two of these drain holes are in the center of your palms—one in each hand. The other two drain holes are on the bottoms of your feet, right near the ball of each foot.
4. Imagine the water beginning to trickle out of these drain holes, and visualize the level of water in your body falling. As the water drains, the level of water falls evenly through the body—front, back, and sides—but does so very slowly.
5. As the water level falls, imagine or visualize it washing away any stress, tension, aches and pains, discomfort, exhaustion and fatigue, or anything that just doesn't feel right. The water leaves behind places that are washed clean, relaxed, refreshed, and calm. (No, we haven't dried out these areas, but just given them a nice bath.)
6. Continue visualizing the level of water falling, until there are only a few drops of water left in your feet. As the drops leave through the bottoms of your feet, follow them with your mind as they sink deeply into the earth.

Now your entire body feels calm, relaxed, and comfortable. Stay with this feeling, and enjoy how calm and comfortable you feel. When you are ready, take a few deep breaths, then slowly open your eyes.

Passive Qigong uses mental techniques to clear ourselves of accumulated stress, and the two mental techniques you've just learned, vocalization and visualization, work almost magically to relieve mental tension, stress, and anxiety. You can use both mental clarity Qigong and falling water Qigong to help you feel your best physically, mentally, and emotionally!

About the Author

Al Simon is the director of CloudWater.com, a Web site for learn-at-home Tai Chi and Qigong. Al learned his first Qigong exercises in 1975 and began Tai Chi in 1984, receiving certification in Yang-style Tai Chi. Al is an in-demand instructor, lecturer, and CEO of his own service corporation for consulting and education, including Tai Chi and Qigong instruction. His articles on Tai Chi, Qigong, and health have been published in *Wholistic Alternatives*, *Natural Health Newsletter*, *The Empty Vessel*, and *Qi Journal*. Visit his Web site for free articles, newsletters, and online courses on Tai Chi and Qigong.

PART FOUR

Fitness & Exercise

Lack of activity destroys the good condition of every human being, while movement and methodical physical exercise save it and preserve it.

-- Plato

39

3 Dimensional Personal Training: Success through Synergy

Craig Burton

The whole is greater than the sum of its parts.

In the field of health and fitness, there are many effective techniques to help us achieve our optimal weight, appearance, and fitness level. When used in isolation, however, many such techniques provide only short-term results and often produce a yo-yo effect (think fad diets). In this article, I would like to show you how such goals can be achieved effectively through a synergistic approach.

A synergy can be described as "the interaction of two or more agents or forces so that their combined effect is greater than the sum of their individual effects." I firmly believe that the success of an individual's health and fitness goals depends on a 3 dimensional synergy that includes the right mental approach, physical training, and supportive nutrition and lifestyle.

Mental Approach

Effective goal setting is where the road to success begins. It is essential to understand where you are now in terms of your personal goals, and where you want to be to obtain clarity and purpose and be able to visualize your ultimate goal. Your goals need to *come alive*, so I encourage you to take the time to complete the following exercise and write down the answers.

1. Be *bold*—What is your ultimate health/fitness dream?
2. Be *honest*—Why do you want to achieve this? what will this outcome get for you and allow you to do?
3. Be *connected*—What will you see, hear, and feel when you have it?
4. Be *courageous*—When will you achieve it?
5. Be *realistic*—What are you willing to give up to get what you desire?

6. Be *creative*—How can you enjoy the process while doing what is necessary to achieve this?

The secret to achieving a positive mental approach lies in how often you can be connected and aligned to these thoughts and feelings.

Physical Training

I believe there are three aspects of physical training that need to be addressed:

1. *The need for muscle.* Muscle is one of your best friends if you want to lose body fat because it is an active tissue that directly increases your rate of metabolism. Unfortunately, around the age of thirty, our muscles begin to shrink, so it is imperative to regularly maintain or build them. When it comes to training, I highly recommend avoiding fixed resistance machines as they allow no freedom for the muscles, literally boring them senseless with the same pattern and decreasing neuromuscular awareness. So choose free weights or cables instead, and try incorporating Swiss balls (also known as Physio Balls) to increase neuromuscular demands. Additionally, think training "movements," not "muscles": pushing, pulling, squatting, lunging, bending, and twisting are the basic movements of day-to-day life, and we should try to mirror these during exercise.
2. *Cardio in moderation.* It is important not to overdo the cardiovascular exercise (e.g., cross training or jogging) as this can lead to a decrease in muscle mass, which reduces your ability to burn fat. I am by no means suggesting that cardio is bad as it allows nutrients to be transported to the cells via the bloodstream. When fat is released from storage centers (adipose cells), it travels through the bloodstream to be burned as energy. However, if there is a decrease in muscle mass, the body's ability to burn fat is also decreased. As such, I recommend short-duration, high-intensity cardio to limit the possibility of losing muscle.
3. *Flexibility.* Not only do our muscles shrink with age, but gravity begins to take its toll as well, drawing us down to earth. Adding to that, our seated culture is a major contributor to the current epidemic of poor posture. Faulty posture can lead to injuries and regular bouts of associated pain. The details can be complex, but suffice to say there are muscles in your body that naturally become short and tight and others that get long and weak by nature. The required response to correct this is to stretch the shorter, tighter muscles and strengthen the longer, weaker muscles. For example, when someone has a posture that resembles the Pink Panther—protruding head and rounded shoulders—the chest is one

muscle that needs a good stretch. However, only stretch what is tight as stretching the long and weak muscles will lead to further imbalances.

Supportive Nutrition and Lifestyle

This part of the puzzle is without a doubt the most confusing and neglected. What you eat and drink daily and the amount of rest you have are vital ingredients toward optimal health

1. *Eat to boost metabolism.* Largely, this means minimizing your intake of simple sugars and refined carbohydrates, but consuming frequent meals (no greater than fours hours between each one) consisting of quality proteins (preferably free-range, chemical/hormone-free animals), fibrous carbohydrates (above ground vegetables), starchy carbohydrates (sweet potatoes, brown rice), and good fats and oils (seeds, fish, olive oil). When it comes to the specific ratios of each macronutrient (especially the amount of starchy carbohydrates), it's a case of listening to your body after each meal to account for bioindividuality and stress levels. I recommend using a food diary and recording after each meal (or at the end of the day) what you ate, including proportions and the respective reactions, for example, satisfied, not satisfied, bloated, hungry, mentally focused, and so on.
2. *Drink plenty of water.* The body is made up of around 75 percent water. Water is crucial when it comes to health by playing a role in nutrient transport, digestion, elimination of waste products, detoxification, and so on. Beware: a dry mouth is not a safe indicator of thirst; it is actually a sign that the body is well into dehydration. How much water should we drink each day? That depends on several factors, including your weight and how active you are. But without complicating it with liters or ounces, my rule is to start the day with two big glasses of filtered water and then take a water bottle everywhere you go, sipping throughout the day.
3. *Get sufficient sleep.* Sleep is another factor that has huge ramifications on the body. I consider sleep a major tipping point as many times I have personally seen clients who are addressing the above points, but only once they get to bed earlier and sleep a little longer do they achieve significant results.

As human beings, we are 3 dimensional, consisting of body, mind, and spirit. Neglecting any one of these three aspects prevents us from truly experiencing our full potential as human beings.

I wish you all the best in your health and fitness endeavors.

About the Author

Craig Burton is the founder of 3 Dimensional Personal Training Systems. For over ten years, his mission has been the "transformation of people to a fitter, leaner and stronger body, full of freedom and confidence to allow full self-expression." Craig's unique holistic personal training methods come from his eclectic experience and training: from freestyle martial arts, a sports science degree, a massage therapy diploma, training at one of Australia's leading physical theater schools, and numerous advanced qualifications from within the health and fitness industry from leading institutions including the National Academy of Sports Medicine and the CHEK Institute. Craig is the author of "The 21 Day Roadmap to Health" (available at http://www.3dpts.com). His online personal training and nutritional coaching programs are available worldwide. Visit http://www.3dpts.com.

40

Discover the Three Key Pillars to Attainable Health and Fitness

Danielle Cardinal

A fallacy is being perpetuated that attainable health and fitness is complicated, impossible, frustrating, or just plain out of one's reach. Individuals are often conditioned to believe that health and fitness require an all-or-nothing approach. You are either super fit or sedentary. Period! You were either born with perfect genes, or you're jinxed. You either dedicate all your energies to improving your health, or you enthusiastically pursue your career. The notion is portrayed as an either-or principle.

Is it any wonder that most feel helpless or discouraged when embarking on their health journeys? They start in a backward fashion, envisioning only a list of hurdles that await them down the track. Their expectations are low, and failure seems much more probable than success. No wonder disempowerment, discouragement, abandonment, and resignation are rampant with potential health enthusiasts.

Enough! Discover what attainable health and fitness can truly embody by shifting your vantage point from an all-or-nothing approach to a more incremental and adaptable strategy. Below are three key components to be reviewed as you embark on your health and fitness journey.

Fun

Unfortunately, the fun factor seems to have been forgotten when creating a health and fitness plan. Energy is often wasted on battling preconceived notions of how hard and arduous the endeavor might be.

First, look for existing strengths and build on those to generate triumphs and helpful associations. Foster opportunities for enjoyment by creating fun fitness environments. Specific strategies can involve choosing a workout buddy you feel is infectiously energetic and positive, signing up for a group fitness activity that will allow you to socialize while exercising, or offer to babysit a child or dog that are guaranteed to keep you moving and active.

Get back to the basics and discover the fun factor in health and fitness. This seemingly simplistic approach allows individuals to rediscover what engages and motivates them at the core. By enjoying the process and creating fun situations, healthy hopefuls are moving toward their goals with reduced effort. Let your imagination and childlike curiosity steer you to try new activities.

There are a multitude of fun exercise options that are waiting to be discovered. Being open can help you discover those untraditional physical possibilities. For example, have you considered getting on a full-size trampoline? Or how about creating an obstacle course you can do with the kids while playing at the park? Get creative! Permanent and positive changes are more easily created and perpetuated by discovering what works best for you. If the thought of going to a gym triggers anxiety, then continue exploring other possible scenarios that will generate fun feelings.

Be a kid again! Forget limiting beliefs and tackle challenges with your imagination, optimism, and enthusiasm. Fundamentally, there is no cookie-cutter, one-size-fits-all remedy. Enjoy discovering the vast opportunities for fun!

Flexibility

Since the frenetic pace of life has everyone training as an athlete competing in the human race, best to take a moment to touch on time. Your schedule is already filled with important tasks, and adding another item can sometimes overwhelm even the most levelheaded individual. Proper time management can alleviate some of the pressure, but even then, life has a funny way of sending surprises our way. Best to stay adaptable and flexible by having some plan Bs in place for those key chaotic moments. If you are bringing your children to a soccer practice, can you walk around the perimeter of the field while they play? Or is there an activity you can sign up for at the same sport facility that coincides with theirs? Are there any other parents that may be interested in creating a fit parent group while your kids play? Have you asked?

Another practical tactic is to increase incrementally your steps during the course of a day by wearing a pedometer. It may sound silly, but walking over to your colleague's desk rather than zipping him or her an e-mail will add considerable steps to your day. Use what you've got around you, and that can be as simple as extra trips up and down your stairs at home. Yes, it can really be that easy while also being effective. Keep adding practical and flexible fitness routines here and there throughout your day, and they will quickly add up.

Focus

State your goals and build your focus like every other powerful muscle in your body. Never underestimate the power of the mind in whatever project you undertake. Consistent focus and action will keep you moving in a direction that will lead you to your objective. Infuse focus into your workouts and action plans, and let it fuel your drive to succeed. Ensure that the intensity of your workouts requires that you stretch yourself slightly beyond your current comfort zone. For example, while weight training, visualize the muscle shortening and working hard, rather than just mechanically lifting without much thought. Regard your body as a fine-tuned machine that is operating at an optimal level. It is on its way to serious improvements in performance and positive results.

The following are suggestions that you can take and customize to your style to maximize focus: affirmations, declarations, visualizations, and inspirational quotes. All or some may be beneficial regularly, or they may come in handy on those days when you feel you need to refocus more intensely.

Simply put, it's not a click or a switch that causes people to improve their lives, but rather an ongoing shift in gaining continued momentum in a positive direction on the health and fitness spectrum. Certain individuals who have transformed their bodies and lives may speak of one event in particular that triggered their quests for health. However, those who are successfully maintaining those changes year after year often highlight that constant action is key. These individuals know that over time, the intensity of action required will reduce significantly. Health and fitness strategies increasingly become habitual, rather than laborious.

Individuals are encouraged to identify their starting point and recognize where they began their health and fitness journey. More importantly, "change challengers" fix their sights on where they are headed. As motivational speaker Denis Waitley states, "Winners dwell on the rewards of success!" What will assist you in winning? What elements of health and fitness can provide you with the feelings of excitement, passion, and curiosity?

The preceding paragraphs have explored three pillars that have proven to be of tremendous value for those looking for great ways to improve their health. Rather than recycle through another fad diet or trend, these tools will incite permanent and positive changes. Start your journey with confidence, and build your healthy foundation with fun, flexibility, and focus!

About the Author

Danielle Cardinal leads the team at FitFleet Fitness, a mobile personal training outfit based in Ottawa, Canada. This dynamo is a self-confessed nutrition nut, exercise enthusiast, and boundary buster. Danielle graduated with honors in 2000 from the Human Kinetics program at the University of Ottawa. Her passion surrounding the enormous potential of the human body and mind encourages her to pursue additional studies. She has explored the following fields: Massage Therapy (Algonquin College), Personal Training (Can-Fit-Pro), Personal Development (Peak Potentials), Nutrition (Precision Nutrition), Wellness (Advivum) and Motivation (Power Within). These acquired abilities and invaluable skills have kept her flexible and eclectic in her approach for improved health. Her continued interest in providing her customers with strategies for attainable health and fitness have fueled and inspired projects such as the Big Audacious Goal Body Challenge, "Outside the Box" Outings, and corporate health initiatives. Danielle enthusiastically invites your feedback at dc@fitfleetfitness.ca.

41

Synergizing Your Hormones for Weight Loss

Joseph Cilea, DC

The world of fitness and weight loss can be extremely confusing and frustrating. Who are you to believe? Low fat. Low carb. High protein. High fat. Zone, Atkins, South Beach. The list seems to go on and on. Then there are the workouts: Pilates, Curves, Cuts, cross-training, cardio, weight training. It is no wonder why so many people have difficulty sticking to a regimen. For many, all of this confusion can impede them from even starting.

Imagine for a moment that there was a pill that could not only cause your body to burn fat but also gain muscle and strength. Blockbuster drug, right? Not quite. While drugs like this exist, the bad news is that, like many, they are linked to a slew of health conditions, including cancer and sexual dysfunction.

But the fact is that your body actually makes chemicals—perfect and natural forms—with no side effects. These chemicals are called hormones. The secret lies in the understanding of how you can naturally stimulate your body to produce more of these hormones to burn fat and build muscle.

Once you understand the physiology of the human body, the need for the quick fix diet or drug will no longer matter. Human physiology has been studied, and the methods I will share are absolute and backed by science. This means that they can work for everyone.

The Big Four

An understanding of four important hormones can help create huge breakthroughs in your body's ability to lose weight. Although there are more hormones involved in weight loss and muscle gains, we will focus on these four major players.

Testosterone

Testosterone is an anabolic hormone. This means it is responsible for building strength and endurance in your muscles. It also allows your body to efficiently use fat as energy. The more intense your workouts are, the more testosterone will be produced, which also stimulates your body to burn fat when you are not working out due to the fact that the testosterone stimulating effects may last up to forty-eight hours after intense workouts.

Growth Hormone

Growth hormone (GH) is responsible for general growth throughout our lives. In fact, there are various genetic disorders that cause low or high levels of GH to be produced, thus affecting normal growth. Growth hormone stimulates muscular growth and is also stimulated when intense cardiovascular training or heavy weight training is performed. These hormonal responses trace back to our primitive origins and were created for survival.

Estrogen

Estrogen, a hormone more dominant in woman but present in men, also plays a role in weight loss and human performance. Estrogen is important for bone formation and allows the body to utilize fat for energy (fat burning).

Insulin

One of the biggest players in your body's fat loss ability is insulin. GH and insulin are inversely related. This simply means that when there are high levels of insulin in the body, GH is naturally inhibited through complicated feedback mechanisms in the body. Insulin is a necessary hormone. It basically acts as the gatekeeper between getting sugar from the blood into the cells, where they are needed for energy production for all cellular functions. All the cells of the body require sugar or fat to perform bodily functions. In fact, the brain can only function on sugar, whereas other tissues can utilize either fat or sugar for energy.

The bad news is that excess insulin production causes fat deposition. This means that in the presence of high amounts of insulin in the blood, the body converts the sugar and stores it as fat. High circulating amounts of insulin can be extremely detrimental to the health of our bodies. Studies have shown that high insulin levels promote atherosclerosis, inflammation in blood vessels, and water retention, all of which lead to high blood pressure.

Now that we understand the harmful effects of insulin, how do we keep appropriate, healthy levels? Insulin is stimulated when the body breaks down the foods we eat into sugar. The faster we convert food into sugar, the quicker insulin production will be triggered. Foods that are processed and refined, including white flours, soft drinks, and even fruit juices, cause unnatural spikes in our sugar levels, prompting our body to produce insulin in a fast and unnatural way. As a result, over time, our body becomes nonresponsive to insulin, which can lead to insulin resistance or type 2 diabetes.

Now that we understand how hormones affect our body's ability to lose weight, what can we do to harness these hormones to optimize fitness, lose weight, and build muscle? How do we apply the knowledge of these hormones to our workouts for maximum muscular gains and fat loss?

Get Intense

Whether it be cardio training or weight training, the common thread must be high intensity. This allows for the greatest hormonal response for muscular gains and fat loss. Studies show that the primary source of your energy during your workout will be the opposite during recovery. In other words, if you burn sugar during your workout, you will be a fat burner during recovery. This is a key concept. For those that enjoy low- to medium-intensity cardio, the body will burn fat during the workout only and will burn sugar for energy during recovery. Don't you want your body burning fat when you are not working out?

Some other negative effects of long-duration cardiovascular work (thirty to sixty or more minutes) are joint injuries as well as the catabolic effects (muscular breakdown) of the hormone cortisol when the body is under stress. Cortisol is also known as the stress hormone. With excessive exercise, including lengthy workouts or lack of recovery time, cortisol levels can be raised, which actually breaks down muscle and causes weight gain.

With high-intensity cardio or weight training, since the primary source of fuel is sugar, at recovery, the body utilizes fat as energy. Understanding this key concept will revolutionize the way you train and allow for real results.

How to Apply the Key Concepts to
Your Workouts and Diet

Testosterone/Growth Hormone/Estrogen
Testosterone, GH, and estrogen are best stimulated with high stress on muscle tissue as well as high intensity to the cardiovascular system (80–85 percent of maximum heart rate). It is best to include sets of heavy weights that utilize multijoint movements.

Insulin
A diet with a low glycemic index will keep insulin levels equally low and GH high, and this will allow muscles to develop and mobilize fat as a source of energy. Keeping sugar levels stable will show up in the form of steady energy levels and a body that is able to tap into fat as a source of energy. Eliminate refined flour and sugar from the diet. Replace with whole grains, fruits, vegetables, and healthy

proteins and fats, including grass-fed beef, bison, lamb, and free-range chicken and eggs, with nuts, avocado, coconut oil, and olive oil for your fats. For weight loss, reduce all sugars and grains, even healthy ones, to a minimum.

Like all exercise and nutrition programs, consult with your physician prior to beginning. This program will maximize your body's natural ability to gain lean muscle and allow you to lose weight and fat, all without overworking your joints and causing injuries. The basis of this program is centered on real physiology and principles; therefore it will work for everyone, excluding those with rare medical conditions.

Bibliography

Pacheco-Sanchez, M., and K. K. Grunewald. "Body Fat Deposition: Effects of Dietary Fat and Two Exercise Protocols." *Journal of the American College of Nutrition* 13 (1994): 601–7.

Pritzlaff, C. J., Laurie Wideman, Judy Y. Weltman, Robert D. Abbott, Margaret E. Gutgesell, Mark L. Hartman, Johannes D. Veldhuis, and Arthur Weltman. "Impact of Acute Exercise Intensity on Pulsatile Growth Hormone Release in Men." *Journal of Applied Physiology* 87 (1999): 498–504.

Pritzlaff, C. J., L. Wideman, J. Y. Weltman, M. E. Gutgesell, M. L. Hartman, J. D. Veldhuis, and A. Weltman. "Effects of Exercise Intensity on Growth Hormone (GH) Release." *Medicine and Science in Sports and Exercise* 30 (1998): abstract 273.

About the Author

In 1997, Dr. Cilea established his chiropractic practice in Marlboro, New Jersey. Throughout the years, his practice evolved to include a broad range of physical therapy and pain management services. To promote wellness and a healthy lifestyle, Dr. Cilea is a frequent guest lecturer, sharing his insights on a broad range of topics. He speaks to local companies, schools, and sports teams about all facets of nutrition, injury prevention, and wellness. A former collegiate athlete, Dr. Cilea understands sports injuries and helps athletes rehabilitate injuries and optimize performance. Dr. Cilea graduated from Villanova University in 1991 and earned his doctorate of chiropractic from Life University in Marietta, Georgia, in 1995.

42

Aging Gracefully with Tai Chi

Carolyn Cooper

Tai Chi chuan, or simply Tai Chi (because there are two translations of the Chinese language, it is also written *Taijiquan*, or *Taiji*), was developed centuries ago by martial arts experts to advance their self-defense skills. Most commonly practiced today for its amazing health benefits, this slow, graceful Chinese exercise simultaneously heals the physical, mental, emotional, and spiritual body. It is performed with a completely focused yet relaxed attitude. Tai Chi forms involve a series of choreographed martial arts poses that flow together like a slow-motion dance. They are done in a precise order to help facilitate energy flow, fitness, relaxation, and mental concentration. Tai Chi encompasses several styles or forms, and over its long history, many interpretations of these styles have emerged, resulting in numerous variations in form. Most traditional forms take twelve to twenty minutes to perform. Although these forms can take up to one year to learn, and many more years of practice to experience all the subtleties of the art, there are also many simplified forms that take much less time to learn. These simplified forms make this ancient exercise more accessible to a greater number of people, and are a great way to get your feet wet while still providing many health benefits. The moves are simple, gentle, and easy to learn. They require no special skill, clothing, or equipment and can be done anywhere: indoors, outdoors, alone, or with a group.

Tai Chi improves overall fitness, coordination, and agility. People who practice Tai Chi regularly tend to have good posture, flexibility, and range of motion. They also tend to have more mental clarity and sleep more soundly at night. Tai Chi goes to the root of most health problems by relaxing the muscles and mind, aligning the spinal posture, and balancing the energy systems that run through the body, providing them with life energy. As a profound self-improvement tool, Tai Chi is one of the most powerful yet soothing things we can do for ourselves. The magic of Tai Chi is found in the unique combination of movement, breathing, and meditation.

Movement

Because Tai Chi involves all the major muscle groups, it improves agility, strength, flexibility, stamina, muscle tone, and coordination. This is of extreme importance as we have a large population of baby boomers. It is reported that one of every three adults sixty-five years or older falls each year, often with devastating results. Hip fractures are the seventh leading cause of death among older adults. If this could be reduced even by 10 percent, we would save over $1 billion a year, not to mention the pain and suffering of the patients and their families.

Appearing in the May 1996 issue of the *Journal of the American Geriatrics Society* were the first two studies involving Tai Chi to be reported by scientists in a special frailty reduction program sponsored by the National Institute on Aging. The studies showed how Tai Chi's attention to balance could increase body awareness, reducing the incidence of falls by up to 50 percent in elderly patients. Results of another randomized trial published in the December 2004 issue of *Medicine and Science in Sports and Exercise* show that Tai Chi reduces falls in the six months after intervention for patients seventy years and older.

Through the postures of Tai Chi, we learn how to move the body correctly, thereby becoming conscious of our physical presence, so along with this increased balance, we are also less likely to lose mobility. Tai Chi rotates all the joints in the body, releasing any blocked energy that could contribute to the aging process. It also stimulates the liquid systems of the body to keep our joints and other tissues suppler, increasing range of motion and reducing any symptoms of arthritis. The many movements performed by turning from the waist work as an internal massage. By stimulating the abdomen, these movements aid digestion and help relieve constipation and gastrointestinal conditions.

Breathing

The deep breathing of Tai Chi regulates the respiratory system, helping to treat ailments such as asthma, bronchitis, and emphysema. Exhaling toxins from the lungs while inhaling fresh air increases lung capacity, stretches the muscles involved in breathing, and releases tension. Symbolically, the exhaling and inhaling remind us to let go of that which is no longer serving us and allow new abundance to enter our lives.

Meditation

Research shows that taking time to slow down the mind and body is not only calming, but also enhances mental acuity and focus, reduces anxiety, and lowers blood pressure and heart rate. Tai Chi's meditative nature is also beneficial for the immune system and the central nervous system, which makes it especially good for people with a chronic illness, depression, or any stress-related conditions. The quiet mindfulness of Tai Chi teaches us to listen to our bodies, thereby helping us become aware of problems before they become acute. This same mindfulness can permeate all other aspects of our lives, helping us find gratitude in each moment.

About the Author

Carolyn Cooper is an A.C.E. certified fitness professional and longtime Tai Chi instructor. She is the founder of Tai Chi Flow, Inc., offering simplified, user-friendly Tai Chi videos/DVDs. The series includes an exercise routine designed for pregnancy, a kids workout, and a program for every-body (http://www.taichiflow.com). In addition, Carolyn is a gifted, intuitive energy therapist and creator of "Calyco Healing". This powerful, cutting-edge vibrational healing realigns energy patterns and releases negative subconscious beliefs. Her clients report profound and life-changing results. Carolyn's seminars attract an international audience (http://www.CarolynCooper.com). Married twenty-six years, Carolyn is the mother of five children.

43

How I Beat Obesity and Insulin Resistance in Ninety Days

Shane Ellison, MS

I have been rail thin, and I have carried more fat than I like to admit. As a collegiate wrestler, I was 4 percent body fat. As time passed into my late twenties, I ballooned to a whopping 30 percent body fat. I felt weak, tired, edgy, depressed, and was haunted by a constant craving for food—usually anything that had sugar. My brain screamed eat, eat, eat, and my body said store, store, store. It was a metabolic nightmare. Disgusted, I was determined to awaken from it and lose the unwanted fat while building more muscle—in the shortest amount of time possible.

As an organic chemist trained in biochemistry and drug design, I scrutinized every fat loss method available. I studied volumes of research available on fad diets, the government-mandated Food Pyramid, and strenuous exercise programs. I mapped out the actions of purported fat loss drugs like Wellbutrin, Phentermine, Xenical, Clenbuterol, Meridia, and amphetamines. I learned that none of these options were for me. They only provided temporary fat loss at best, while putting me at risk for worsening health.

Digging deeper into science, I discovered that I could lose excess fat and gain solid muscle by adhering to key lifestyle habits that controlled a single hormone in my body: insulin. Insulin is the nutrient taxi. It escorts blood glucose (a.k.a. blood sugar) and other nutrients into the muscle cells to be used for fuel. This keeps us alive and energized. Too much insulin, however, can be detrimental.

Excess insulin tells the body to store fat and instead use glucose for fuel. In addition, many hormonal systems that regulate appetite, mood, muscle growth, and even fertility are thrown out of whack by excess insulin. This imbalance is usually secured long-term by a sugar addiction that accompanies excess insulin. Soda, juice, cereal, beer, and candy manufacturers have built empires around such addictions.

Since the body is burning glucose for energy and storing fat, it screams for more sugar as glucose is converted into energy. This is the metabolic nightmare our parents innately feared when they told us, "Don't eat too much sugar."

As adults, most of us have ignored the warning not to eat sugar. We pay more attention to how many calories or grams of fat we put into our bodies. This is a deadly mistake. Most low-calorie and low-fat foods are loaded with sugar or sugar mimics. These include sucrose, glucose, high-fructose corn syrup, monosodium glutamate, hydrolyzed proteins, trans-fat, and milk sugars such as lactose and maltose.

Looking at my own eating habits, I was consuming sugar every time I put something into my mouth. Whether I was drinking a so-called sports drink, eating a so-called health food bar, or slurping Campbell's soup, I was consuming some type of detrimental sugar. Little did I know that I was headed toward more treacherous health problems than just obesity.

If habitual sugar consumption continues, the metabolic nightmare can turn into a living hell. Over time, high insulin levels lead to a medical condition known as insulin resistance or Syndrome X.

Similar to those who consume excess alcohol and develop resistance to it, excess insulin numbs the cells. Our muscles no longer react to it. Unable to gain entry into muscle cells, glucose remains in the bloodstream. Blood sugar skyrockets. Recognizing the rise in blood glucose, the pancreas attempts to curtail the danger with yet more insulin production. Insulin resistance begins to take its toll on the body. Insulin and glucose overload leads to hypertension, polycystic ovarian syndrome, heart disease, diabetes, and cancer. Aging accelerates so fast among those who suffer from insulin resistance that they can erase ten years from their lives!

Alarmed with what I learned, I became wildly motivated to control my insulin. It wasn't that difficult. I never starved. I never counted calories. I never suffered in the gym. I learned how to control my insulin by adhering to simple lifestyle habits. Doing so allowed me to burn fat day and night. My body innately knew when to eat and how much to eat.

By controlling my insulin, I descended from 30 percent body fat to a lean 12 percent body fat in ninety days! During that time, I gained six pounds of muscle. I had abundant energy all day. My mood was consistently upbeat. My physical and mental endurance was at an all time high. My productivity quadrupled. I felt like my newfound habits were the Holy Grail for effortless fat loss.

I awoke from my metabolic nightmare and freed myself from the impending health crisis that eighty million Americans are now faced with. Here are the simple steps I took:

- I had to learn how to exercise properly. Proper exercise and insulin resistance cannot coexist. I did interval training with weights for forty-five minutes three times per week. This consisted of short bursts of intense exercise separated by short rest periods. I attained the best results when I exercised first thing in the morning, before breakfast.

- I had to quit sugar and sugar mimics. I scrutinized every food label to ensure that there were no sugars. If something tasted sweet, I didn't eat it—not even fruit for the first ninety days. I abstained from all artificial sweeteners. I only used the natural sweetener known as Stevia. I quit all soda and fruit juice and replaced it with purified water, water with squeezed lemon, or green tea. I limited wine consumption to at most one glass per week.

- I avoided dieting. Lowering food intake and dieting teaches the body to store fat. I ate a meal every three to four hours until I was totally full. My meals focused on healthy fat, vegetables, and protein. Sources of food were grass-fed beef (London broil, sausage, New York strip, and so on), eggs (the whole egg), pork, tuna, whey isolate (free of sugar and artificial flavors), beans, rice, chicken, organic salads at least every other day, steamed vegetables, blueberries, coconut oil, fish, organic bread with REAL butter, cashews, almonds, sunflower seeds, and avocados.

- I got more sunshine. I exposed at least 80 percent of my body to sunshine for ten to twenty minutes per day. This helped control my appetite and mood while normalizing insulin and blood glucose levels[1].

- I drank more water at the right times of the day. Drinking water activates your body's natural ability to burn fat (i.e., thermogenesis) by up to 30 percent. I drank sixteen ounces of purified water on waking in the morning and five minutes before every meal.

- I used supplements. As a drug chemist, I always knew that nutritional supplements could be useful. After all, the vast majority of drugs are derived from nutritional supplements. It wasn't until I fully embraced their proper use that I was able to experience their powerful benefits. To mobilize my fat from fat stores and intensify my workouts, I used a thermogenic aid. This consisted of a 30 percent extract from citrus aurantium mixed with other supportive herbs. To increase my insulin sensitivity, I used green tea (Provantage) or a 1 percent banaba extract with cinnamon and red ginseng. To help with digestion and circulation, I supplemented with cayenne pepper. To mitigate my intense sugar cravings, I utilized the essential amino acid L-tryptophan. Dosage and timing were important factors that ensured the effectiveness of these supplements.

- I cheated. To ensure that I could stick to my habits long term, I cheated once per week. During this time, I did whatever I wanted to.

---

[1] Sullivan Krispin, "The Miracle of Vitamin D," *Wise Traditions in Food, Farming, and the Healing Arts*, 2000, http://www.westonaprice.org/basicnutrition/vitamindmiracle.html. Sunshine stimulates the production of vitamin D and melanocyte stimulating hormone.

As others learned of my findings and applied them, they too had the same success, perhaps even greater. Consider Frank Dannenberg. At five foot four inches, Frank weighed 205 pounds. He was a three-time heart attack victim and type II diabetic. At a mere fifty-eight years old, Frank was planning his own funeral. After following the habits for ninety days, Frank lost twenty-three pounds of fat, gained ten pounds of muscle, and reversed his diabetes! With his newfound health, he abandoned nine prescription drugs!

Without a doubt, the benefits of controlling insulin via the habits used above go beyond fat loss. Insulin control is the long-awaited panacea that Americans have been searching for. Physician David Katz, director of the Prevention Research Center at Yale Medical School, summed it up best. He suggested that learning how to regulate insulin could be the master control of *all disease*, not just obesity.

About the Author

Shane Ellison, also known as The People's Chemist, holds a master's degree in organic chemistry and has firsthand experience in drug design. Abandoning his career as a medicinal chemist for a major pharmaceutical company, he is dedicated to stopping prescription drug hype. He is an internationally recognized authority on therapeutic nutrition and author of *Health Myths Exposed*, *The Hidden Truth about Cholesterol-Lowering Drugs*, and *The AM-PM Fat Loss Discovery*. He is also the lead scientist for Health-FX (http://www.health-fx.net), a leader in health education and targeted nutrition for fat loss, insulin resistance, and sports performance. His books and free offers can be found at http://www.healthmyths.net.

44

Weight Training for Longevity

Rick Kampen

My intention in writing this article is to pass along the most fundamental, but equally most important information I can about resistance training using weights. While there are a great many authors on this subject, my purpose is to guide you in this theater in accomplishing a strong, flexible, and functional body well into old age.

Use It or Lose It

Our muscles and skeleton provide a frame of reference for each other. As our need for strength increases, even if modestly, our frame or skeleton will also strengthen to provide a frame of reference. In other words, as our muscles grow and strengthen, our bones will have to as well to deal with the stress. If a person does little in the way of exercise, the muscles will stay in a weakened state, and consequently, so will your bones. As we age, this becomes more of an issue in being able to withstand the most basic of physical stresses and only hastens our physical demise and potential for injury. Weight training can and will stave off the ravages of time and decreasing hormonal output and keep our bodies strong and better able to repair themselves, and we will maintain increased physical and mental vigor.

While it is never too late to begin such a program, the earlier you start in life, the better your discipline and training will become. I have been weight training for over thirty years as well as incorporating body weight training and what Charles Atlas used to refer to as dynamic tension. As I now have the opportunity to interview many people at gyms, I have come to see how little they really understand of what they're doing and how little endurance most of them have.

Frequency Is Most Important

There is a plethora of information on types of exercise and routines to use. The single most important thing in all these is frequency of training. Most folks will never win a marathon or become a champion fighter by only training once a week.

With regard to weight training, I diverge from the crowd. Most of the people I speak to train each muscle group only once per week. I train each group three times per week. For years I stuck with twice a week, until I came across a program from the Soviet Bloc in 1989 that advocated training three times per week; this program created a fundamental change in my whole approach. I realize I am hard-core and wouldn't ask the average person to try this as it is very taxing in terms of effort and time. So many people tell me that they are too sore to train twice a week per muscle group and that I must have good genetics to be able to recover so well and still train like this at the ripe old age of forty-six. This is hogwash. Any and all training routines are about discipline first. Nothing will be gained without effort and dedication. I was born a chronic asthmatic, and if I can manage a two-day split, then anyone can manage a three-day split (the entire body worked out in three days).

Frequency also applies to the amount of repetitions per set. Using a higher number of reps (the number of times you press or pull the weight before failure) will build strength and endurance. Endurance is just as or more important than strength alone. Remember the joke Robert Duvall told Sean Penn about the bulls in the movie *Colors*? Strength means very little if you've blown yourself away after only sixty seconds of effort.

If It Hurts, Don't Do It

Sounds pretty simple, doesn't it? You wouldn't believe how many people do exercises in a fashion that is unnatural for the body. Getting hit by a car years ago showed me pretty quickly what works and what doesn't for my back. I have known so many people who are in constant pain because of constantly performing the same exercises because they were told they should. Listen to your body. Pain is your body telling you that something is wrong. Figure it out. Change the way you do the exercise, and see if that makes a difference. If you keep pushing through the pain, you will be headed for surgery or incapacity. This will be counterproductive to achieving a strong body. Whenever possible, use dumbbells. These allow for a broad range of motion and certainly task the muscles more effectively than any bar can do. If you experience pain when pressing a bar overhead, you may find this goes away by simply using dumbbells and rotating your hands ninety degrees. Simple, but it works.

Isolating the Muscle Isolates the Joint

Again, I will break precedent with so many in the weight lifting field. Your limiting factor in weight training or any other form of exercise is how well your tendons and ligaments deal with the stress. Connective tissue takes much longer to strengthen or repair if damaged. Your body was never meant to push or pull in an isolated manner. When you pick up a child or push a wheelbarrow, your body works as a cohesive unit. If you use equipment that isolates a particular muscle group, such as a preacher bench for bicep curls, you also focus undue stress on your elbows. Most folks who use a preacher have ripping pain in their elbows as they curl. And yet they continue as they love the pump. To what end? When you can't pick up your kid anymore because of shoulder or elbow pain, how are you better off? Use exercises that allow your body to support what you're doing.

A good many of gym exercises and the equipment to perform them are a waste of time and can lead to debilitating injury.

Slow and Steady

To stay healthy and continue to build strength and endurance, you should always focus on style and never speed. I know all about the speed training techniques and the reasoning behind them. I also know all about ripped muscles and, worse, detached or torn tendons. Fast twitch muscle, if trained strong enough, is capable of overcoming the associated tendons. It is all too easy to cause injury when you move a weight too fast.

When you have to push a car, you apply yourself in the correct manner automatically. If you took a good run at the car and slammed into it, the car probably wouldn't budge, and you would be the worse off for trying.

No Excuses

Now I know there are a great many people who will say that they can't afford the expense or time of a gym or any training program that keeps them from home. I'd like to think I've heard all the excuses. Buy a pull-up/dip station for your home. Weight training is not limited to iron weights. You carry around the best tool possible: your body. Most weight lifters will never accomplish ten reps of pull-ups, but with a little time and work, you will be able to perform twenty to twenty-five of these nonstop. The same goes with dips. Several sets of these two or three times a week will give you incredibly strong shoulder, back, and chest muscles. Look at the bodies of gymnasts. Again, endurance is key to overall strength and longevity.

There is a gentleman by the name of Matt Furey who has numerous publications about body weight training. These are definitely worth looking into as you will be challenged to perform even a few reps when you first get started. The only equipment you'll need to bring to the party is your body. Now you have no excuse not to get started.

Stretch, Stretch, and Stretch

Ever marvel at the power and speed of cats? Watch their stretching routine. The joints are opened, never compressed. This allows power to flow effortlessly. Look at how many people are stooped and inflexible in their older years. This is due to inactivity, both muscular contraction and expansion or stretching. Stretching will keep the tendons and joints flexible and impart greater strength to the body than resistance training alone. I know too many people who are broken down in their prime due to too much strain on their bodies without the counterbalance of stretching. This is probably the most overlooked area of strength building. Yoga is a marvelous adjunct to any training routine.

Vary Your Workout

Routine: the word implies dull and dead-end. In my program, I have two light days with high reps, two medium days with more weight and moderately high reps, and two power days with lower reps and heavy weight. Don't always start with the same body part. Change the type of exercise for each body part every two weeks or so. Stay on high reps (up to twenty) for a month, and then switch to lower reps with greater weight for a month. Your body will continually respond and adapt. If you become bored, your training—and consequently, your results—will reflect this.

Last but Not Least

Whatever you do, do it for you. If you wish to alter your being because somebody else is pushing your buttons, you won't last long. Make it a lifelong commitment for a long and healthy life. My personal motto here is "And the weak shall inherit the girth."

About the Author

Rick Kampen lives just outside Charlotte, North Carolina. He is forty-six years old and has been weight and resistance training for thirty-one years. He owns a nutritional supplement store in Charlotte with an up-and-coming Web site. Rick has taken the best of twenty-six years of self-defense training with various styles and is developing his own style with the fulfillment of his ambition to perfect the two-hit fight. Married with six kids and living on a small farm that houses his wife's mobile petting zoo, Rick is the lucky one who gets to roll the thousand-pound round bales of hay as far as three acres' distance out to the animals as he is too poor to afford a tractor.

45

Qigong and the Ageless Woman

Shoshanna Katzman, LAc, CA, MS

The Chinese have studied ways of creating and maintaining healthful longevity for thousands of years. One of the jewels coming out of this quest for everlasting youth is the gentle, life-enhancing exercise practice of Qigong (pronounced chee-GUNG). Commonly known as Chinese yoga and Feng Shui for the body, Qigong is an ancient form of Chinese medicine exercise that retards the aging process by cultivating and strengthening the vital energy (Qi) in the body. It is an easy-to-perform exercise practiced to self-create medicine naturally within the body and is suitable for people of all ages and physical abilities, especially older people and those recovering from illness or injury.

Qigong is a key to healthful longevity because it balances emotions, promotes serenity, and strengthens the body. A typical Qigong workout includes stretching and strengthening exercises, breath work, creative visualization, self-massage, vocalization of sounds, and meditation through both movement and stillness.

Practiced for twenty minutes on a regular basis, Qigong tones not only the body, but also the mind and spirit.

Practice of this ancient art of self-healing and fitness is often likened to giving yourself acupuncture because it opens the flow of Qi, releases Qi blockages within the energy pathways (meridians), and promotes blood flow. This is nourishing, protecting, and balancing to the body because it provides ample vital energy and blood flow. This is beneficial to the physical structures of the body, creating sustenance and maintenance for life. The result is youthful skin, bright eyes and shiny hair, enhanced sexual vitality, fortified bones, flexible muscles and tendons, balanced hormones, abundant energy, and a clear mind and vibrant spirit.

Qigong can be practiced anywhere by anyone and is especially helpful to women who desire to be ageless. In ancient China prior to 500 b.c. and the dynasties led by kings, it is believed that it was the mature women shamans who created the art of Qi cultivation through their magical powers. The ideogram for women, *wu*, is even thought to originally mean "to heal." As modern women, we, too, can benefit from the healing power of Qi to keep ourselves healthy, vibrant, and beautiful for as long as we live.

According to Chinese medicine, good health occurs when there is a balance maintained between the two opposing, yet intimately related and attracting energies of yin and yang. Each person is made up of a predominance of either yin or yang energy; however, women tend to be more yin, whereas men tend to be more yang. This is because women tend to be more cold, soft, deep, wet, internal, and contracting, which are yin qualities, whereas men tend to be more hot, hard, superficial, dry, external, and expanding, which are yang qualities. Qigong practice creates a healing process, where the goal is to move more toward the center of the yin-yang continuum so that there is no longer a preponderance of yin or yang creating imbalance within the system.

True health exists when the body is adjusted according to the principles of yin and yang as well as synchronized with the yin and yang of nature, namely heaven and earth. An imbalance in the forces of heaven leads to tornados, hurricanes, and other natural disasters. An imbalance within the earth causes earthquakes and rivers to change directions. So, too, an imbalance in the forces of yin and yang energies within the human body causes illness to take hold.

The relative balance between these yin and yang energies also waxes and wanes, depending on various factors such as the energetics of foods eaten, weather conditions, temperature and dampness of one's dwelling, emotional states, and hereditary factors. For example, ingesting cold, wet food creates more yin, whereas hot, dry foods create more yang energy.

Women can enhance themselves and become ageless through the practice of Qigong as it creates body warmth without too much heat and adequate blood flow to counteract the tendency toward dryness. In practical terms, this explains how Qigong practice maintains healthy skin, nails, and hair. Qigong practice also reduces hot flashes, insomnia, depression, pain, anxiety, and diminishing vital fluids that so often accompany a woman's life changes.

Qigong helps women to cope emotionally through nourishing the spirit as it promotes feeling up and provides the energy necessary to be creative, achieve goals, and manifest dreams and aspirations. Practice of these empowering exercises helps women speak their minds freely and express themselves in a loving, gentle way that others can accept and honor.

The ultimate goal in Chinese medicine is to return to one's true self—to nourish one's destiny. This is done through searching for your true self in life through virtuous deeds. An initial step toward this goal is to be quiet with yourself on a daily basis by practicing these simple and gentle exercises. This will bring us back to the basic, true nature of peacefulness and oneness within ourselves.

An Exercise

Here is a Qigong exercise to help you connect with yourself. Calm down, release tension, and open the flow of energy throughout your body. Look deep within yourself and realize what the bottom line of importance is for you. Connect with yourself, and find that inner peace and wisdom.

- Open your mouth wide and feel if there is tension in your jaw.
- Massage the point called "Yintang," which is located in the middle of your forehead between your eyebrows, commonly known as your third eye.
- Place your hands over your heart and do self-acupressure on the point called "Sea of Tranquility," located at the center of your chest.
- Take three slow, gentle, and rhythmic deep breaths into your lower *dan tian*, located two inches below your navel. These breaths are done with your mouth closed and your tongue resting gently on the roof of your mouth. Inhale, and blow your belly up like a big balloon. Exhale, and deflate your belly.
- Open your mouth again, and compare the amount of tension in your jaw from before.

This simple Qigong exercise opens and nourishes the heart energy of the body. Creating and cultivating wonderful, nurturing relationships in life is of utmost importance, especially for promoting a healthy flow of heart energy. The heart energy must be nourished to be able to receive and give love to yourself and others. By creating a harmonious working of your heart through these simple life-enhancing exercises, spiritual and mental strength can be claimed in life. Life begins to flow, just like the movements flow. Life experiences become infused with peace, self-knowledge, intuition, balance, vibrancy, and focus—all great things in creating coping mechanisms to counteract the daily stress and pressures in modern life.

Qigong is a key to becoming an ageless, happy, and healthy woman who looks and feels younger. It softens and helps women to go inward and draw from their natural feminine power. Yet, at the same time, it creates an internal strength that helps women be heard and accepted in a clear and centered manner. Give yourself this glowing gift of Qigong so that you may truly enjoy this and many future years of looking gorgeous on the outside and being filled with vibrant Qi and serenity on the inside.

About the Author

Shoshanna Katzman, LAc, CA, MS, MA has been director of the Red Bank Acupuncture and Wellness Center in Tinton Falls, New Jersey, since 1988. As a licensed acupuncturist, herbalist, Tai Chi/Qigong professional, massage therapist, and energy medicine specialist, Shoshanna has been involved in the field of Oriental medicine for over thirty years. She earned her master's degree in sports medicine from San Francisco State University, CA. in 1981 and her master's degree in Acupuncture from the Tri-State College of Acupuncture, NYC in 1999. Shoshanna also has her master's certification in energy body medicine from Deutsche Schule fur Angewandte Energiekorper Medizin in Hamburg, Germany, in 2007. As author of *Qigong for Staying Young: A Simple 20 Minute Workout to Cultivate Your Vital Energy* (Avery Penguin Group, 2003), Shoshanna has produced a companion DVD. She has been featured in numerous magazine and newspaper articles and has appeared on radio and television, including programs on the Food Channel and America's Health Network. Visit http://www.healing4u.com and http://www.qigong4u.com.

46

Know Your Exercise Type

Carole Taylor

Forget about the so-called exercise experts who all say that everyone should run, or everyone should walk, or do aerobics, or lift weights, or whatever the fad exercise du jour is.

Each of us has a unique mind and body, and we should pick exercises that fit our mental and physical characteristics. By picking exercises that fit us in mind and body, we become more motivated and enthusiastic about making exercise part of our lives.

So do you know your exercise type? Exercise typing correlates certain physical, emotional, and mental characteristics with appropriate types of exercise.

Exercise typing comes from the medical principles of Ayurveda, an Indian system of preventative health care. Ayurveda recognizes each person's unique physical, mental, and emotional traits and chooses the best health plan based on those traits. Derived from the three *dosha* (mind-body types) of Ayurveda, exercise typing has identified three basic exercise groups.

Energetic Types

Energetic types are people who have high burst energy, but low endurance, when it comes to exercise.

Energetic types tend to have high energy in short bursts but tire easily and can easily overexert themselves. As such, energetic types do better with exercises that are brisk, without being exhausting. Exercises for this type should involve high energy but not a lot of strength or stamina. And if it is a new exercise, the movements should be easy to learn and remember.

You might be an energetic type if

- your body frame is thin or bony
- you have a hard time gaining weight, no matter how much you eat
- your skin tends to be dry, rough, cool, chaps easily, or has prominent veins
- your hair is coarse, dry, curly, and/or scant

- emotionally, when things are going well, you are full of joy and enthusiasm, but when things go badly, you become fearful, anxious, or worried
- when learning something new, you tend to grasp it quickly but soon forget what you've learned
- you enjoy being very physically active, especially in activities like gardening or hiking
- when engaged in physical activity, you have lots of energy but little strength or endurance and can tire easily.

Walking, especially for short periods of ten minutes or less, is one exercise that works well for energetic types. Walking is relaxing, especially if it can be done outside in nature or even around one's neighborhood. (Treadmill walking, though, is boring for energetic types and should not be done unless there is no other option.)

If walking is kept to less than ten minutes, it will not be exhausting. If energetic types need or want to walk for longer periods, they should divide the walk into ten to fifteen minute periods, with a short break for each period.

Other exercises that work well are

- aerobics (low impact, with softer music)
- archery
- badminton
- baseball/softball
- bicycling (with frequent breaks)
- bowling
- dancing
- golf
- hiking (light backpack, with frequent breaks)
- horseback riding
- ice skating (indoors away from cold)
- step-training (softer music)
- swimming
- Tai Chi or Qigong (easy styles)
- table tennis
- walking
- yoga.

Endurance Types

Both physically and mentally, endurance types have the most overall energy, but it is not explosive energy like the energetic types; rather, it is steady and enduring energy. They have high endurance but low burst energy—just the opposite of energetic types.

Owing to their low burst energy, endurance types often dislike exercise. They have a hard time getting started with an exercise since getting started often requires burst energy. So with their strengths and weaknesses in mind, endurance types do best with exercises that help stimulate them physically and mentally at the start. Activities that require quick bursts of energy should be avoided. Instead, they should look for activities that take advantage of their stamina and strength.

You might be an endurance type if

- your body frame is large or heavy-set
- you gain weight easily, even if you eat very little and exercise regularly
- your skin tends to be thick, cool, and/or prone to acne
- your hair is thick, shiny, and/or lustrous
- emotionally, when things are going well, you are stable, reliable, forgiving, and nonjudgmental; when things are going poorly, you become overly attached, resistant, and depressed.
- when learning something new, you learn slowly, but rarely forget what you've learned
- you tend to be less physically active, even lethargic, and don't especially enjoy activity
- when engaged in physical activity, you have lots of endurance, but little energy—you find it hard to get started but can keep going once you do.

Walking, especially for long distances, works well for endurance types. They can walk for twenty- or thirty-minute periods (or even longer) without breaks. They especially like to walk outdoors because the sights and scenes help stimulate them.

Other exercises that work well for endurance types are

- aerobics (low impact)
- basketball
- bicycling (slow pace, long distance)
- calisthenics (slow pace)
- cross-country skiing
- football
- ice skating
- jogging (slow pace, long distance)
- racquetball
- rock climbing
- rollerblading
- rowing
- shot-put
- skiing
- stair climbing

- Tai Chi or Qigong (forms with repetitive movements)
- tennis
- walking (slow pace, long distance).

Athletic Types

Athletic types have equal amounts of burst energy and endurance. If they are in good physical condition, they will have high amounts of both. If they are in poor physical condition, they may have low amounts of both. But either way, they have approximately equal amounts.

To capitalize on their strengths and compensate for their weaknesses, athletic types do best with exercises that engage their active minds and involve both burst energy and stamina. They often thrive on exercises that are competitive and/or involve concentration.

But excessive competition brings out the worst in athletic types, so much so that they may risk injury while competing. As such, activities where the athletic type competes against herself or himself (such as improving on past performances or skills) are often better than head-to-head competition with someone else.

You might be an athletic type if

- your body frame is medium or muscular
- you are average weight or muscular, though you might gain weight without proper nutrition or exercise
- your skin tends to be oily, warm, sensitive, reddish, and/or inflamed
- your hair is thin, oily, and/or has premature gray or hair loss
- emotionally, when things are going well, you are assertive and confident; when things are going poorly, you become aggressive, angry, or frustrated
- when learning something new, you enjoy challenges, tend to quickly grasp it, and remember it easily
- you enjoy being very physically active, especially in competitive sports or learning complex physical skills
- when engaged in physical activity, you have moderate to strong amounts of both energy and endurance and don't like to take breaks

Swimming, especially swimming a given number of timed laps in a pool, works well for athletic types. It involves concentration, strength, and competitiveness. Athletic types also do well with learning complicated movement patterns, such as yoga, Tai Chi, and karate sets or forms.

Other exercises that work well for athletic types are

- basketball
- bicycling (moderate pace, long distance)

- field hockey
- football
- gymnastics
- ice hockey
- ice skating (in/outdoors)
- kayaking
- karate
- mountain biking
- mountain climbing
- rollerblading
- skiing
- soccer
- Tai Chi or Qigong (highly detailed styles)
- tennis
- surfing
- water skiing
- windsurfing
- Yoga
- walking/jogging
- weight-lifting

Exercise That Fits You!

Start to exercise with your mind and body, and not against them! Exercise typing helps you find exercises that fit your unique physical, mental, and emotional traits. Use the above guidelines to find your type and the activities that best fit you. If you do, you'll become more motivated and enthusiastic about improving your health and making exercise part of your life!

About the Author

Carole Taylor is the director of YoungAfter50.com, a Web site for helping people develop a customized approach to health and longevity. Carole holds certifications in nutritional advising, neurotransmitter balancing, and Tai Chi exercise instruction. A living example of what she preaches, Carole is nearly seventy years old, but with the energy, vigor, and looks of someone in her forties. Carole helps clients over the Internet develop personalized plans for health, nutrition, and longevity. Her Web site contains nutrition and diet profiling tools, an exercise typing tool, and free articles and newsletters on health, diet, nutrition, and mind-body wellness.

PART FIVE

Hidden Health Dangers

How much today is still hidden?
How much will be uncovered tomorrow?

-- David Riklan

47

My Experience with Mercury Toxicity

Chuck Balzer, MSc

After dissolving into tears of frustration, pain, and perplexity, I went to a local emergency room (ER) in March 2002. Approximately six months prior to my ER visit, I had begun feeling slowly progressing lower leg pain and discomfort that grew to searing pain on standing still for more than a few minutes. At first, I had self-diagnosed this pain as Achilles tendonitis and accepted it as an inevitable fact of life that accompanies an active lifestyle in an aging body. As it progressed and was joined by other symptoms, I became concerned and frightened.

My primary complaints upon ER admission included bilateral lower leg pain, exacerbating arthritis, fatigue, and a feeling that I can only describe as my legs feeling unstable under me. I was greeted with the same perplexity I had been receiving over recent months from various physicians across the medical discipline spectrum. These opinions varied from a rheumatologist's demoralizing diagnosis of depression-induced fibromyalgia to an ER physician questioning me about the use of hard street drugs. One kind ER physician recommended that I be evaluated by the hospital's chief of neurology. I again felt a swell of frustration building as I had recently been evaluated by a neurologist whose treatment plan was to give me a prescription for Darvocet, along with a pat on the back. As she was leaving the room, I mentioned to the ER physician, "For what it's worth, I'm also having strange bodily twitching." An inquisitive look came over her face, and she stated that she wanted to test my mercury level. I did not think much of it and was released on advice to rest, medicate for pain as needed, and follow up with a neurologist. Three days later, an ER nurse phoned me and stated that my serum mercury level was elevated. I called poison control and was met with a response that if I had consumed seafood within 72 hours prior to testing, the result was meaningless. My general practitioner (GP) also assumed lab error or recent ingestion of seafood and had the test repeated. This time, I had been seafood-free for ten days, but again, the results were an elevated level of mercury. My life, knowledge, and perspective on many issues ranging from medicine to the environment would never be the same.

Mercury: The Toxic Metal

Mercury (Hg) is an extremely toxic metal, second only to cadmium as the most poisonous on earth.[1] This toxin has an affinity for the human nervous system, with deleterious neurological effects extremely well documented in medical history.[2] Mercury's multiple physiological capabilities include, but are far from limited to,

- altering and damaging the cardiac, renal, and immune systems[3]
- elevating oxidative stress and depleting/disrupting antioxidant protection[4]
- peripheral nerve damage[5]
- altering calcium homeostasis[6]
- interfering with enzyme functions.[7]

How Does One Become Mercury-Toxic?

Coal-burning power plants dump approximately forty tons of mercury into the atmosphere per year.[8] This vaporized Hg eventually finds its way into lakes, rivers,

---

[1] H. B. Gerstner et al., "Clinical toxicology of mercury," *Journal of Toxicology and Environmental Health* 2 (1977): 491–526.

[2] Ibid.; C. Sanfeliu et al., "Neurotoxicity of organomercurial compounds," *Neurotoxicology Research* 5 (2003): 283–86; K. Eto et al., "An autopsy case of minamata disease (methylmercury poisoning)— Pathological viewpoints of peripheral nerves," *Toxicology and Pathology* 30 (2002): 714–22; A. F. Castoldi et al., "Neurotoxic and molecular effects of methylmercury in humans," *Reviews on Environmental Health* 18 (2003): 19–31.

[3] E. Guallar et al., "Mercury, fish oils, and the risk of myocardial infarction," *New England Journal of Medicine* 347 (2002): 1747–54; W. L. Mortada et al., "Mercury in dental restorations: Is there a risk of nephrotoxicity?," *Journal of Nephrology* 15 (2002): 171–76; J. Bartova et al., "Dental amalgam as one of the risk factors in autoimmune diseases," *Neuroendocrinology Letters* 24 (2003): 65–67; L. D. Koller, "Immunotoxicity of heavy metals," *International Journal of Immunopharmacology* 2 (1980): 269–79; S. H. Kim et al., "Cytotoxicity of inorganic mercury in murine T and B lymphoma cell lines: Involvement of reactive oxygen species, Ca(2+) homeostasis, and cytokine gene expression," *Toxicology In Vitro* 17 (2003): 385–95.

[4] Sanfeliu, "Neurotoxicity"; Castoldi, "Neurotoxic"; M. Mahboob et al., "Lipid peroxidation and antioxidant enzyme activity in different organs of mice exposed to level mercury," *Journal of Environmental Science and Health B* 36 (2001): 687–97; M. Pizzicini et al., "Influence of amalgam fillings on Hg levels and total antioxidant activity in plasma of healthy donors," *Science of the Total Environment* 301 (2003): 43–50; Kim, "Cytotoxicity"; J. T. Salonen et al., "Intake of mercury from fish, lipid peroxidation, and the risk of myocardial infarction and coronary, cardiovascular, and any death in Finnish men," *Circulation* 91 (1995): 645–55

[5] Eto, "Autopsy case"; C. C. Chu et al., "Chronic inorganic induced peripheral neuropathy," *Acta Neurologica Scandinavica* 98 (1998): 461–65.

[6] Sanfeliu, "Neurotoxicity"; Castoldi, "Neurotoxic"; Kim, "Cytotoxicity."

[7] Sanfeliu, "Neurotoxicity"; Mahboob, "Lipid peroxidation."

and oceans. Bacteria in water and soil convert mercury to its most toxic methylated form.[9] Contaminated food sources are then ingested by aqueous creatures, thus increasing their bodily mercury levels in accordance with their place on the food chain.[10] This modern biological fact has recently prompted the Food and Drug Administration (FDA) to advise the general public to limit their intake of specific species of fish.[11] In addition, pregnant women have been advised not only to limit, but avoid consuming fish high on the food chain. The species of fish included in this warning are swordfish, shark, mackerel, and tuna.[12]

A controversial source of mercury is from dental amalgams. *Amalgam* is a generic term for so-called silver dental fillings, which contain up to 50 percent liquid metallic mercury. The scientific research is clear that the more amalgam fillings one has in his or her mouth, the higher the person's level of systemic mercury.[13] In fact, mercury amalgams are the primary source of systemic mercury in the human population.

Actions and habits such as chewing, brushing, and inordinate mouth breathing increase both the vapor release of mercury from amalgam and subsequent inhalation.[14] Scientific research supports the connection between amalgam placement and pathological alterations.[15] The Environmental Protection Agency (EPA) has set a safe limit of 0.1 micrograms of methylmercury per kilograms per

---

[8] U.S. Environment Protection Agency, *Plant by Plant Mercury Emission Estimates* (Washington, DC, 2000); U.S. Environment Protection Agency, *Mercury Study Report to Congress* (Washington, DC, 1997).

[9] Ibid.

[10] U.S. Environmental Protection Agency, *Mercury Study*.

[11] Ibid.

[12] Ibid.; E. C. Evans, "The FDA recommendations on fish intake during pregnancy," *Journal of Obstetrics, Gynecology, and Neonatal Nursing* 31 (2002): 71520.

[13] Pizzicini, "Influence"; Mortada, "Mercury"; J. Leisteuo et al., "Dental amalgam fillings and the amount of organic mercury in human saliva," *Caries Research* 35 (2001): 163–66; N. Galic et al., "Elimination of mercury from amalgam in rats," *Journal of Trace Elements and Biology* 15 (2001): 1–4; S. W. Lindow et al., "Maternal and neonatal hair mercury concentrations: The effect of dental amalgam," *British Journal of Obstetrics and Gynaecology* 110 (2003): 287–91.

[14] T. W. Clarkson et al., "The prediction of intake of mercury vapor from amalgams," in *Biological Monitoring of Toxic Metals* (New York: Plenum Press, 1988), 247–64; J. E. Patterson et al., "Mercury in human breath from dental amalgam," *Bulletin of Environmental Contamination and Toxicology* 34 (1985): 459–68.

[15] Pizzicini, "Influence"; Mortada, "Mercury"; Bartova, "Dental amalgam"; I. Sterzl et al., "Mercury and nickel allergy: Risk factors in fatigue and autoimmunity," *Neuroendocrinology Letters* 20 (1999): 221–28.

day.[16] Other toxicology authorities maintain that there is no threshold level of mercury exposure that can be considered totally harmless.[17]

The Road to Detoxification

My options were multiple, but my goal was clear—detoxification. My GP, who is, for the most part, conventional in his medical approach surprised me by saying that he felt that my twenty-two amalgams should be removed. Along with removal of my amalgam fillings, a seafood-free diet, and an array of self-researched nutrition supplements, I was treated with chelation therapy for systemic mercury removal.

Initially, I was treated by my GP with 2,3-dimercaptosuccinic acid (DMSA), or Chemet, a prescription medication commonly used for lead poisoning in children.[18] After three weeks and slight clinical improvement, I consulted with an integrative physician, whose approach was 2,3-dimercapto-1-propanesulfonic acid (DMPS) intravenously, followed by a vitamin and glutathione drip. He tested my mercury body burden with what is called a DMPS challenge test.[19] The results had me excreting urinary mercury at a level five times the upper range of normal. This was after three weeks of the first-line treatment with DMSA!

Mercury is a tenacious poison, thus making the process of detoxification long and arduous—one that I can only analogize as a roller-coaster of good and bad days. I knew this would be the case prior to initiation, through my own research and from the health care practitioners treating me. Although expected, it was nonetheless challenging and frustrating.

Today

As of this writing, I have been symptom-free for over two months. I am very active, alternating between biking ten miles, walking three miles on the beach, ocean kayaking, and playing beach volleyball. I have had days where I've done all four in one day! This is an unimaginable progression from being unable to stand for three minutes without burning pain.

One of my primary concerns is the deleterious effect that Hg poisoning has had on my cardiovascular health. With my subpar genetic history in this area, I make a

---

[16] U.S. Environmental Protection Agency, *Mercury Study*.

[17] Ibid.; National Institute for Occupational Safety and Health, *A Recommended Standard for Occupational Exposure to Inorganic Mercury*, Rep. PB-222 223 (Washington, DC: U.S. Government Printing Office, 1973).

[18] H. V. Aposhan, "DMSA and DMPS—Water soluble antidotes for heavy metal poisoning," *Annual Reviews in Pharmacology and Toxicology* 23 (1983): 193–215.

[19] Ibid.

special effort at strictly controlling my cholesterol and blood pressure. I have chosen a diet that is virtually seafood-free, supplementing with omega-3 fatty acids, rather than the generally advised intake of two to three servings of fish per week. Recent research is citing that not only is Hg toxicity deleterious to cardiovascular health, but the mercury content of many species of fish may negate the natural cardioprotective components contained therein.[20] In addition, I take broad-spectrum antioxidants to aid in the healing and maintenance of systems that were likely altered by mercury toxicity.[21]

Conclusion

As for those reading this, I would recommend that you take caution in your seafood intake—both amount and species. In addition, ask your dental practitioner why the second most toxic metal on the planet has been implanted into the bodies of most reading this article. Don't gently succumb to intimidating responses such as that the mercury is rendered harmless when amalgamated with other materials. After reviewing the American Dental Association's (ADA) position statement on the safety of amalgam, and scouring the (global) research on the subject, it is my opinion that the ADA has been far from unbiased, balanced, and forthcoming in their position on this issue. This stance has put both the professionals within this organization and the public whom they serve at risk of ill health. At the very least, it should be mandatory that patients be informed about the content of the material being implanted in their mouths. Dental professionals are strongly mandated to carefully discard of unused or removed amalgam as to protect the environment.[22] Intriguing that according to regulations, amalgam is safe when placed in the mouth, but not into ordinary garbage.

On the political and environmental fronts, I would advise self-education and activism on this issue. Much legislation is presently under way and needed to protect the general public from both environmental and medically induced risks of mercury poisoning.[23]

---

[20] Guallar, "Mercury"; Salonen, "Intake"; "Heavy metals test heart's mettle: Mercury and lead may contribute to heart disease and hypertension," *Harvard Heart Letters* 13 (2003): 6–7.

[21] Sanfeliu, "Neurotoxicity"; Castoldi, "Neurotoxic"; Mahboob, "Lipid peroxidation"; Pizzicini, "Influence"; Kim, "Cytotoxicity"; U. Lindh et al., "Removal of dental amalgam and other metal alloys supported by antioxidant therapy alleviates symptoms and improves quality of life in patients with amalgam-associated ill health," *Neuroendocrinology Letters* 23 (2002): 459–82; Salonen, "Intake."

[22] American Dental Association, "Best management practices for amalgam waste," http://www.ada.org/prof/resources/topics/amalgam bmp.asp (accessed March 12, 2004).

[23] Arizona Mercury Amalgam Fillings Act, HB 2467, 46th Legis., 1st sess., 2003 (see http://www.azleg.state.az.us/legtext/46leg/1r/bills/hb2467p.htm); Connecticut Public Act 03-72. See also http://www.mercurypolicy.org.

About the Author

Chuck Balzer, MSc, BSc, is a nutritionist and nutra/pharmaceutical consultant with over ten years of experience as a clinical registered dietitian and college instructor. He has had multiple published commentaries in medical journals, in addition to having presented internationally on the subject of vitamins and minerals in health and disease. He can be reached at ChuckMSRD@aol.com. More of his commentaries and articles can be accessed at http://EverettLabs.com.

48

Thinking outside the Box: Your Coffin

James E. Hicks, DC, FIAMA, DAAPM, NMD

Nutrition is a vital part of good health, and with the current epidemics of obesity and heart disease being experienced in the United States, Americans need to begin "thinking outside the coffin" to prolong life and avoid early disease or death. The following are some quick tips on how to jump-start your health and stay ahead of the pervasive toxicity that surrounds us.

1. *Eliminate trans fats from your diet.* One of the best health measures you can do for yourself this year is to eliminate all man-made trans fats from your diet. These make you fatter, and it takes about three months to get these bad fats to metabolize out of your body.

   Obesity is now a disease, and we need to think outside the coffin. One thing that clearly contributes to early death is the consumption of bad fats—like trans fats—in foods such as snacks, prepackaged foods, margarine, deep-fried foods, and French fries.

   There is no safe level of trans fats in your diet. They interfere with fat metabolism, which is essential to health—our bodies cannot naturally process these artificial fats. You need good fats for your skin, hair, nails, arteries, immune system, and hormones. You can get these from essential fatty acids found in fish oil, eggs, nuts and seeds, sunflower and olive oils, and poultry.

   The food industry uses trans fats to prolong the shelf life of packaged products. Keep in mind that if a product does not decompose, it probably shouldn't be eaten!

2. *Boycott monosodium glutamate, aspartame, and high fructose corn syrup.* One of the contributing causes of obesity is the consumption of corn products like corn chips, corn dogs, and all high fructose corn syrup (HFCS) products. HFCS is in abundance in sodas, packaged sushi, cookies, yogurt, and many processed foods. The key is to read the labels.

   Monosodium glutamate (MSG) products and aspartame are toxic to the brain. They are considered excitotoxins. These products excite or vibrate the brain neurons to death. MSG adds flavoring to many products such as Ramen noodle soups. Aspartame is a known carcinogen found in products like diet sodas and—unbelievably—popular children's vitamins.

Anyone trying to lose weight, or anyone suffering from tremors because of diseases like parkinsonism, multiple sclerosis, or amyotrophic lateral sclerosis, should be off these products immediately and completely. You may need to be detoxed from these substances if they have compromised your health.

3. *Supplement with omega-3 fish oils.* A tremendous benefit to promoting and supporting good overall health is fish oil (omega-3) essential fatty acid (EFA) supplementation. EFAs are found in flaxseeds, nuts, and avocados. Omega-3s are great for children with learning disabilities, ADD/ADHD, self-destructive behavior, and oppositional defiance disorders and for adults with chronic pain, disc herniation, osteoarthritis, cardiovascular disease, diabetes, autoimmune disorders, Alzheimer's, colitis, multiple sclerosis, asthma, allergies, dermatitis, psoriasis, inflammation, and depression. Omega-3s are critical for proper brain and nervous system function. Fish oils work because they contain the two unsaturated flexible fatty acids—eicosapentaenoic and docosahexanoic—that comprise all our cell membranes and influence a variety of other cellular functions.

Eating fish (sockeye salmon, wild Atlantic salmon, cod liver, tuna) may be another way of incorporating these oils into the diet. You just cannot eat enough of it, though, and therefore supplementation is strongly recommended. The safest form is a pharmaceutical grade omega-3 fish oil. In addition, minerals provide for proper absorption and utilization of the omega-3 oils in addition to improving heart function.[1]

4. *Drink plenty of good-quality water.* Water is the elixir of life! Simply put, your body requires water to function as it was designed. It is a good idea to have bottled spring water delivered to your home. It's more economical, about five dollars for a five-gallon jug. Get a stainless steel or high-density plastic container to hold your water from a local health food store. It will have a number 7 on the bottom encircled by a triangle. This type of container will prevent leaching of plastic into the drinking water. Drinking water should be at room temperature—not ice cold.

There is a proverb that states that you can never clean dirty water. The tap water you receive has probably gone through several commodes before you reconsume the water. Tap water for consumption should generally be avoided. There can be a certain level of arsenic, chlorine, fluoride, lead, and total dissolved solids or impurities in tap water. Your shower should also have a filter to help

---

[1] P. C. Calder, "Immunoregulatory and Anti-inflammatory Effects of n-3 Polyunsaturated Fatty Acids," *Brazilian Journal of Medicine and Biology Research* 31 (1998): 467–90.

remove chlorine—otherwise, your body will become a sponge for these contaminants. Also, drinking distilled water for long periods of time may rob your body of good minerals.

If you are trying to lose weight and are hooked on sodas, switch to a sparkling water to wean yourself away from sugared drinks and aspartame. The carbonation in sparkling water still has to be processed by your body but is much better than soda. Eventually, get off the sparkling water and begin drinking spring water.

5. *Start a heart healthy diet.* Major hospitals are constantly building specialized wings to take care of heart patients. We all know that the number one killer today is heart disease. However, with all our technology, we are not able to keep our citizens out of the hospital, and we cannot keep them from having a sudden death heart attack. We have little control over our family history but have the power to choose a diet that is heart healthy.

Typically, heart patients are told to go on a low-fat diet and eliminate salt. The body, however, needs fat, especially healthy fats like omega-3 essential fatty acids. It is the trans fats (hydrogenated or partially hydrogenated) that are dangerous for human consumption. Again, there are no safe levels of these fats!

A heart healthy diet should be the healthiest diet in the world—the Mediterranean diet (try a sampling of a Greek salad) coupled with the blood type diet. A sample of the Mediterranean diet may include asparagus, broccoli, carrots, feta cheese, garlic cloves, chicken breasts, extra virgin olive oil, olives, red wine, brown rice, spinach, tomatoes, tuna, turkey, fresh fruits and vegetables, balsamic vinegar, walnuts, onions, and mushrooms. A sample of the blood type diet is best resourced in Dr. Peter J. D'Adamo's book *Live Right 4 Your Type*.[2] Look up your specific blood type, and see which foods are most compatible with your makeup.

Your diet should also include good spring water, Celtic sea salt, whole food nutrition that helps repair the heart and circulatory system, CoQ-10, bioflavonoids, fruits, veggies, B complex, and an omega-3 supplement, like a fish oil or a tablespoon of raw flax oil daily. Avoid synthetic, man-made fractionated vitamins. These will do more harm than good. Avoid smoking, and minimize alcohol. Of course, an exercise routine of yoga, Qigong, or Tai Chi is always heart healthy, as is frequent infrared sauna usage with supervision.

We are slowly killing ourselves with our poor food choices. There is a natural solution. We should not feel that we have a death sentence of lifelong heart medication. Most of the medications deplete vital minerals and nutrients. We do not need bigger hospital wings, special heart walks, or more contributions for heart research—we simply need to make whole food nutrition our mainstay diet.

---

[2] Peter J. D'Adamo, *Live Right 4 Your Type* (New York: Putnam's, 2001).

About the Author

Dr. James E. Hicks graduated from the U.S. Military Academy at West Point with a bachelor of science degree and graduated with a doctorate degree from Cleveland Chiropractic College. While in the U.S. Army Reserves, he became a certified U.S. Army master fitness trainer. Dr. Hicks has been the clinical director of Hicks Chiropractic & Healing Arts Center in Reynoldsburg, Ohio, since 2000. He has specialized and advanced training in whiplash and spinal trauma, auricular therapy, acupuncture, detoxification, nutritional and laser therapies, and pain management in the treatment of compulsive disorders and addictions, treatment for balance and dizziness disorders, and metabolic stress and nutritional assessments. Visit http://www.doctorhicks.com.

49

Blood Testing for Achieving Optimal Health

Ed Jones, CN

Blood testing has been traditionally used for diagnosing diseases; however, some health professionals now realize its vital importance in optimizing health, instead of just in diagnosing disease. I have been counseling clients on how to improve their health for almost thirty years, and I strongly insist that clients receive complete blood work to be able to evaluate their health prevention plans. I will tell you how you can utilize this phenomenal method of building your health and save hundreds of dollars at the same time.

When you go to the doctor for a physical, you will most likely receive blood work that will measure your cholesterol level, white and red blood cell count, liver function, kidney function, and sometimes thyroid function. These tests are good for diagnosing medical problems; however, to improve your health in the future, you must be able to receive additional blood tests that more accurately reveal the direction your health is going and what you can do about it.

The problem in the past was that very few physicians were knowledgeable about which tests to order for preventative health, and also, the price of these special tests were normally cost-prohibitive. Now all blood work can be ordered through Internet companies that cut out the middleman profits, and the labs are the same ones that your doctor uses! Your blood is drawn at local labs that are found in every major city in the United States.

The tests that are needed after age forty to achieve optimal health are usually not paid for by insurance companies because these companies will often not reimburse for preventative health. This is a responsibility that must be assumed by each individual.

The first step is finding the proper lab. I recommend using any reputable Internet blood testing company; however, I have found DirectLabs.com or Lef.org to be very reliable. When you log on to these Web sites, you will be able to choose any tests that your doctor can order; however, since most people do not have knowledge of blood work, the easiest method is to choose the blood test panels that are offered such as a male or female panel. Additional tests that I feel are absolutely necessary to be included in your panels are the following: homocysteine, high-sensitivity C-reactive, fasting insulin, and 25 hydroxy vitamin D. I find that to truly receive the combination of blood work necessary to give you this information, the cost would be approximately three hundred to four hundred dollars. These same tests would cost you over one thousand dollars if you paid for them at your doctor's office.

Once the results are received from your blood work, consultation with a nutritionally oriented physician is important to completely interpret the results. It is important to find health professionals who are willing to work with you on your goals of achieving superior health.

Traditional physicians may lack the expertise to know how to evaluate blood work from the aspect of knowing the difference between reference ranges and optimal ranges. Reference ranges in blood work values apply to the majority of people and are used only for diagnosing disease; however, optimal ranges are where you want to find yourself on blood values to achieve the best health. The optimal values are much narrower, and these values can be found at Lef.org or from BloodChemistryAnalysis.com. Dr. Weatherby, author of *Blood Chemistry and CBC Analysis*, offers entire courses for the public and health professionals on the importance of optimal blood analysis and long-term health.

The final importance of personal blood testing is that you can follow trends in your year-to-year blood work, and this may be the most accurate way of indicating which way your health is heading. Most people think that when a doctor diagnoses them with a chronic disease, they just got sick, when in fact, they were probably heading toward the diagnosis for many years. Doctors usually only diagnose from blood work when red flags are shown on the tests; however, many times, this is a process that could have been altered if the trends were viewed earlier with proper blood work. One problem, however, is that few traditionally trained physicians ever observe year-to-year trends of patients to follow the direction in which the person's health is going.

Blood testing by the individual is yet another example of the need to take responsibility for one's own health. This responsibility requires some effort and expense; however, the long-term benefits to your health could be tremendous.

About the Author

Ed Jones, CN, has been involved in natural health since opening his first nutrition store in 1979. Ed Jones has been a part of every aspect of natural health, ranging from formulating state-of-the-art nutritional products to speaking and consulting. He has been advising clients on natural health for over twenty years and continues to grow by owning a wellness center in Chattanooga, Tennessee, that is focused on integrative health. Ed Jones is a member of the Institute for Functional Medicine, the Natural Products Association, and is a graduate from American Health Sciences University. For more information, log on to http://www.nutritionw.com.

50

Posture and Pain: From the Feet Up

Linda Mac Dougall, MA

The ideal body has a framework of curves and arches that, with the joints, support and balance the body's weight. When spinal curves or foot arches flatten or are exaggerated, our center of gravity is shifted. The result? Pain!

The more self-imposed problems often come from poor ergonomics when using the computer or doing some other activity repetitively over a long period of time that disturbs the balance of the body's structural components. Even worse is doing an activity incorrectly and repetitively.

The body is all about balance. If the bones are in their proper places, joints meeting as they should, then the muscles are not fighting against each other or against misaligned or stuck bony elements to facilitate movement. A balanced body is a body with fluid, painless movement.

Imbalanced, strained muscles pull on bones, joints, and ligaments, rotating and tilting skeletal components throughout the human form. Rippling upward from our foundation, improper foot structure or use can cause symptoms all the way up to the head. The problem may appear small and insignificant, but the cascade it can initiate can be damaging.

We don't tend to think of our feet until they exhibit some problem. These trusty, pyramid-shaped stabilizers of the body do their job virtually unthought of as we go about our tasks from day to day. But your whole body knows it when your feet hurt. Their pain is radiated to other areas disturbed by the awkward gait or tentative foot strike of the injured area.

Whenever there is an injury to an area, other areas compensate for the lost movement. If you limp, the other leg attempts to take up the slack. In so doing, it is strained and more easily injured itself. In protecting the original site of pain, the body is brought out of balance and into a state of strain and dysfunction.

To illustrate, let's consider the common problem of flat feet. The normal foot has nearly the same arch when it is bearing weight and when it is not. Flat feet have various degrees of arch degradation when the body's weight is on them.

195

As the arch rotates inward, the foot also rotates forward. The tibia or lower leg bone descends and turns internally with the flattened arch, pulling the entire skeletal frame with it. The toes point outward, and the leg becomes functionally shorter. The Achilles tendon at the heel bows inward. The tibia's rotation takes with it the knee. The body's center of gravity is forced forward to the forefoot, as is the body's weight.

If the condition is unequal or unilateral, the body will lean to one side. If the lean is slight, it may easily go unnoticed. That side will experience compression. Muscles and fascia will become habitually shortened and tight. Organ function may eventually be compromised. Blood and nerve supply is impaired. Joints of the compressed side can lose their range of motion.

On the other side, the bony structures are drawn toward the compressed side, while the muscles are stretched tight trying to right the body. With this torquing of the body, a functional scoliosis is created. One shoulder is tugged downward with the short side, bringing with it the neck and head.

This chain of events can cause foot, ankle, knee, hip, sacroiliac, back, and neck pain. Several disorders of the foot itself will emerge over time. And as ever so far away it may seem, jaw dysfunction can occur.

Pain can be from inflammation where stresses on the framework cause dysfunction such as joint misalignment, muscle fatigue, spasms, restricted blood flow, and disturbed enervation to the muscles. Myofascial trigger points in leg muscles can disrupt the proper function of the foot. Over time, these issues wear down the joints.

The foot itself can develop callus buildup, bunions, neuromas, and so on, which can all be signals of alignment problems. Where do you find calluses on your foot, if any? This tells you where there is pressure on the foot. Are the toes straight or turned in or out? Does your arch flatten when you stand? Are there toes turning under others? Do the toe joints bend easily, or are they stiff and claw-like?

Surgery is often the chosen solution for many problems that can often be avoided or minimized. Surgery also often has its own set of problems once it is done. It is our responsibility to take care of ourselves. It is our responsibility to be as informed as possible on our choices. Surgery should be a last option, not a first reaction.

Our feet were not designed to be cooped up in shoes or to walk on mostly hard, flat surfaces. By imprisoning these ingenious tools, we have robbed them of their strength. No longer do the muscles of the legs and feet have to constantly adapt to changes in the surfaces on which they travel. Adaptation is what made them and our core strong.

On uneven surfaces, bare feet adjust with each step. When the arch is pressured, its reflex is to withdraw by contraction. Each contraction strengthens the arch and its support system. Modern life has weakened both the arch and the several leg muscles that assist in arch functioning. Shoes made more for fashion than for functionality have also increased foot disorders.

The first step is to correct the foot's stance and thereby bring better balance to the body. This alone can ease pain and inflammation. Supportive footwear, muscle retraining, and sometimes orthotics can all help in regaining balance. Podiatry or chiropractic consults are a good place to start.

Working with your chosen health care provider, a good massage therapist can then deal with the involved muscles. Trigger points in the lower leg and foot muscles need to be defused through gradual, deep pressure. An example of a trigger point would be when a pressed calf muscle refers pain to the heel.

If a trigger point is less reactive, a muscle stripping or deep lengthwise stroke can be effective. Kneading the muscle can also bring some relief. This work must be done to your level of tolerance, so be sure to communicate with your therapist throughout your session.

Long-held fascial tissue restrictions also need to be worked out. Muscle fiber adhesions can then be released through pressure and stretching. All this work stimulates the circulatory and nervous systems and gives relief to the tissues and joints.

Your professionals are working to make your life better. Not too much can be permanently accomplished without you as a participating partner. Your job is to work on strengthening the arch and muscles supporting it.

Pick up small objects with your toes. Roll a small ball under your foot in the arch. Write a short sentence in the air with your toes. Put your weight on the outside of your feet and contract your toes a bit. Feel that position for ten or more seconds where the arch is lifted. Relax and repeat. Keep your feet busy—use those joints to keep them flexible.

So now it is up to you. If you suspect that feet may be at least part of a problem that you or a loved one has, get a professional opinion or two. Make yourself a full partner in the process. This could also mean improving your diet to support muscles, joints, bones, nerves, and circulation.

In our hectic lives, we tend to tune in to the external and tune out the body and all it is warning us about. We need to pay attention for our own health as well as that of our children. A proper and early diagnosis can help prevent a lifetime of pain.

About the Author

Linda Mac Dougall is a holistic health practitioner/massage therapist in Port Hueneme, California. She holds a MA in psychology and has a long history of working with people with disabilities and senior populations. Linda currently acts as a researcher and conduit of information on alternative therapies for her holistic health and massage clients so that, with their doctors, they proceed with their decision making processes more fully aware of the options available to them. She works with select nutritional companies and enzymatic therapies to better the health of her clients. Visit her Web site at http://www.ilresources.com/MacDougallConsulting.htm or e-mail her at drgnstar@earthlink.net.

51

Positive Is Bad, Negative Is Good

Eric Madrid, MD

Are you fatigued, depressed, or constantly sick? Negative ions may be of benefit. Sounding like Orwellian doublespeak, the statement "positive is bad, negative is good" is scientifically backed. Hundreds of research articles over the past thirty years have shown evidence that negatively charged air ions are actually good for our health, while positive air ions are not. Unfortunately, household conveniences have created environments where many are now surrounded by an excess of positively charged ions and therefore lack the benefits of negative ions. Negative ionizer machines can help restore the balance.

What Is a Negative Air Ion?

A negative ion is a molecule with a negative charge assigned to it. Negative ions occur commonly throughout nature and can create an overall sense of well-being. Negative ions are found after a rainstorm, near waterfalls, in forests, and after lightning strikes. The refreshing smell in the air generated after a storm is due to the presence of negatively charged air ions.

What Is a Positive Air Ion?

Positive ions are positively charged molecules (such as carbon dioxide) and are believed to have negative health effects on humans, both physically and mentally. When pollution, dust, or smoke is present, positive ions are found in high concentrations and can have adverse affects.

Is Your Computer Monitor Harming You?

We all enjoy the conveniences of modern technology, but at what cost to our health? Many of our homes, offices, and autos are inundated with pollution and an excess of positive air ions while lacking the beneficial negative air ions. Negative ions are neutralized when air goes through ducts or by exposure to tobacco smoke, cleaning chemicals, furniture or carpet glues, and even electronic devices like TVs and computer monitors. The positively charged monitor neutralizes the negatively charged air ions.

Air Pollution

The dangers of indoor air pollution have become well known to many over the last ten years, and the term *sick building syndrome* has become a common topic on national morning news programs. However, few focus on actually restoring negative ion concentrations as the benefits are seldom realized.

Exposure to outdoor pollution can be just as harmful. With commuters spending record time on freeways and highways, exposure to auto exhaust is unavoidable, as is exposure to harmful positive ions when in traffic. These ions leave many of us feeling angry, frustrated, and irritable by the end of our drive. Perhaps lack of negative ions are partially responsible for the road rage phenomenon?

Effects of Positive Ions on Human Health

- Depression
- Fatigue and irritability
- Poor memory
- Difficulty concentrating
- Increased risk of colds, bronchitis, and other lung or sinus infections
- Chronic cough
- Allergy symptoms
- Delays in wound healing

Benefits of Negative Ions

Negative ions have air cleaning properties. Airborne dust, pollens, and other common pollutants are positively charged. If the concentration of negative ions is increased, the air will be cleaned. Simply, the negatively charged ion molecule binds to the positively charged pollutant, causing the air impurity to fall to the ground surface and out of one's breathing space. Routine cleaning removes the impurities from the carpet or floor.

What Can Air Ionization (Negative Ions) Do for You?

- Evidence shows that negative ions clean the air of dust, molds, bacteria, soot, and household odors.
- Air ionization minimizes allergies and asthma by eliminating common triggers.
- Air ionizers have been reported to be helpful to people with seasonal affective disorder by regulating hormone levels and minimizing depression symptoms.
- Air ionizers clean the air of pollen, therefore being helpful for those with hay fever and other seasonal allergies.
- Air ionizers have been reported to help relieve tension and improve sleep. (I can personally attest to negative ionizers helping one sleep better. As a matter of fact, I used to turn my negative ionizer off before tests in college so I would not sleep too deeply.)

Reported Physiologic Effects of Negative Ions[1]

- Decreased respiratory rate (indicating relaxation)
- Decreased blood pressure (not a substitute for current medical therapy)
- Increased feelings of well-being
- Increased vital capacity
- Decreased blood inflammation (as measured by erythrocyte sedimentation rate)
- Increased wind pipe (trachea) cleaning by stimulating ciliary activity
- Increased resistance to infection by minimizing exposure to germs
- Suggested adjunctive therapy for chronic rhinitis, sinusitis, migraines, insomnia, wound and burn healing, asthma, hay fever, emphysema, bronchitis, and more

How Can You Generate Negative Ions in Your Home?

Every day, when we shower, we are generating our own negative ions in our home. Falling water is a great negative ion generator, and this likely explains the popularity of home and desktop fountains. Furthermore, fountains are known for creating a calm and gentle environment. Obviously, allowing a shower to run for the purpose of creating negative ions would not be practical. However, use of a home fountain or a commercial negative ion generator would.

---

[1] As reported in Felix Gad Sulman, *The Effect of Air Ionization, Electric Fields, Atmospherics and Other Electrical Phenomena on Man and Animal* (Phoenix, AZ: Thomas Books, 1980).

Late night infomercials have made ionizer machines more accessible, usually with three easy payments. However, when choosing a negative ion generator, it is important to choose a manufacturer that not only has a solid warranty, but also a machine that has scientific studies to back up its effectiveness. Unfortunately, there are only a few of these high-density negative ion generators available. It is important that one does research and investigates the various high-density negative ion generators on the market before making a choice. Units can cost anywhere from ninety-nine to over five hundred dollars. I personally do not recommend combination ionizer/HEPA filter models if the goal is to benefit from air ionization as these ionizers are usually more of a marketing ploy and are usually of low concentration.

Overall, evidence shows that negative ions and exposure to them have numerous health benefits. Likewise, positive ions have negative effects on our health. In this fast-paced society, where our mood can be affected by our external environments, it becomes apparent that restoring balance should be paramount.

Bibliography

Goel, N. "Bright Light, Negative Air Ions and Auditory Stimuli Produce Rapid Mood Changes in a Student Population: A Placebo-Controlled Study." *Psychology Medicine* 36 (2006): 1253–63.

Grinshpun, S. A., A. Adhikari, B. U. Lee, M. Trunov, G. Mainelis, M. Yermakov, and T. Reponen. "Indoor Air Pollution Control through Ionization." In *Air Pollution: Modeling, Monitoring and Management of Air Pollution*, edited by C. A. Brebbia, 689–704. Southampton, UK: WIT Press, 2004. Study used the Wein VI-2500 Negative Ionizer.

Sulman, Felix Gad. *The Effect of Air Ionization, Electric Fields, Atmospherics and Other Electrical Phenomena on Man and Animal.*

Terman, Michael, and Jiuan Su Terman. "Treatment of Seasonal Affective Disorder with a High Output Negative Ionizer." *Journal of Alternative and Complementary Medicine* 1 (1995): 87–92. Study used the Wein VI-2500 Negative Ionizer.

Wein Products. *VI-2500 High Density Negative Ionizer Product Manual.* Los Angeles: Wein Products, 2000.

About the Author

Eric Madrid, MD, is a board-certified family physician who practices in Temecula, California. In addition to seeing patients, he conducts product research and development for eHealthSupplies.com, an online retailer of negative ionizers, air purifiers, water filters, and other home health products. He personally uses the Wein VI-2500 High Density Negative Ionizer in his home and the Wein Auto-Mate 1250 auto ionizer in his car as they have numerous scientific studies to back their effectiveness. E-mail drmadrid@ehealthsupplies.com with any questions.

52

Acid Blockers and Malnutrition: Your Prescription for Osteoporosis, Visual Disturbances, Heart Disease, Dementia, and So Much More

Juliana Mazzeo, MS, CDN

Acid blockers or proton inhibitors range from the mild antacids, which neutralize stomach acid, to the powerful proton pump inhibitors that prevent stomach cells from producing stomach acid. We know them as the little purple pill, Nexium®, Pepcid®, Aciphex®, Protonix®, or as calcium supplements, for example, Tums®.[1]

What Is Acid Reflux?

Acid reflux is plain old indigestion. Because of the pricey medicines advertised to patients, acid indigestion was give a new name: acid reflux.

What Is the Cause of Acid Reflux?

There are many causes of indigestion, the main ones being poor diet, structural problems, obesity, hypochlorohydria (inadequate stomach acid), processed foods, consumption of vegetable oils, specifically foods fried in rancid vegetable oils that have been hydrogenated (cottonseed, soybean, corn, Crisco, and other vegetable shortenings), consumption of sugar, excess alcohol intake, smoking, loss of digestive enzymes, inadequate chewing, and large meals.

How Do These Factors Cause Hyperacidity?

Let's say we just consumed a huge processed meal such as French fries, an extra large soda, and two hot dogs on white buns. The arrival of this large bolus in the stomach contains foreign chemicals and preservatives that the stomach does not

---

[1] *H. pylori* and Barrett's syndrome will not be discussed in this article.

recognize. Let's add to that insufficient chewing (digestion of foods starts in the mouth by proper chewing and salivary enzymes) and insufficient enzymes (which anyone eating the standard American diet has), which will cause this mass to lie in the stomach, giving rise to fermentation and bacterial action. Fermentation expands and gives rise to gas and distension. As these gases rise, they are trapped in the esophagus, causing distension and mimicking chest pain. This pull and tension of the overloaded stomach insults the gastroesophageal valve to the point where it is pulled open. This overstretched valve allows stomach acid and its contents, along with the gases, up into the esophagus. The esophagus, unlike the stomach, does not contain acid-secreting cells, and thus it is very sensitive to this acid. This action causes a burning sensation in the esophagus, which can mimic signs of a heart attack.

Consequences and Side Effects Associated with Use of Acid Blockers

Long-term health complications related to acid blockers are many and very severe. They include nutrient deficiencies, increased risk of stomach cancer, low immune function, poor digestion of proteins, osteoporosis, heart disease, depression, pernicious anemia, poor eye sight, paralysis, severe neurological problems, and dementia, to name a few. We will briefly discuss some of the consequences of these medications.

Low Immunity

Immune cells are made of immunoglobulins, which are made up of protein from the food we eat. Failure of protein digestion results in inadequate protein to produce a strong immune system. A poor immune response can lead to any health problem, from a simple cold to cancer and anything in between.

Osteoporosis

Calcium plays a major role in bone remodeling and is dependent on the presence of stomach acid for absorption. Taking Tums for calcium supplementation is absurd. Tums is nothing but calcium carbonate (lime stone/dirt), chalk that neutralizes stomach acid. If the acid is neutralized, how is the calcium absorbed? It's not.

Arthritis

Poor protein absorption causes the body to steal protein from joint surfaces, with the end result being arthritis. Glycoaminoglycans found in cartilage are composed of proteins. Thus no protein digestion or absorption and no glycoaminoglycans results in arthritis.

Pernicious Anemia

This is a very prevalent condition in the elderly. Active B_{12} known as methylcobalamin is the key nutrient to treat dementia. B_{12} absorption is dependent on intrinsic factor. What is intrinsic factor? Intrinsic factor is a protein made by the parietal cells in the stomach, the same cells that secrete stomach acid and the same cells destroyed by acid blockers. B_{12} and several other vitamins are protein-dependent and protein bound. In other words, once this nutrient is ingested, it does not travel by itself in the body, but it is escorted by protein. So if you don't digest protein because it is putrefying in your gut because you are blocking stomach acid, how can B_{12} absorption take place? B_{12} deficiency is a very serious problem because it can mimic dementia. B_{12} deficiencies also cause irreversible paralysis and neurological disorders. An important point to remember is that B_{12} is only found in animal products. There is no such thing as B_{12} from plant foods. Those are B_{12} analogs, which only increase the need for more B_{12}.

Heart Disease

Dr. Kilmer McCully, a pathologist from Harvard, first identified homocysteine in 1969. Unfortunately, Dr. McCully got kicked out of Harvard for suggesting that homocysteine causes heart disease and not cholesterol. Dr. McCully lost all his funding, and it took him thirty years to get his name back. Just goes to show how politically motivated science is, and how in the interim people suffer from improper diagnosis and dangerous treatments. So what is homocysteine? It is a byproduct of methionine. Problems occur when there is a deficiency of B_{12}, B_6, folic acid, betaine, and stomach acid.

Folic acid, like B_{12}, is also protein bound and requires protein transport. In a stomach with no acid, folic acid suffers the same fate as B_{12}. Folic acid deficiencies cause neural tube defects,[2] heart disease, cancer, osteoporosis, and Alzheimer's disease due to elevated homocysteine levels.

Poor Vision

Lack of stomach acid inhibits absorption of protein. The eyes rely heavily on protein for proper function. Thus one of the first organs to respond to lack of protein are the eyes, and thus acid blockers are directly related to poor vision and blindness.

Acid Rebound

Continued use of acid blockers leads to a rebound effect of making excess acid when medication is discontinued.

---

[2] It took the Food and Drug Administration thirty years to admit this fact and to finally recommend supplements for women of childbearing age, at the expense of thousands of babies born with birth defects and spinal deformities, not to mention their immeasurable suffering and the suffering of their parents.

Side Effects of These Drugs

Owing to their cholinergic effects, some of these medications interfere with nerve function. This can lead to EKG abnormalities, potentially fatal ventricular tachycardia and ventricular fibrillation, nausea, constipation, anxiety, joint pain, hypertension, blood clots, impotence, headaches, and abdominal pain, to name a few.

Conclusion

A clean diet, free of processed foods and rancid fats, is a must. Eating fast and inadequate chewing must be addressed. Reducing excess weight will help. I always recommend digestive enzymes for anyone eating the typical diet. Vital enzymes are only found in raw or fermented foods. The average person rarely consumes fermented cultured vegetables or raw dairy, which enhance digestion and absorption of nutrients. So every time we eat, we use up precious enzymes to digest food. That is why constant eating/grazing and chewing gum are a waste of precious enzymes. Enzymes have thousands of functions, including searching for and destroying cancer cells that can only be detected by pancreatic enzymes.

Health starts in the digestive tract, and death starts in the colon. Our basis for eating food is for it to give us energy to support life. The inability to digest our food and assimilate its nutrients is a sure prescription for many diseases. These Western conditions are preventable. According to the National Academy of Science, 95 percent of all disease is caused by diet, the environment, and lifestyle. Only 5 percent can be attributed to our genes. In essence, we cannot blame our parents or grandparents for certain conditions. This is a way of shunning responsibility for our health. Our health is in our hands. Don't wait for the government or your doctor to take care of your health, and don't wait for HMOs to take care of you once you are sick. There is no day but today to take charge of your health and restore your vitality so that you may live a productive, healthy, and long life.

About the Author

Juliana Mazzeo, MS, CDN (http://www.nymedicalnutrition.com), holds a BA in psychology and an advanced MS in clinical nutrition. She has maintained both a private practice and worked in the field of cardiovascular medicine with prominent local physicians. She is a guest speaker and lectures in many settings. Juliana is published in the *American College of Nutrition*.

53

I Survived the Upcoming Bird Flu Pandemic . . . or Hoax . . . and You Can, Too!

AmyLee, Medicine Woman

I am headed to the Avian Influenza Preparedness Symposium—my fifth. As a state and federally licensed wildlife rehabilitator for the past quarter century, I come in daily contact with ailing birds of prey. During the recent reign of the West Nile virus, it rained hawks and owls! They dropped like the Centers for Disease Control predict we humans will be dropping when the avian bird flu hits our shores.

Bird flu news comes in waves. Communities have been gearing up for a pandemic by hosting so-called preparedness programs. Political warriors are trying to take prisoners: some politicians want us to line up like sheep to be inoculated, while others smell a scam and want to warn us of senators who own controlling interest in the vaccine company. Some predict a global pandemic taking unimaginable tolls, while others decry the whole thing to be a shameless hoax, an attempt to further line pharmaceutical giants' pockets with our hard-earned fear-money.

Many prognosticators are focused on the data predicting numbers of people who would become stricken. I find it equally important to examine who is likely to *survive* a pandemic, *why* they are the likely survivors, and *how* we can emulate their immunity and endurance. Herein is a starting place, with the understanding that having a strong immune system may prevent any and all viral or bacterial infections—and in the event one does contract the flu, or any other disease, a strong immune response provides the best chance for speedy and thorough recovery.

The first question for most: to inoculate or not? This is a question each and every autumn as we head into so-called flu season. While people should retain personal autonomy in such decisions, I offer this information in support of their choices for themselves:

- Vaccinations get a lot of high-profile press coverage, most of which is based on the flawed presumption that the shots are effective and that everybody should get one . . . if they can (enter the scarcity mentality, which fuels fear and drives people to the legalized drug peddlers).

- Long before the flu virus hits the human population, drug companies play a form of casino roulette, attempting to guess which strain of which virus will be the active one for the next year's upcoming flu season.
- Their guesses are then grown on human or animal tissue that has been harvested for scientific study. The *Physician's Desk Reference* lists some of the forms of tissue for vaccine cultures as coming from lung cells of aborted fetuses and monkey kidneys. Each and every time a virus is transferred from even one tissue to another, it mutates to varying degrees.
- Then that already mutated viral strain is attenuated. That means the virus is altered and weakened in the hope that it will not give the flu to the person receiving the inoculation.
- The body's immune system, however, now has a harder time identifying the new assailant via this inoculation because it has been disguised. Unable or slow to identify the altered virus, the body's own immune response is compromised, confused, and may react ineffectively to this virus—and *future* viral and bacterial assaults!
- To counteract your body's impaired immune response, impaired by the flu drug vaccine, the drug company then adds chemicals to boost the immune system's ability to recognize the virus. As listed in the *Physician's Desk Reference*, the boosting agents, also called "adjutants," for this year's flu shot include mercury (in the form of Thimersal), aluminum, formaldehyde, and ethylene glycol (one of the primary ingredients of radiator fluid).
  o Mercury is a known neurotoxin and is considered to be the third most harmful and lethal substance known to mankind. (Wherever the old-style mercury thermometers are still used, a haz-mat team must be called in to handle disposition of even a single broken thermometer.) There are strong indications, through scientific studies, that mercury exposure is a factor in the current surge of autism. Where are our children exposed to mercury most often? Vaccines, including those mandated by law prior to admission to the U.S. school system.
  o Aluminum is also a neurotoxin associated with developing Alzheimer's disease. Reliable sources claim that if you had five consecutive flu shots in any decade, your chances of getting Alzheimer's disease are ten times higher. This is, in part, due to mercury and aluminum buildup in the brain, which then suffers cognitive dysfunction.

o   Formaldehyde is a known carcinogenic used in embalming and forensic work.

o   Ethylene glycol, when it is in radiator fluid, is listed as lethal if ingested.

The side effects of flu vaccines mimic the flu itself, with the added stress of low-level chemotherapy. The trusting person accepts the vaccine. Shortly thereafter, he or she breaks out in a sweat. Why? The body is trying to purge itself of the toxic invaders. Numerous cases of vomiting and nausea accompany flu vaccines. Why? The body, in its wisdom and cellular memory, knows to defend itself from foreign, hostile invaders. The wise body wants those drugs out of its system, and *now*!

• When the body is attacked by a virus in the typical manner—via our noses or mouths, then into our throats—there is a gauntlet of protection activated by the body. At the first sign of a sore throat or headache or sneeze, the body mounts a counterassault on the invading virus. If one does not suppress the symptoms and instead boosts the immune system with nutrition, rest, and herbal supplements, the body also produces antibodies to that virus. Hence you won't catch that one again!

• However, when you ingest the vaccine, taking it directly into your digestive track in one swallow, bypassing the entire gauntlet of natural defenses, or when you get a shot directly into your body, through the skin barrier of protection, the front lines of defense are bypassed altogether. You now have the virus and its accompanying host of toxic chemicals more deeply in your body than if someone with the flu were to sneeze and cough on you repeatedly! You have just wheeled a Trojan Horse into your domain, with the hope that it will defend you against the same enemy it comes from and not, instead, turn on you and kill you.

• There are no accurate statistics for how many hundreds, or thousands, of people die each year from complications induced by flu shots.

• There is a growing body of scientific evidence indicating that various diseases are caused by or worsened by the use of vaccines.

Whether you opt for inoculations or another protocol, or adopt a combination, the key is to *make yourself too tough to kill!* Whether one is facing an oncoming epidemic, a lesser flu du jour, or their own genetic destiny, building the immune system hones the body's self-defense response by maintaining continual detoxification. Then you, too, can wear your own T-shirt announcing, "I survived the upcoming bird flu pandemic . . . or hoax. Ask me how!"

About the Author

Born to Haudensauenee (Iroquois) parents, AmyLee apprenticed under her respected Grandmother for twenty-one years. The last in her lineage of Medicine Women, AmyLee has devoted her life to the care and protection of Nature and Native futures. She founded http://www.HerNativeRoots.com as an interactive alternative health and healing Web site featuring her own line of Native American Indian Herbals. AmyLee has been an invited contributor to numerous publications, including the 2007 release of Dr. Judith Boice's book *Menopause with Science and Soul.* Her lecture circuits include universities, corporations, PBS and syndicated television, women's studies associations, and First Nations collectives. The article appearing in this book is an excerpt from "The Medicine Woman's Guidebook" at http://www.MedWom.com. AmyLee may be contacted by e-mailing Answers@HerNativeRoots.com.

54

Conscious Care of Your Nervous System Can Mean Life or Death

Dr. Kyle D. Morgan

As youngsters, we were taught strategies to prevent illness such as washing our hands, not sharing drinks with friends who have the flu, and wearing a coat when it's cold outside. These habits have served us well; however, they are not the whole story. They don't tell us why we get sick. In this chapter, we will look at the *real* reason we lose our health and how to regain it optimally.

Why We Get Sick

My experience as an integrative medicine family practice physician has taught me a lot about why we get sick. When we are conceived, most of us are as close to a Pure—unaltered and completely balanced—Self as we are ever going to be. All our experiences in life are then stored in our bodies, both positive and negative. The negative experiences, such as physical or emotional injuries, toxins, and bad feelings, thoughts, and relationships, accumulate like layers of an onion and move us further and further away from our original Pure Self. Our positive experiences move us back in toward our center, our Pure Self.

Furthermore, we have what I call a "sickness threshold" located some distance out from our center. When we cross this threshold, negative experience has built up in our system to the degree that a dysregulation happens at the level of our autonomic nervous system.

Our autonomic nervous system is responsible for what goes on inside our bodies. It has two components: the sympathetic, fight or flight nerves and the parasympathetic nerves that help us chill out. When we're driving and a car pulls out in front of us, it's the autonomic nervous system that causes an increase in our heart rate and sweat on our palms. The autonomic nervous system regulates all our body's internal functions. It is the accumulation of negative experience that causes an imbalance between the sympathetic and parasympathetic nerves. With enough negative buildup, we cross the sickness threshold and acquire a disease category—anything from headaches to diabetes to thyroid problems, or even cancer.

"But," you may ask, "what about my genes?" Our genes are not static. They change in response to our environment. Numerous medical studies done on identical twins have revealed that though these twins possess the same genes, their health issues can vary greatly. Just because your mom and her brother had diabetes and heart disease does not mean that you will. Why? Because it is your nervous system and the care you give it that determine what happens genetically in your body. Therefore, taking care of your nervous system is crucial to improving and maintaining your health.

How We Heal

Healing is quite straightforward. It requires that you simply reverse the process of moving further from your Pure Self and cross back over the sickness threshold to a place of balance. As we'll soon see, there are many ways to do this, but basically, it is a combination of cleansing your system of negative experiences and drawing in positive experiences that will assist you in regaining your health. Here are a few fundamental strategies to help you care for your nervous system.

Become Conscious

Develop an awareness of past and present negative experiences and consider their impact on your health. Consider traumas and negative relationships or emotions and thoughts that others have inflicted or that you harbor about yourself. Choose positive experiences and work toward discarding or working through negative experiences.

You'll find that different negative experiences impact you on different levels and with different intensities. Some you can shrug off. Others continue to cause emotional and physical reactions in your body. The ones that continue to affect you are the ones that need attention. But instead of dwelling on the negative experiences in life, find ways of moving through and beyond them. Transform the negative into positive by ridding your system of them. We'll soon see a variety of ways to remove negativity from your life. Ultimately, you'll attend to the negative experiences in life by making every moment a positive one.

Hold Intention for Health

Intention goes beyond positive thinking. Intention is a unifying power that we all possess that links us to the Source beyond ourselves. Through intention we can trust that our link creates an avenue to solving our problems—even health problems. So create an intention for optimal health—see yourself completely healthy, full of joy and happiness. Spend time actually visualizing and feeling how it feels to be well and freely functioning. Plant the seed of wellness through these feelings, and revisit them often. Believe that optimal health is easily attainable.

Dr. Wayne Dyer, in his book *The Power of Intention,* writes, "An exceptionally positive emotional response indicates that you are summoning the divine energy of intention and allowing that energy to flow to you in a non-resistant manner."[3] Feeling good about health invites it in. The combination of being conscious and holding intention attracts a positive, stress-free pattern that balances our nervous systems and encourages optimal health.

Maintain the Pursuit of Better Health

Focus on what is available rather than on what you don't have. Embrace the notion that no matter where you are on the path toward health, you can improve it. Set your intention on continually pursuing new means of seeking positive changes in your life. It's not about doing a one-time purge in your life, but about continually walking forward in new, positive ways, seeking greater healing.

A Means to an End

101 Great Ways to Improve Your Health is filled with many ideas that will balance your nervous system such as acupuncture, Reiki, Tai Chi, and other energy-based modalities. These are subtle methods that align your energy, creating a balanced flow in your system. With energy medicine, you may experience your nervous system effortlessly slipping into balance, providing you with a renewed template for your experience. An added bonus of the energy-based modalities is that they can be infused with a spiritual component, which often accelerates healing.

Since your body's structure and functions are interrelated, methods that realign your physical body support your nervous system in its balance. Chiropractic and osteopathic adjustments work to align the muscles and bones, which allows proper function and ease of motion. Additionally, because your nervous system is housed in your spine, spinal adjustments allow for optimal blood flow to your nerves, increasing the opportunity for balance. Other body work modalities, including massage therapy, cranial-sacral, and reflexology, also help balance your nervous system.

If you are harboring negativity from past or present experiences, you may want to find a practitioner who can assist you in releasing those negative experiences. There are a variety of practitioners, from traditional psychotherapists to hypnotists and practitioners of Eye Movement and Desensitization and Reprocessing, Emotional Freedom Techniques, and PSYCH-K, who are trained to help. If your negative experiences include trauma or abuse, you may want to seek a professional

---

[3] Wayne W. Dyer, *The Power of Intention* (Carlsbad, CA: Hay House, 2004, 180).

trained in somatic experiencing, a technique that effortlessly releases the trauma from your body.

Finally, seek some spiritual connection. It can be a traditional connection to God through a religious or spiritual community, or it can be through personal spiritual practice like meditation or yoga. Carrying a spiritual connection through your days intensifies your intention toward health and healing.

Truly caring for your health goes beyond the age-old adages of exercising, eating right, and washing your hands; continually and consciously caring for your nervous system keeps you pointed in the direction of optimal healing and health. The way you will do this is as unique as you are as an individual. Thankfully, you don't have to go it alone, and optimal health is yours for the asking.

About the Author

Kyle D. Morgan is a doctor of osteopathy in the Ann Arbor, Michigan, area and is board certified in family medicine. Her integrative medicine practice employs osteopathic manipulation, acupuncture, homeopathy, bioidentical hormone replacement, energetic medicine, and detoxification. For further information, visit http://www.Doctorkyle.com. In Dr. Morgan's upcoming book, *Brain Detox: The Healing Secret*, she details a self-administered technique, rooted in ancient healing practices, that transforms our mind-body well-being and physical health. Unlike hypnosis and other mind-body practices, this technique replaces negative subconscious thoughts permanently and immediately by entering positive mind-body statements into "whole-brain looping," a process which activates the right and left hemispheres, as well as the conscious and subconscious mind, simultaneously. This technique ultimately clears the subconscious of negative thoughts, thereby restoring balance to the autonomic nervous system. The healing of physical symptoms is then a natural outcome of a balance nervous system.

55

The Yeast-Fungus Link to Most Modern Diseases

Jane Remington

As a lifelong student and advocate of natural healing and alternative medicine, I have read, studied, and tried almost every diet ever published. But the diet I found to have by far the most power to *heal* is called the yeast-free diet.

This is the diet that cleans, renews, and restores the human immune system, thereby allowing the body to heal *itself*. It is simple, effective, and powerful. Everyone can use this tool to chart a path to wholeness during any stage of disease, or simply as a preventive measure.

I personally have witnessed amazing turnarounds from cancers, allergies, asthma, upper respiratory diseases, COPD, depression, Alzheimer's, mental disorders, fatigue, PMS, arthritis, and rheumatoid arthritis. The list also includes autoimmune diseases such as diabetes, fibromyalgia, colitis, Crohn's disease, hypothyroidism, multiple sclerosis, ALS, and lupus. Also helped have been weight problems, skin diseases, chemical sensitivities, chronic fatigue syndrome, headaches, digestive problems, addictions, ADD, ADHD, autism, cravings and mood swings, heart and circulatory disease, elevated blood pressure and cholesterol levels, ear, nose, and throat problems, hormone problems, and urinary tract and sinus infections! The list goes on and on.

It is becoming recognized that there is a fungal link to all these conditions!

My personal experience with the diet came years ago when I developed a systemic yeast infection (also called *Candida albicans*) after taking antibiotics. In my search for a natural solution, I found a wonderful and gifted naturopath and medical intuitive who correctly diagnosed a mild systemic yeast infection and gave me a copy of her yeast-free diet. In a few days, I started to feel healthy again. The fatigue, aching, brain fog, and digestive complaints began to fade, and in three weeks, I felt totally renewed. Truly a miracle.

After that, I started working with this naturopath as her appointment secretary and was privileged to work with her for the next nine years. During that time, I saw most of her patients use the yeast-free diet and gradually heal their immune systems and themselves—just as I had. In an effort to guide and help her patients stay on the yeast-free diet, I began to collect and modify recipes to be yeast-free. Eventually, the first edition of *The Yeast-Free Kitchen* was published, then a second edition, and two years ago, a third. I continue to see and hear about healings of all diseases (especially chronic ones) from people who use it.

What is yeast? How did we become so infested with its overgrowth? Yeasts are benign organisms that live normally in harmony with the friendly bacteria in our intestinal tracts. They were designed to stay there in proper balance with each other, each contributing to the digestion of food and providing population control for each other. They were also designed to wait until our death, at which time they are programmed to proliferate all over the body to break it down and decompose it, thereby keeping our planet clean. Think about what the earth would be like without them! We'd all be hopping over dinosaurs and everything that died since the beginning of time!

But two things happened. First was the introduction of antibiotics, steroids, hormones, and birth control pills at the end of World War II. Fungal infections were rare before their advent. Second came the meteoric rise and increased use of processed and highly sugared foods.

Because yeast loves to feast on these items, it was stimulated prematurely to break out of the normal confines of our digestive tracts and travel through the bloodstream and lymph channels (where they were never intended to go). It circulated throughout our bodies, establishing new colonies in our hearts, lungs, pancreas, kidneys, ovaries, prostates, brains, and doing what it was designed to do: *decompose.* Now, instead of waiting to go to work at our deaths, it is trying to decompose our bodies *while we are still living!*

What happens during this process? As huge colonies of yeast burrow through the colon walls and escape into the bloodstream (creating leaky gut syndrome), yeast turns vicious and morphs into its fungal stage—its most dangerous, aggressive stage. It then begins to colonize all over the body, eating tissue to remain alive. As it lives and dies, it gives off mycotoxins (yeast poisons) and an alcohol called ethanol, which circulate in the bloodstream. Then whole hosts of symptoms begin to emerge, from just feeling lousy, to allergies, to digestive complaints, to asthma.

As yeast continues to grow and the immune system becomes more compromised, more serious diseases develop. A terrible downward spiral begins as more symptoms appear and more antibiotics, steroids, hormones, birth control pills, and drugs are prescribed. As our internal terrain becomes more and more unbalanced and unhealthy, the opportunistic yeast/fungi go into a feeding frenzy and can cause death.

The only way to stop their progression is to *stop feeding them!* That is where the yeast-free diet comes in.

When you remove what feeds and stimulates yeast to grow, they literally starve to death. Eventually, balance is restored in the colon and digestive tract. When that happens, the immune system is relieved of its burden of supporting huge colonies of fungal overgrowths and can function as God intended. When the immune system is restored, health is restored.

What feeds or stimulates the growth of yeast? Unfortunately, the answer is found in many things that have become ingrained in our culture and lifestyles. Beside the already mentioned drugs, the top culprit is refined sugar. Americans are woofing down over one hundred pounds a year of the stuff—per person—in the twenty gallons of ice cream, three hundred cans of soft drinks, and fifty pounds of cakes and biscuits we consume each year. Yeast loves it first and foremost. The diet banishes it first and foremost.

Medical research is proving that cancer cells are notorious sugar junkies. The cells multiply frantically when glucose is present, and conversely, they self-destruct when glucose is removed.[1] Glucose elimination is the Achilles' heel of cancer cells and has always been the cornerstone of the yeast-free diet.

Next, our love affair with dairy products and caffeine has produced uncountable crops of yeasts and fungi to torment us, so the yeast-free diet excludes them. Alcohol (which is pure yeast mycotoxin) produces untold misery for us through bumper crops of yeast and so is forbidden. Mushrooms are fungi and feed the fungal population in the gut, and so these are also eliminated. Yeast breads must go. (Since yeast makes bread swell, it also makes *us* swell with yeast.) High-sugar bananas and grapes and all dried fruit are on the no-no list. Since vinegar is fermented and contains mold, it is not allowed. Beef, veal, and pork, since they contain steroids, hormones, mycotoxins, and antibiotics, are banned. All artificial sweeteners such as Aspartame, NutraSweet, Equal, and even Splenda should be banished from your diet forever. They are dangerous, and yeast loves them all.

But, don't panic—there is *plenty* of good food to eat. You will dine happily on chicken, turkey, lamb, wild game, eggs, beans, rice, potatoes, pastas (in moderation), veggies, salads, some grains, fruits, soups, seeds and nuts, tortillas, yeast-free breads, nuts and nut butters, honey and maple syrup (in moderation), popcorn, muffins, cornbread, biscuits, pancakes, tortilla chips, a few desserts and smoothies—all while the yeast beasts die.

One of the best features of this diet is that it isn't a life sentence, but a sentence to life. A minimum of twenty-one days on the program will kill a majority of yeast colonies—if you have a mild condition. You can then ease into a more varied diet.

---

[1] H. Shim and C. Dang, "A Unique Glucose-Dependent Apoptopic Pathway Induced by c-Myc," *Proceedings of the National Academy of Sciences of the United States of America* 95 (1998): 1511–16.

For most major diseases, three to six months is advised, and for major diseases of the brain, a year might be needed. Thereafter you should live closely to the diet, with occasional forays into no-no land.

I hope you will feel motivated to add the yeast-free diet to your game plan for health. It will require resolve, discipline, perseverance, and patience, but you are worth it. Your life and your health are worth it. Your future may depend on it. Now go get well. Godspeed!

<u>About the Author</u>

Jane Remington is a lifelong student of holistic medicine and natural healing therapies. After her introduction to the yeast-free diet and the subsequent restoration of her immune system, she continued to study and research the subject, eventually publishing *The Yeast-Free Kitchen*. It can be purchased from Amazon.com or from the publisher at http://www.Trafford.com. You can also visit Jane's Web site at http://www.JaneRemington.com.

56

Nine Truths Parents Can't Ignore

Rene Schooler

I have found myself standing at the bus stop listening to other moms talking about sickness, trips to the doctor, and which antibiotics their children are taking, and I realize that I don't fit in. I have not taken my five children to the doctor in three years. I try to talk about nutrition, and I feel alienated. Every minute of every day, we breathe in pollutants, eat chemically engineered foods, drink liquid toxins, and then go to the doctor for a chemical injection (antibiotics) that shorten the life span of a common flu or cold. Because of these toxins, our children face chronic illness such as allergies, digestive ailments, asthma, cancers, and learning and behavioral difficulties. As parents, we have control over what goes into our children's bodies, and below I will cover nine major areas of concern and what we can do to keep our kids healthy.

Are Our Children Getting Fat?

The Centers for Disease Control have reported that the percentage of children under twelve years of age who are overweight or obese has doubled in the last twenty years, and among our teenagers, it has tripled. An overweight child is a perfect breeding ground for diabetes, heart disease, high cholesterol, and blood pressure. How do we save our children from this? Get rid of soda consumption completely, limit your fast food and processed foods, and incorporate fresh fruits and vegetables and lots of water.

A Sweet Tooth!

Sugar steals our children's lives, and according to U.S. Department of Agriculture data of 1999, we consume over 150 pounds per person per year. We find ourselves and our children addicted to this sweet drug available in so many forms, most of which are not natural and cause damage to the body, one of the worst forms being high fructose corn syrup (HFCS). Natural fructose can be found in most fruits and vegetables. Natural fructose can be easily digested, unlike HFCS, which causes great stress on the body, depleting mineral stores and causing your child's blood levels to roller coaster. HFCS is also highly addictive, the reason it is added to so many foods and drinks. The best way to avoid this drug is to read labels, buy organic evaporated cane juice in place of sugar, and use honey.

Why Use Artificial Sweeteners?

There is a growing amount of negative support showing damage that man-made chemical-based sweeteners (aspartame, Splenda, acesulfame k) have on the body. The problem with these are simple: they are chemical based. They react in the body as an enemy, causing havoc. When you buy products with these fake sugars, you are in fact giving your child aspartic acid (linked to causing lesions and tumors in the brain), phenylalanine, and methanol (which converts to formaldehyde in the retina of the eye), causing numerous health issues. There are Web sites to help you cleanse the toxic effects of these sweeteners.[1] Your best sweetener choices are natural and unrefined.

Milk—Does It Really Do a Body Good?

We have been taught that milk is a great source of vitamins and calcium. However, what we have not been told is that due to pasteurization (a heating process that eliminates all the enzymes), our bodies cannot metabolize it, which means it is useless to our bodies. But it prevents osteoporosis? Then why is the United States, with its high level of milk intake, ranking among the top of the charts with osteoporosis? This is shown in a few studies such as the Beijing Osteoporosis project of 1996 and in the World Health Organization Program on Aging in 1999. In August 2000, *Discover Magazine* had an article titled "Worrying About Milk," where these very threats and others were made against milk consumption. The National Osteoporosis Foundation states that 55 percent of people over the age of fifty are in danger of developing this disease.
It is my personal opinion that if you are going to serve milk to your child, try organic raw milk, not the pasteurized, man-made version.

What's in the Water You Drink?

Water is the life force that keeps our bodies moving. It hydrates us like no other liquid. Sports drinks and sodas, loaded with high fructose corn syrup, do the direct

---

[1] See, e.g., http://www.holisticmed.com/aspartame/detox.html.

opposite, despite what the advertisements say. Your body needs lots every day just to flush out toxins and keep the brain functioning properly. But if your water comes from a municipal source, you more than likely need to check into purifying it. Water coming out of your tap is not likely fit for drinking and cooking. Find out what really is in your water. What's the lead content? How many chemicals are being added such as fluoride and chlorine? Check for bacterias and heavy metals.

More Additives, Please!

The more processed our diets get with factory-made foods, the more chemical additives become part of our lives. These additives are mostly all the words on the label that we cannot pronounce. But other additives are sugar and salt. The ones to avoid are aspartame, Splenda, acesulfame k, saccharine (now found in most toothpastes), sodium nitrite (found in most packaged meats and linked to pancreatic cancer), and all artificial colorings, especially red dye 40. These are all cancer-causing chemicals according to the National Institutes of Health, the Centers for Disease Control and Prevention, and many articles published worldwide such as in the *New York Times* and *The Pulse*.

Why Focus on Fiber?

Studies show that as a culture, we do not eat enough fiber. The average American adult gets between ten and fifteen grams a day, according to the American Heart Association. This is less than half the fiber intake we need, as stated by the American Dietetic Association. Fiber is responsible for cleaning out our intestinal linings and our colons. By doing this, fiber also helps in the absorption of important nutrients that otherwise would just pass through our bodies unused. In recent studies, it has been shown that fiber is also a benefit in reducing cancers and fighting fatty buildup in the bloodstream. In other words, fiber keeps the arteries clean. The best places to get fiber are from vegetables, fruits, and whole grains. I suggest not settling for less than eight grams of fiber in a serving of cereal or three grams in a slice of bread. The closer to thirty-five grams of fiber a day you get as an adult, the better for your entire body's health. A simple rule for children's fiber intake is the age-plus-five rule (take the child's age and add five grams of fiber to it). This will give you a good starting point, as shown in the *Journal of the American Dietetic* in 1998.[2]

---

[2] J. S. Hampl, N. M. Betts, and B. A. Benes, "The 'Age+5' Rule: Comparisons of Dietary Fiber Intake Among 4- to 10-Year-Old Children," *Journal of the American Dietetic Association* 98 (1998): 1418–23.

That's Too Salty!

Even though sodium is essential for maintaining bodily fluids and proper nerve function, as a whole, we consume too much. How much is too much? The recommended daily amount is 1.25 teaspoons of salt. Most sodium comes from the seasoning and ingredients of the foods we eat such as MSG, soy sauce, and mayonnaise. Other high-sodium contributors are canned soups, lunch meats, fast foods, and chips. Sodium is mainly responsible for raising blood pressure to unhealthy levels.

Is It a Real Cure?

It has been shown that if antibiotics are used too much, our bodies actually become immune to their positive effects, and at that point, if they are ever needed, the body will not react to them. Our children are being overdosed with one antibiotic after another. Taking our kids to the doctor every time they cough, sneeze, or have an ear or stomachache results in the abuse of antibiotics. Another thing to realize is that antibiotics are a primary reason for yeast overgrowth in the mucous membranes, causing numerous health problems. Some of these are thrush, vaginal yeast infections, dandruff, athlete's foot, acne, muscle pain, fatigue, digestive disorders, and respiratory problems. So lay off the antibiotics, and let your child work through his everyday cold with natural remedies. Instead of running to the doctor, look at your local health food store for immunity boosters. Try garlic oil in warm olive oil to treat an ear infection instead of antibiotic drops.

Conclusion

As children, we ate what our parents fed us. We were told that milk builds strong bones, when in fact exercise does more for bone density than calcium from milk.[3] This is just one mistruth that has been passed on through the generations. As a concerned parent, I keep coming back to what matters most: healthy children. Our children are our future, and paying attention to these nine truths can save your child from a life full of health complications and ensure them a vibrant, healthy future—a future where they have learned to make nutritional choices.

---

[3] Tom Lloyd, Vernon M. Chinchilli, Nan Johnson-Rollings, Kessey Kieselhorst, Douglas F. Eggli, and Robert Marcus, "Adult Female Hip Bone Density Reflects Teenage Sports-Exercise Patterns but Not Teenage Calcium Intake," *Pediatrics* 106 (2000): 40–44.

About the Author

Rene wanted to learn Japanese and become a corporate attorney living in Japan. She was never going to have children. She fell in love with Paul, got married at eighteen, and is today the mother of five beautiful children: Samantha, Rebekah, Zachariah, Juliana, and Levi. Rene finds her purpose in raising healthy children in a highly processed country and is in the process of writing a book on just how to do that titled *Elephant in the Kitchen*. Rene and her family live in the Salt Lake City area. Aside from trying to cook with fresh, natural products, she supplements through a company that she belongs to called ITV Ventures (http://www.itvventures.com/goodinbadout. The book Web site is http://www.elephantinthekitchen.com. She can be reached at goodinbadout@yahoo.com.

57

Are You a Walking Time Bomb?

Stephen Sinatra, MD, FACC, FACN, CNS

Some of you may have read a recent front-page article in *The Wall Street Journal*. It was titled "Medical Ignorance Contributes to Toll from Aortic Illness." The reporters discussed how all too often, the medical community is incompetent when it comes to diagnosing aortic aneurysms; not enough physicians and care providers are sufficiently knowledgeable about this precarious problem. Countless autopsies, performed on individuals whose sudden deaths occurred after a bout of chest pain, have revealed that an aortic aneurysm was the true culprit, and not a heart attack.

This was the case with someone I loved deeply. I was devastated and grief stricken when I failed to resuscitate my own father on the floor of my childhood bedroom. Can you imagine, with all my training, to lose one of the people to whom I owed my life and education? An autopsy revealed that no one could have saved my dad that day; his aorta had ripped open suddenly. He was seventy-six years young. He was so bright and vital, we'd never dreamed anything like this could be wrong. But there he was. He denied any chest pain. He had an abrupt onset of weakness, dizziness, and leg paralysis. How many times have I asked myself if there were any earlier, telltale signs that his physicians, and I, may have missed? Though I've written of this event and warning signs before, it's a subject I'd like to revisit and update.[1]

The recent unexpected loss of actor John Ritter, only fifty-four years old, was the alarm clock that reawakened my own feelings of loss and made me aware of just how many people continue to walk around with undiagnosed aneurysms, just like my dad. You may have caught some of the media interviews that followed Ritter's

---

[1] Symptoms of TAA include constant, nagging, or intermittent pain in the neck, chest, or upper back; blood in the mucus; persistent coughing, or a "goose cough" with a brassy quality; and difficulty swallowing and hoarseness. Symptoms of abdominal aortic aneurysm include persistent or intermittent pain in the lower abdomen and lower back and a throbbing sensation in the abdomen, which sometimes can be seen or felt as a throbbing lump, and may be accompanied by weight loss or loss of appetite.

death, during which doctors described dissection (a weakened portion of the aorta that begins to tear) as rare and undetectable. Hearing such comments was, quite frankly, unsettling for someone like me. In my professional life as an interventional cardiovascular specialist (that's one who does invasive procedures), I've seen my fair share of thoracic aortic aneurysms in all age groups. Some are slow tears, when there is time for intervention if the correct diagnosis is made. Blood leaks between layers of the arterial wall but can be repaired. But sometimes, the tear happens too quickly and forcefully for it to be repaired.

My first experience with this catastrophic situation was with a twenty-five-year-old fellow whose aortic wall tore apart during a free-fall parachute jump. Although emergency surgery saved this young man, he later went on to die of a second dissection when he was only in his mid-thirties. When this happened, twenty-five years ago, we lacked the technology or knowledge to predict it.

I recall with deep sadness another case. A fifteen-year-old girl had passed out while she was working at a nursing home. She was at the top of her school class, bright, alert, and engaging. I thanked God that day that I was able to diagnose her symptoms very quickly in our community hospital's emergency room. I had high hopes that she would be fine if we acted fast. She was resting comfortably when I called the closest heart surgery hospital to mobilize the open heart team. When the chief of cardiac surgery challenged my diagnosis, I was firm and confident and stood my ground. His team scrambled to the operating room as the ambulance pulled in to transport her there. But we lost our race against time. As I explained what was happening to her and her parents that day, she smiled in acceptance. She looked so peaceful. We would learn afterward that her aorta had clotted itself and stabilized at that point. A moment later, she sat up. Looking startled, she exclaimed, "Oh!" and died in my arms as a secondary tear ruptured her entire aorta. It will always be a painful memory.

Some of you may recall another case from my book *Heartbreak and Heart Disease.* I shared the story of an older gentleman in a similar emergency situation. He was sixty-four years old and had just experienced an episode of intense emotional distress. His aorta began to dissect during a fit of rage. By the time I met him in the emergency room, he was hanging onto life by a thread. He was in cardiogenic shock, with profoundly low blood pressure and respiratory depression. Fortunately for him and his family, a quick diagnosis and early surgical intervention ended happily.

So you must be asking yourself by now, how common are thoracic aortic aneurysms (TAAs)? As I mentioned, a large number of TAAs are not apparent until an autopsy is performed. TAAs are also found in people who have died of other causes, lurking like a potential time bomb, just ticking away until it explodes.

Epidemiology and Genetics of Thoracic Aortic Aneurysms

It's imperative that you understand how common TAA can be and the hereditary risks involved so you can seek evaluation if you, like me, are at risk. You see, it's actually been estimated that aortic aneurysm is the thirteenth most common cause of death in the United States. Every year, there are approximately 5.9 cases of TAA for every 100,000 people, and the average age at diagnosis is fifty-nine to sixty-nine.

Cases of thoracic aortic dissection in young people, like the two I have shared with you, are usually due to a genetic vulnerability. Individuals with a predisposition to TAA develop premature necrosis, or cell death, of the medial (middle) layer of their aorta. In this condition, a loss of elastic fibers and smooth muscle cells leads to the accelerated aging of the aorta, rendering the artery weak and vulnerable to dissection.

We also know that there is an association between aortic aneurysms and two uncommon medical disorders: Marfan's and Turner syndromes. Even with this knowledge, patients who have these conditions still have undetected and undiagnosed TAAs. So if you have one of these conditions, have yourself checked for TAA risk.

More commonly, we see a phenomenon known as familial, nonsyndromic TAA in about 19 percent of patients who have it. In other words, it runs in their families but is not associated with another medical syndrome. These patients are younger at the time of diagnosis (mean age 56.8 years) than those with sporadic TAA (mean age 64.3 years).

In sporadic TAA, some factor has provoked an episode of aortic dissection, such as extremely high blood pressure—this may have been the cause for the sixty-four-year-old enraged gentleman I mentioned. Preexisting high blood pressure is a contributing factor that's been observed in 73 percent of cases of familial nonsyndromic TAAs and 75 percent of sporadic cases.

Early Detection Is a Must If You're at Risk

Remember, awareness can be curative for many conditions, and TAA is one of them. My dad's brother, my dear uncle Ben, also endured the pain of a growing aneurysm for many years before he died last year of unrelated causes. But he knew he had one, and he monitored it closely. With our strong family history, I've advised all my siblings and cousins that they be checked and that we check our kids and grandkids.

For those of you with a family history of aortic aneurysm, it is absolutely mandatory that your children, and even grandchildren, be assessed for thoracic aortic aneurysm. This is where knowing your family history can be life saving.

Remember, *The Wall Street Journal* article said it all. Most doctors won't think of ruptured aortic aneurysm if you find yourself in the emergency room, so you may have to be the one to raise the red flag. People with TAA can look perfectly fine when their arterial blood gas is checked. The electrocardiogram won't show any changes either, leaving physicians perplexed as to why there is so much pain. Many thoracic aneurysms won't even show up on a routine chest X ray, and rarely, folks like my dad won't have any chest pain at all. The leg paralysis, dizziness, and weakness, like my dad had, are also atypical symptoms.

A high-resolution computed tomography (CT) scan will, however, provide a clear image of the aortic pathology in TAA. I'm going to repeat my own CT scan soon. Magnetic resonance imaging (MRI) is also frequently used, particularly for people who have poor kidney function that contraindicates the injection of contrast material. MRI is especially useful for complex cases, where imaging from multiple angles is key to diagnosis. In this regard, MRI can give you vital information. If the definition of branch vessel anatomy is required, some physicians will also order a magnetic resonance angiography. Angiography is performed to evaluate the need for surgery.

Other simple diagnostic tools that can detect a large number of dissections—and even dilatation of aortic root—are the aortic ultrasound and the transesophageal echocardiography, where the definitive anatomy of the aortic valve and ascending aorta can be displayed. Again, the problem with aortic dissection is that most physicians don't recognize it or even think about it. Once the aorta tears, death can happen within two hours, if not sooner. So the importance of a correct diagnosis cannot be overstated.

Think of a Zebra

Thirty years ago, my interns nicknamed me "Zebra." Why? I had an expression that went like this: "When you hear the hoof beats, what do you think of? The common answer is horses. But a good diagnostician must always think of zebras," the less obvious, unexpected condition. TAA is a zebra diagnosis.

So I advise you to get your own doctor thinking about zebras. If you have any family history of TAA, or any undiagnosed chest pain, plant the seed for your concern about an aortic aneurysm with your MD, PA, or nurse practitioner. Acute dissection is a situation that you do *not* want to find yourself facing. If they won't cooperate, or reject the idea, stand firm and insist on testing.

And What If You Know You Have an Aortic Aneurysm?

If you're one of the unfortunate individuals who are diagnosed with an aortic aneurysm, it's important to understand the natural history of thoracic aortic aneurysms and how it applies to you. First of all, thoracic abdominal aneurysms grow an average of about 0.1 cm a year. So have checkups and diagnostic evaluations at least annually, and more often should your symptoms change. And you'll also want to know at what point surgery is indicated and the risks of that surgery compared to the risk of not having it. In my uncle's case, his risk of dying during surgery was excessively high, and so he endured the discomfort of a growing aneurysm that limited his lifestyle rather than run that risk. Let's look at research that can help sway your decision.[2]

The Yale Experience

Here in my home state of Connecticut, a ten-year study was conducted at Yale University, where both my wife and I did some training. Yale developed a large database of patients with thoracic aneurysms and dissections. Specialized statistical methods were applied to an accumulated population of 1,600 people with TAA dissection and included 3,000 serial imaging studies and 3,000 patient years of follow-up. It is really good data.

The major cutoff points for natural complications of aortic aneurysm (rupture or dissection) were found to be 6 cm for the ascending aorta (which comes right out of the heart) and 7 cm for the descending one (the portion that leads through the diaphragm and into the abdomen). Yearly event rates suggest that anyone whose thoracic aorta reaches a 6-cm maximal diameter faces significant risks for a devastating cardiac event: a 3.6 percent rupture rate; a 3.7 percent dissect rate; and a 10.8 percent mortality rate.

Their reported surgical risk of death from aortic surgery of thoracic aneurysms was 2.5 percent for the ascending aorta and the aortic arch and 8 percent for the descending and abdominal aorta. In fact, the Yale report of a 2.5 percent for the ascending aorta is a conservative estimate. Most centers predict a 5 to 10 percent mortality rate for this population. Interestingly, genetic analysis in the Yale study revealed that 21 percent of patients with TAA have a first-family member with some arterial aneurysm. This is similar to previous data reporting a 19 percent occurrence rate.

---

[2] Some excellent cardiac centers for TAA repair in the United States follow: (1) Cleveland Clinic Foundation, 9500 Euclid Avenue, Cleveland, OH 44195, (216) 444-2200; (2) Mayo Clinic, 200 First Street SW, Rochester, MN 55905, (507) 284-2511; (3) Massachusetts General Hospital, 55 Fruit Street, Boston, MA 02114, (617) 726-2000; (4) Brigham and Women's Hospital, 75 Francis Street, Boston, MA 02115, (617) 732-5500 or, toll-free, (800) 294-9999; (5) Duke University Medical Center, Erwin Road, Durham, NC 27710, (919) 684-8111; and (6) the Johns Hopkins Hospital, 600 North Wolfe Street, Baltimore, MD 21287, (410) 955-5000.

My Surgical Guidelines

What does this all mean to you? On the basis of these findings, I set guidelines for my own surgical recommendations. In asymptomatic people, I suggest surgery only if your thoracic aneurysm is 5.5 cm or greater or your abdominal aorta measures 6.5 cm or more. If you are symptomatic with chest pain, or have a tear or dissection, then you must be operated on, regardless of the size of your aneurysm. Remember, anyone who has an aortic aneurysm, but doesn't know it, is at risk for sudden cardiac death. You don't want that to be the first sign that you have a problem. This large Yale trial is reaffirmation that anyone with a family history be evaluated.

I immediately thought of this disorder when my sister experienced severe chest pain, but imaging studies of her aorta showed that she did not have an aortic aneurysm. Who knows if the tragic and unexpected death of John Ritter as well as many others might have been prevented with early diagnosis and intervention? One thing is quite reassuring: we know that nonemergency surgical repair of aneurysms has clearly had a positive impact on the natural history of the disease.

The Wall Street Journal said it all. Many physicians may not consider this diagnosis, so your awareness of it can be life saving. We now have the science to easily diagnose TAA with simple, noninvasive imaging techniques, so we can treat it successfully.

Most importantly, if you do uncover this life-threatening condition in yourself or a loved one, please be vigilant about it. Wear a Medic Alert bracelet. If yours is a family history of thoracic aortic aneurysm—or even a sudden death for which a cause was not clearly defined at autopsy—you must be proactive and get evaluated. Should you recognize the symptoms, take yourself or any of your family members to an emergency room for a medical assessment, and remember to tell them about zebras.

Bibliography

Coady, M. A., R. R. Davies, M. Roberts, L. J. Goldstein, M. J. Rogalski, J. A. Rizzo, G. L. Hammond, G. S. Kopf, and J. A. Elefteriades, "Familial Patterns of Thoracic Aortic Aneurysms," *Archives of Surgery* 134 (1999): 361–67.

Coady, M. A., J. A. Rizzo, L. J. Goldstein, and J. A. Elefteriades, "Natural History, Pathogenesis, and Etiology of Thoracic Aortic Aneurysms and Dissections," *Cardiology Clinics* 17 (1999): 615–35.

Coady, M. A., J. A. Rizzo, G. L. Hammond, G. S. Kopf, and J. A. Elefteriades, "Surgical Intervention Criteria for Thoracic Aortic Aneurysms: A Study of Growth Rates and Complications," *Annals of Thoracic Surgery* 67 (1999): 1922–26.

Elefteriades, J. A., "Natural History of Thoracic Aortic Aneurysms: Indications for Surgery, and Surgical versus Non-surgical Risks," *Annals of Thoracic Surgery* 74 (2002): S1877–80.

About the Author

Over twenty-five years ago, Stephen Sinatra, MD, FACC, FACN, CNS, realized that his patients' best interests were served by a broader perspective, encompassing both a wide array of traditional medical expertise and a serious, objective study of alternative and complementary medicine. Dr. Sinatra's mission is to integrate conventional medical treatments with the best complementary nutritional, antiaging, and psychological therapies that help heal the heart. Board certified in internal medicine, cardiology, nutrition, and antiaging medicine, Dr. Sinatra is not a slave to conventional or alternative medicine. Instead, he uses his vast medical training to identify the best cures, period. For more information, visit http://www.DrSinatra.com.

PART SIX

Holistic Health

Oh, the powers of nature!
She knows what we need...

- Benvenuto Cellini

58

The Root Cause of All Cancer

Leonard Coldwell, NMD, PhD

My childhood memories are filled with feelings of desperation as I listened to my mother's screams, emergency doctors coming and going from our house. In fact, every day, the first thing I did when I came home from school was run to my mother's room to check that she was still alive. She had been diagnosed with liver cancer in the terminal stage and told that there was no hope. She was given two years maximum to live. I was petrified. My fear fueled my ambition to find a cure for my mother's cancer. And so began the driving force that led me to become one of the leading experts on cancer and stress-related illness. It took years of trial and error, studying every kind of therapy imaginable, but in the end I cured my mother, who is alive and well thirty-six years later. Unfortunately, in the meantime, I watched my beloved grandmother, father, and seven siblings of my mother die from cancer or some other so-called incurable disease.

I started my quest to find the answer to cancer by studying every successful healing technique worldwide, and I learned about all the alternative or natural forms of healing available. I discovered why people got cancer and how they got healthy after they had it, and why others just died. And so I became one of the leading experts for cancer in Europe long before I graduated from medical/naturopathic medical school.

I then specialized as a general physician in cancer with a particular emphasis on cancer patients who had been deemed incurable by their physicians. Working with these people, I learned that there is always hope, there is always a way, and there will always be patients that will regain their health, no matter what the diagnosis or obstacles. Most importantly, I learned that I was not the healer, I was only the conduit for my patient to pass on the knowledge and tools and training he or she needed to reactivate the immune system and stimulate self-healing powers so that the patient could achieve optimum health.

The bottom line, and the most important lesson I learned from working with over 35,000 patients with so-called incurable diseases, is that nobody can cure anybody; only the sick can cure themselves.

There is no magic bullet or fountain of youth, nor are there any shortcuts to lifelong health and happiness. We must take charge of our health. We are responsible for our past decisions, actions, or lack of action. Most of us are challenged looking at the health situation we created, but it is never too late. It is only important to act now, before it gets tougher.

We are not failures because we are sick, unfit, or overweight. We just learned to use the powers of our brains, bodies, and immune systems in the wrong way. All too often, we are brainwashed by the media or misled by people to believe or do the wrong thing. But the good news is that there is always hope. From now on, you just need to act smarter. Make the decision to take charge of your life, happiness, and health right now! Make the commitment to live up to your potential and create the health you deserve.

The Dr. Coldwell System

In my opinion, all illness comes from lack of energy, and the greatest energy drainer is mental and emotional stress, which I believe to be the root cause of all illness. Stress is one of the major elements that can erode energy to such a large and permanent extent that the immune system loses all possibility of functioning at an optimum level.

I am referring to the mental and emotional stress that is caused by continuous and/or long-term compromises against yourself. These vary from person to person, but some examples include living in unbearable relationships and marriages, doing jobs you hate or hating your boss, or experiencing problems with family, all of which lead to you compromising your sense of self. Emotional and mental stress comes from living with feelings of constant fear, doubt, hopelessness, lack of self-esteem, worry, and, most of all, always compromising your inner feelings, instincts, and personal needs.

The solution is to start by defining what it is in your life that keeps you from feeling happy. Can you answer the question of why you don't respect yourself enough? Or love yourself? Now identify what needs to change or happen in your life to make you feel good about yourself and your personal environment. What is it that you don't want to do, accept, or take anymore from yourself, your spouse, your children, your boss, or your coworkers? Is there someone in your life that makes you feel badly that needs to go? What are your wildest dreams and goals? Looking at your life, what is it that always takes away your energy, and where do you compromise your personal needs and feelings? Identify everything in your life that keeps you from being your true self, and start working on the development of the true you! This is the first and most important step toward achieving optimum health and happiness. And remember that happiness and hope are the most powerful healers and energy creators in your life. Pay attention to your instincts, listen to your inner voice, and start loving and respecting yourself so that you behave according to your true personality.

If you do not live your life according to your needs, you will get or stay stressed, which will reduce your energy and eventually produce an illness. You are the only one who can change your life and improve your health. So start today by defining, creating, and living your life the way you believe is right and good for you.

Create your own self-healing system:

1. Identify life situations that drain you, make you feel uncomfortable, and make you feel stressed, weak, or unhappy, and find a way to change these negative situations.
2. Breath effectively into your stomach below your belly bottom. Inhale four seconds through your nose, and exhale eleven seconds through your mouth ten times in a row and at least three times a day. Also, inhale four seconds, hold your breath for sixteen seconds, and exhale eight minutes though your mouth ten times in a row at least three times a day.
3. Create your own destressing program. Escape twice a day for ten to fifteen minutes mentally to a place in nature where you feel free safe and comfortable. Break the daily stress cycle because stress is not the problem; rather, it is ongoing stress that is causing the damage.
4. Get detoxified twice a year with a good colon, liver, kidney, heavy metal, and chemical cleanse, and use essiac capsules or tea once a year if you don't feel right.
5. Drink a gallon of water a day, and have half a teaspoon of sea salt with it. Also, take good coral calcium.
6. Do aerobic exercise for at least twenty minutes three times a week (just walking is fine).
7. Eat as many fresh vegetables and fruits as possible, and get a juicer—and use it.

In love and respect,

Dr. Leonard Coldwell

About the Author

Dr. Leonard Coldwell, NMD, PhD, is considered Europe's leading expert on cancer, stress-related illness, and educational self-help and self-healing systems. He is the author of eight best-selling books and of the most sought after newsletter for self-help education in Europe, and he is also a consultant, trainer, and speaker for some of the largest companies in Europe. The Dr. Coldwell system has produced unmatched results in transforming people's lives and health. He is the founder of the Foundation for Drug and Crime Free Schools and Health for Children. Dr. Coldwell's best-selling books will be available in English in the fall of 2007. His Web site is http://www.drcoldwellsystems.com, and his e-mail address is dr.leonardcoldwell@gmail.com.

59

Your Strata Zone

Courtney Findlay

Your skin is your largest organ and a part of your immune system, containing a variety of nerve endings, sensitive to your environment, providing an excellent barrier against viruses and pathogens, regulating body temperature (by dilating blood vessels for heat loss or constricting blood vessels to retain heat), providing insulation and waterproofing, controlling fluid loss, storing and synthesizing vitamin D, releasing toxins, reversing UV damage with DNA enzymes, absorbing small amounts of oxygen, and allowing the easy administration of time-release medications. Made up of multiple layers (or stratas) protecting underlying muscles and organs, your skin has the largest surface area of all organs as well as weighing more than any other, contributing to about 15 percent of your body weight.

This epidermal layer is also capable of letting you know if your bodily systems are unbalanced through symptoms such as flushing, itching, rashes, dermatitis, psoriasis, and eczema. Some skin disorders are caused by an unknown origin, but even more are caused by allergic reactions. A skin disorder is already telling you that something somewhere is misbalanced, and controlling the symptoms by using yet more possible allergens in skin care products or treatments actually adds to the toxic overload that your immune systems is already trying to keep in check.

Widely prescribed for skin conditions and their uncomfortable effects are the unpleasant pharmaceutical options that include steroid creams and medications, tar shampoos, topical antibiotics, hormones, systemic antibiotics, and corticosteroids, among other numerous unnatural remedies that always include side effects. Any ongoing treatment of a skin condition could easily cost you hundreds of thousands of dollars in prescriptions and doctor and hospital visits! I know that some of these treatments appear to be working by controlling the symptoms, but the actual source of the inflammation is merely camouflaged, waiting patiently to make a rapid reappearance. A must-try-first remedy is one I have personally seen work over and over again to relieve skin conditions, and it is simply a bar of natural soap.

Keeping your skin clean is part of keeping yourself healthy. Your skin can perform its many functions when its dead cells, dirt, and sweat are routinely cleansed away. Millions of micro-organisms live on your skin, keeping it in balance for optimum protection.

The amount of chemical exposure from our environment is constant. Twenty-four hours of every day, we are bombarded with chemicals, some that are practically impossible to avoid, some that are avoidable but may require some lifestyle changes, and some that we invite into our homes and into our bodies day after day.

Two products that most of us use every day are soaps and lotions. And because we want to provide the healthiest best for our families, we often look for words such as *organic, pure, allergy tested,* and *fragrance-free.* Sadly, none of these words actually ensures that the product is just that. Company marketing executives phrase their advertising copy extremely carefully to mislead you into believing that their merchandise will improve your life. There are no Food and Drug Administration regulations in place to protect you from this.

Initially, soap started with the simplest natural ingredients of oils, water, and lye. With time and accurate measuring, this formulation evolved to allow for a gentle and effective cleanser. Truly natural soap will contain vegetable oils (coconut, olive, canola, palm), nonchlorinated, untreated spring water, and sodium hydroxide (an electrolysed salt). This method creates naturally occurring glycerine, which is moisturizing to the skin. For a scented or extra moisturizing soap bar, look for additions such as therapeutic essential oils (naturally from plants) or butters such as cocoa or shea for extra replenishing.

But the soap bars you buy today are not actually soap—they are a detergent, and detergents are often manufactured with animal fats and/or mineral oil, a petroleum product derived from crude oil. From this "soap," the glycerine is removed and sold separately, sometimes as the base for melt and pour soap. Store-bought brand name soap can be drying and can contain numerous chemicals. A well-known, brand name body wash product with the words *moisturizing, naturals, aloe vera,* and *vitamin E* on its label does contain aloe vera and vitamin E, but it also contains twenty other ingredients, eighteen of which are chemicals. One of the ingredients is stearamidopropyl PG-dimonium chloride phosphate, added for its conditioning abilities, yet this chemical is an ammonium known to cause tissue death at a 0.1 percent solution.

Another part of our daily cleansing routine is to moisturize, especially after using our brand name soap. Another international brand name moisturizer containing the words vitamin C and absolutes (a term used with expensive essential oils) has sixty-three ingredients, including the stated vitamin C, fifteen other recognizable ingredients (two extracts, but no absolutes), and forty-eight chemicals. Listed is lauramide diethanolamine, used to give the moisturizer a creamy texture, yet this chemical is from a family of chemicals known to increase the risk of cancer.

There are always alternatives to mass-produced synthetic products. Create or find a truthfully natural skin care routine that adds to your health and doesn't take away from it. Three fundamental ingredients are all that is needed for a moisturizer. Any basic and honest all natural lotion will have ingredients such as jojoba oil (which closely resembles our skin), sweet almond oil or apricot kernel oil (both skin loving and nutrient-rich), bee's wax (to solidify), and spring water (for a less oily consistency). Look for skin-rejuvenating ingredients such as green tea, glycerine, honey, carrot tissue oil, cocoa butter, and essential oils (not synthetic fragrance oils). One supereasy, all natural alternative is a few drops of rose hip oil applied with a damp cloth.

Check your local reputable health food store for skin care products that are far less toxic than brand name products (see the National Products Database) or, with a few ingredients, create your own. Customize a skin care routine specific to your needs and skin type, celebrating this step to a healthier lifestyle.

About the Author

Courtney Findlay is a professional soapmaker, having started and later sold a successful soap and bath products business on the west coast, and who still makes her own natural soap and lotions at home. Courtney is now the creator of the thriving Indigo Earth, an online company that provides newsletters and information on health issues, product evaluations, and watchdog reports. Visit this enlightening and educational Web site at http://www.theindigoearth.com.

60

Eye Care If You Care: Proven Methods to Improve Your Vision

Kevin D. Geiger, OD

Do you want to have clear and comfortable vision for many years? Whether you are a student, a computer user, middle-aged, or a senior, the following information will help you maintain the good eyesight that you presently enjoy.

Healthy Body, Healthy Eyes

The most basic and easiest advice is what each of my patients receive: "Take care of your body, and your eyes will follow." This most fundamental ideal is very profound. Our eyes are connected to the brain and possess an abundance of blood vessels. In fact, the retina (back of the eye) is the only place in our bodies that we are able to observe arteries and veins at the same time without having to cut into tissue. It is for this reason that your eye doctor can see the effects of diabetes, hypertension, systemic lupus erythematous, AIDs, and so on. Therefore I recommend annual routine eye examinations. Remember, you are not going to your eye doctor just for a new eyeglass or contact lens prescription—you are being examined to make sure your eyes (and body) are healthy!

What is good for your body is also good for your eyes. Make sure to get plenty of rest and aerobic exercise, and eat healthy. A healthy diet consists of minimally processed carbohydrates and lots of fresh produce. Two of the best foods for your eyes are spinach and fish from cold, deep waters: salmon, mackerel, sardines, herring, and so on contain lots of omega-3 fatty acids, which are great for your body and eyes. Spinach is very high in lutein and has been shown to help those who have macular degeneration.

Of course, *don't smoke!* Smoking has been shown to be a risk factor in cataracts, macular degeneration, and glaucoma.

- Rule 1: Take care of your body, and your eyes will follow.
- Rule 2: Make sure to schedule annual, routine eye examinations.

Dry Eyes

Dry eyes is one of the most common conditions treated by eye doctors, affecting more than 10 million Americans. The most common symptoms of dry eyes are burning, watery eyes, or the sensation of having grit or sand in the eye. Whereas perimenopausal women are affected the most by dry eyes, anyone at any age may experience dry eyes. Systemic illnesses, such as Sjogren's disease, may also cause/exacerbate dry eye symptoms. Various occupations or work environments that are dry, dusty, or smoke filled can also cause/exacerbate dry eye symptoms.

Anyone with symptoms of dry eyes would benefit from slow, conscious blinking. A good blink (and often) is very soothing and can really help those who are suffering from mild dry eyes. As often as you can remember, close your eyes gently and slowly. Keep your eyes closed for two to three seconds. Try this. It is very soothing. This is very helpful to computer users who tend to stare at their monitors and blink at a rate that is much less than we normally do.

Many individuals have clogged oil glands that line the eyelids. These glands are very important for keeping our ocular surfaces wet. Simple cleansing of the eyelids often can bring dramatic relief. Wrap a wash cloth around your index finger, put the wash cloth under hot water, and then rub your finger with the hot wash cloth over it along your eyelids. The glands are along the rim of your eyelids, just behind your eyelashes. This needs to be done twice a day on both your upper and lower eyelids of each eye. Relief is usually felt within two weeks, although some people need to continue with the lid scrubs once a day, especially during the cold winter months. If your eyelid glands are severely clogged, your eye doctor may need to prescribe an oral antibiotic to relieve your symptoms.

A healthy way to improve dry eyes is to increase or supplement your diet with omega-3 fatty acids. These can be found in deep, cold water fish such as mackerel, sardines, and herring, or in flax seeds or flaxseed oil.

Over-the-counter eye lubricants will help but should not be overused. I only recommend preservative-free lubricants. There are over twenty different brands on the market; ask your eye doctor or pharmacist for a brand they prefer. I also recommend *not* using eye drops that minimize redness in the eyes—the chemical that reduces redness does *not* help relieve dryness.

If you are a computer user, lowering the height of your desktop monitor will reduce symptoms of dry eyes. The top of the screen should be at eye level or below.

Moderate or more severe dry eyes can be helped by your eye doctor. Your eye doctor can prescribe the prescription Restasis. Restasis has been clinically shown to *increase* tear production. While this is great, the drug does not work immediately, requiring you to use drops twice a day, with relief not usually being felt until after two months or more.

Another option that your doctor can use is punctal plugs. These plugs help keep your tears on the surface of your eyes by plugging the drains that your tears normally drain through.

Oral antibiotics, Restasis, and punctal plugs can all be employed by your eye doctor. Consciously slow blinking, increasing your fatty acid intake, and cleaning your eyelids can all be done by *you*!

* Rule 3: Dry eyes is a common condition. Simple lifestyle adjustments can bring relief.

Visual Hygiene

Visual hygiene is a fancy term used by the eye care community to describe good habits that allow our eyes to feel comfortable and work efficiently and stress-free. Bad visual hygiene (bad eye habits) cause our eyes to feel tired, dry, and tense and can lead to nearsightedness.

Good visual hygiene consists of
1. good lighting
2. taking frequent rest breaks when doing near activities
3. breathing when doing near activities
4. placing reading material on a work surface that is angled twenty degrees
5. using counterstress or stress-relieving eyeglasses when doing near activities.

The good visual hygiene habits are mostly common sense. Good lighting means that the lighting is proper for the activity being performed; the light should not be directed into your eyes, and reading should not be done in dim lighting. The sun's light is better than artificial light.

Whenever you read, do deskwork, computer work, sew, or any other nearpoint activity, the muscles in your eyes are working. There is no muscle in the body that wants to work for a half hour straight. Neither do your eyes. Take frequent rest breaks. Every fifteen minutes of close work, take a two-minute break. Look far away into the distance. When you look up close, the muscles in your eyes are working; when you look far away, the muscles in your eyes are relaxed.

Nearpoint work is very stressful to our visual systems. Stress causes shallow breathing, among other things. Remember this, and breathe slowly and deeply while doing computer work, reading, or other nearpoint, concentrated tasks.

It has been shown that when we read, we are more comfortable and efficient if our eyes are perpendicular to the plane of our reading material. Therefore, if our reading material (homework) is on a table, that table should be tilted upward about twenty degrees so that when we bend our heads downward at our reading material, it is perpendicular to our line of sight.

Counterstress or stress-relieving eyeglasses would be prescribed by your eye doctor. After probing your eyes through nearpoint testing, your eye doctor may find a prescription that makes reading and nearpoint work easier and less stressful to your visual system. These same eyeglasses can help to stop or slow down the progression of nearsightedness for you. These eyeglasses have made a tremendous difference to many of my patients as well as myself. I am proud to say that I am one of the few eye doctors that does not require eyeglasses or contact lenses to see clearly in the distance.

- Rule 4: Humans were not meant to read. Good visual hygiene, such as proper lighting, frequent rest breaks, and breathing, can help you do nearpoint activities comfortably.

About the Author

Dr. Kevin D. Geiger received his OD degree from the SUNY State College of Optometry. He is a practicing optometrist in Perth Amboy, New Jersey. He is the past recipient of the Frederick Brock Memorial Award for his clinical expertise in working with patients requiring vision therapy and other visual interventions for a multitude of ocular conditions relating to binocular and perceptual deficiencies. Dr. Geiger's book *Rx for Computer Eyes* discusses the stresses computers have on our eyes and body and contains easy-to-follow suggestions that computer users of all ages can implement to reduce these stresses. Dr. Geiger has also been featured on NBC's television show *Inside Stuff* for his expert knowledge on the eyes' role in basketball and athletics in general. To learn more about Dr. Geiger, visit http://www.drkevingeiger.com.

61

Newton, Einstein, and Antiaging

Jane G. Goldberg, PhD

Everyone knows the story of the man who goes up in a spacecraft and comes back to earth years later. His wife, who was in her prime when he left, is now old and decrepit. The space traveler, however, has only aged a few years. So goes aging in space. As speed of travel increases to the speed of light, aging begins to go very, very slowly. So goes the theory of time and space by Einstein.

As we ourselves get older, we want to defy, like the space traveler, the aging process. And thanks to another scientist who predated Einstein by three hundred years, we know how we can. We all know Newton discovered gravity. But what may not be so obvious (and it was a question Newton himself never thought about) is the way in which gravity contributes to the aging process. We don't often think about how much energy we exert fighting gravity. Yet, when we feel tired, we are sensitive to the effects of gravity and feel compelled to lie down to ameliorate some of gravity's inexorable pull. When we walk or run, we're putting all the gravitational pressure of our entire body on one small spot, creating thousands of pounds of pressure per square inch. Many biologists now feel that gravity plays a significant role in the cell's loss of ability to replicate itself, thus contributing directly to aging and death. Well-known nutritionist Dr. Bernard Jensen has said that there is not a single disease in which gravity does not play a part.

If we could reverse the force of gravity on our bodies, we would look and feel younger. But we can't. Gravity is a fact of life that is inescapable, and short of space travel at the speed of light, there is no way that we can escape its effects. What we can do, however, is find ways to allow gravity to work for us instead of against us.

What's wonderful about the last 20 years is that the health movement has made working with gravity (and thus aging reversal) so accessible. There are several methods, each thoroughly enjoyable, and you will see and feel the effects almost immediately. They are rebounding, skipping, using the slant board, and floating.

Rebounding

Rebounding is unique as an aerobic exercise because it stimulates, strengthens, and cleanses every cell in the body. This is because it uses vertical motion, rather than the horizontal motion that is used in all other forms of exercise. When you bounce up and down, your entire body goes through repetitive vertical acceleration and deceleration, working against gravity. At the bottom of every bounce, your entire body stops for a split second. At this moment, the force of gravity shoves down on every cell in your body. Then your body shoots back upward, again stopping for just a split instant. This is your moment in space; for this instant, you are weightless and gravityless. Because of the repetitive pushing and pulling on all your cells, the tissues and fibers and muscles in your body all grow stronger. Also, flushing out metabolic waste is increased by 300 percent by rebounding. The compression/decompression of cell membranes that occurs in rebounding significantly boosts the diffusion of fluid into and out of the cells, carrying in fresh oxygen and nutrients and flushing out the toxins. Rebounding can also substantially boost the immune system by increasing the activity of lymphocytes within the bloodstream. There is literally no other form of exercise that has this same capacity for total cellular cleansing.

Skipping

Of course, you remember skipping. You may also remember how happy you felt when you skipped. I don't mean content, or satisfied, or feeling good or nice. I mean happy. The health benefits of skipping are the same as rebounding. Skipping is more aerobic than running, with none of the disadvantages of running. It's all done on your toes and the front of your feet, and this area has great padding. This cushions all the bones and joints in your legs as well as your back, so you will not get injured the way runners do.

The Slant Board

Yoga discovered the importance of being upside-down five thousand years ago. The slant board is the shortcut version of the yoga postures of head and shoulder stands.

Brain anemia may not be a medically recognized disease entity, but many of us have it. If muscle tone or circulation is not good enough, then the blood can't travel uphill to the brain sufficiently to feed the brain. Without sufficient blood to the brain, virtually all of our functions will be weakened. The cerebellum, the back part of your brain, is where every physical organ is regenerated. You cannot breathe; you cannot hear, see, or taste; and you cannot think properly or move any part of your body without your back brain getting enough blood flow. This is, as well, the first part of the brain to be adversely affected by gravity.

Many animals instinctively feed their brains the blood that is needed by how they sleep. (They don't need slant boards.) The animal is always in a prone position during sleep, and its head falls lower than the rest of its body.

Lying on the slant board puts your head at a forty-five degree angle below your feet. It repositions all of the internal organs. Gravity pulls the organs upward, thus creating space between the organs so that the oxygen can reach the organs more easily.

Floating

It was a rave in the 1970s. Most major cities still have at least one float room. Floating is an antigravity experience like none other. You float peacefully in the water that has been saturated with eight hundred pounds of Epsom salts, thus experiencing both buoyancy and weightlessness (like in space—or like the Dead Sea). Because there is little sensory stimulation in the chamber, you enter a state that is like the meditative state—both extraordinarily quiet and intensely conscious. Because the water is heated to the precise degree of skin temperature, there are no nerve transmissions traveling from the skin to the brain. As a result, the relaxation induced is utterly profound. The rejuvenating effect on the body and brain is shown to be equivalent to five hours of sleep. Research shows the physiological effects from floating:

- it creates a drop in blood pressure
- it slows the pulse rate
- it allows the blood to circulate more freely throughout the body
- it increases alpha and theta waves in the brain
- synchronous and symmetrical rhythms are achieved throughout the cortex
- it decreases levels of hormones associated with stress, the fight or flight hormones
- pH levels and electrolytes are balanced
- heavy metals can be released from the body.

If you can't find a float room, then just fill your bathtub with water and add five pounds of Epsom salts. You won't float, but you will still derive the considerable benefits that the Epsom salt confers. It is a powerful detoxifier, and skin elasticity is improved.

Doing All of Them

Combining all of these techniques in one's life gives an unsurpassed boost of rejuvenative energy. Skip in the morning and skip at night (five minutes). Float (or take an Epsom salt bath) once a week. Rebound for ten minutes every day. And snooze (or do leg lifts) on the slant board for twenty minutes every day (preferably between 3:00 and 5:00 p.m.—the time when the sun and moon change their configuration in relation to each other, and when we feel the most tired). Incorporating these health techniques into our lives not only makes us feel better, but we look better, too.

Bibliography

Brooks, Linda. *Rebounding to Better Health*. Lincoln, NE: KE, 1995.

Carter, Albert E. *The New Miracles of Rebound Exercise*. Fountain Hills, AZ: A. L. M., 1988.

Hutchison, Michael. *The Book of Floating*. New York: Quill, 1984.

Jensen, Bernard. *Nature Has a Remedy*. Escondido, CA: Bernard Jensen, 1979.

Walker, Morton. *Jumping for Health: Guide to Rebounding Aerobics*. Garden City Park, NY: Avery, 1989.

About the Author

Jane G. Goldberg, PhD (DrJaneGoldberg.com) is known widely in both the psychoanalytic and holistic health communities. She is the owner of two New York City day spas; in addition, Dr. Goldberg is a practicing psychoanalyst and author. Dr. Goldberg has specialized in working with cancer patients and has successfully integrated her psychoanalytic work with the field of holistic health. Dr. Goldberg is a prolific writer, having authored numerous articles in the fields of psychological oncology and mind-body health as well as six books, including *The Dark Side of Love* (Tarcher/Putnam, 1993), *Deceits of the Mind (and Their Effects on the Body)* (Transaction, 1991), and *Psychotherapeutic Treatment of Cancer Patients* (Free Press, 1981). Dr. Goldberg has made appearances on most talk television shows, including *The Donahue Show, Sally Jesse Raphael, Jane Whitney, Rikki Lake, The Maury Povich Show, The Morton Downy Show, Maureen O'Boyle*, and others.

62

Naturopathic Physicians: Doctors Who Understand Health as Much as Disease

Colleen Huber, NMD

Naturopathy is essentially an eclectic system of medicine using the most natural and least invasive methods of treating disease. Yet it is not so much a collection of treatment strategies as it is a philosophy of treating. Naturopathic physician Kenneth Proefrock, NMD, says, "What defines naturopathic physicians is not so much the substances we use, but how we use them. Naturopathic doctors will even at times prescribe pharmaceuticals if it will help restore some sense of balance so that the patient can then go on to achieve a higher level of health."[1]

The biggest difference with conventional so-called allopathic medicine is this approach to the patient. *Allo* (opposite) *pathy* (disease) fights symptoms with substances that are opposite in function and suppress those symptoms. Naturopathic physicians, in contrast, are far more interested in how a person got to feel ill in the first place, and identifying that first cause of disease and correcting that cause, so that the resulting symptoms are then eliminated. Sometimes symptom suppression is necessary regardless of the form of medicine, but naturopaths see that as only a means to an end. For example, if patients are in so much pain that they can't function or enjoy life, then pain relief would be appropriate until the underlying cause of the pain is eliminated by other means.

The six defining principles of naturopathic medicine further illustrate this philosophy and approach:

1. First do no harm.
2. Nature has the power to heal.
3. Treat the whole person.
4. Treat the cause.
5. Prevent disease.
6. Doctor as teacher.

---

[1] Kenneth Proefrock, NMD, personal communication, January 19, 2006.

"First do no harm" was Hippocrates's instruction to physicians and may be thought of as an application of the Golden Rule. Whatever intervention a doctor can make in a patient's health and life, the only acceptable action is one that will do no further damage to the patient's health. It doesn't get much more sensible than this rule first learned as toddlers: don't hurt anybody.

Second, naturopathic doctors rely on the healing power of nature to help restore patients to complete health. The really excellent naturopath is one who knows how to work the modalities, that is, to be able to draw from the vast materia medica of natural materials as appropriate for specific patients and to be able to apply them to the great variety and complication of illnesses that are common today, and better yet, to offer the patient a choice among multiple effective treatments.

Another principle is to treat the whole person. Naturopaths know better than to give you a medication that will calm your arthritis but leave you blind or that will clear up the skin while skewing your hormones out of balance. Naturopaths are trained to consider the whole patient, not just the one part of the body with obvious symptoms. The job of the naturopathic doctor is to make sure that what you get is helpful and completely benign for all of you.

The fourth principle is to treat the cause. For example, you may have chronic inflammation that has caused joint stiffness and imbalanced immune function. The naturopath goes to the cause of the problem and treats the inflammation and its cause because when you remove the cause, the joints move more easily, and the immune system improves. So that way, you resolve all three problems, instead of just one.

To prevent disease is another naturopathic principle. The improved lifestyle of naturopathic patients is what enables the body to regain homeostasis and better deflect the constant stresses and toxic conditions that a heavily trafficked industrial society imposes.

Perhaps the last principle is most important of all: it is even more important for a doctor to be a teacher than a healer. In accordance with the idea that if you give someone a fish, he may eat that day, but if you teach him to fish, he may eat for a lifetime, *the doctor must teach how to heal* and how to live comfortably long term with good-quality food; sound sleep; stress reduction measures; and a fun, feasible exercise program. Ultimately, the most successful patients learn to take responsibility for their own health, with the doctor acting as a resource and tutor toward that goal.

Naturopathic physicians are naturopathic doctors (ND) or naturopathic medical doctors (NMD). After graduation from a four-year college or university, naturopaths are trained in four-year medical colleges, just as other physicians are. The difference is that in naturopathic medical school, in addition to learning such basic medical sciences as anatomy, physiology, biochemistry, microbiology, pathology, pharmacology, immunology, histology, neuroanatomy, and genetics, naturopathic students also attend full courses in specific clinical sciences over the next two years: obstetrics, pediatrics, gynecology, urology, geriatrics, neurology, eyes-ears-nose-throat, pulmonology, cardiology, gastroenterology, endocrinology, dermatology, rheumatology, and oncology. Naturopathic students take courses in standard medical procedures: physical diagnosis, laboratory diagnosis, and clinical procedures (multiple courses of each) as well as emergency medicine and minor surgery. Of course, naturopaths also learn the naturopathic therapies. These include clinical nutrition (i.e., nutrition as both a healing therapy and applied biochemistry), botanical medicine (nutritive and therapeutic plants), homeopathy, and Oriental medicine such as acupuncture and herbs as well as environmental medicine, physical medicine, and hydrotherapy. Naturopaths are trained both in the classroom and in a variety of clinical settings.

Throughout the naturopathic medical curriculum, naturopaths are required to take board exams to ensure that both training and skills meet the standards required across North America for the naturopathic profession. Just as for medical doctors and osteopathic physicians, naturopathic physicians are required to take continuing education courses periodically to stay at peak competence.

Just be sure that you ask for a licensed ND or NMD because licensed naturopaths are the ones who are both classroom and clinically trained to practice medicine. There are some health care practitioners who call themselves "naturopaths" or "traditional naturopaths" but who have never enrolled in a medical school. They may have purchased their diploma online and may have never treated anyone before you. Such people may have good intentions and want to help their fellow humans but are at a serious loss regarding the necessary knowledge and experience to be trusted with your health. Licensed naturopathic physicians, on the other hand, have graduated from a four-year, on-site medical school and have worked with several hundred patients at minimum before graduating. A naturopathic doctor's license to practice medicine is issued by one of fourteen states plus the District of Columbia, although naturopathic physicians may be found in all fifty states and abroad.

Naturopathic medicine is still only sometimes covered by medical insurance, and then as out-of-network providers. However, as many people have happily discovered, the out-of-pocket costs to a naturopath's patients are often much less than the out-of-pocket costs (i.e., deductibles and uncovered services and products) for fully insured people who go to conventional physicians and who need pharmaceuticals and/or hospital care; that is, a naturopath's tools, which are basically materials found in nature—often plant materials—are so much less expensive than patented prescription drugs that many people end up paying less, even without insurance. These savings are magnified as time goes on, considering the much greater relative improvement in overall health of the naturopathic patient over the average person.

About the Author

Colleen Huber, NMD, is a naturopathic medical doctor and primary care physician in Tempe, Arizona. Dr. Huber graduated from Southwest College of Naturopathic Medicine in Tempe. Many of her health articles have appeared on Mercola.com, the most visited natural health site. Her own Web site, Naturopathyworks.com, contains more than eighty of her articles in a free newsletter on the topics of health, nutrition, and natural lifestyles. Colleen Huber's book *Choose Your Foods Like Your Life Depends on Them* was published in 2007. Her academic writing has appeared in *Lancet* and other medical journals.

63

Naturopathy

Parthenia S. Izzard, CNHP, ABD

This article focuses on alternative medicine therapies: what they are, why they are, and what difference that should make to you and yours. There might be some who do not know much about naturopathy and the alternative medicine therapies it employs. Wisdom dictates that you contact your physician before trying any of the therapies discussed herein. This article will lay a good foundation for future interactions with alternative medicine. If there are therapies or issues that are of personal concern or mere curiosity, feel free to contact me through the information at the end of this article, and I will address them. I want this to be a fun journey, but certain basics must be known first, so buckle your seat belt.

Naturopathy was the earliest known healing system.[1] Foods, water, and whole herbs were used by many cultures for a wide range of problems before surgery and the synthetic isolation of chemical substances.[2] Many cultures used a variety of naturopathic therapies, ranging from kelp for thyroid health (Chinese), liver for night blindness (Egyptians), and various herbs to promote healing (Native Americans and most others).[3] Is there any wonder that there are still many who make naturopathy an integral part of their lives?

In the United States, the term *naturopathy* is posited to have been coined by Dr. John Schell in 1895, describing his approach to health.[4] There are presently two primary views of naturopathy with respective different agendas. The first view is that naturopaths should be licensed as physicians and are a type of medical doctor who uses herbs, homeopathy, manipulation, nutrition, isolates, counseling, prescription medications, injections, and sometimes minor surgery.[5] This view tends to be one shared by those endeavoring to require a medical degree of some sort for one to be a naturopath. The second view purports that naturopathy is in the public domain and that its practitioners are not medical doctors and should employ only those modalities that are natural, and should not perform surgery or write prescriptions.[6] This latter view I share in as much as it describes

---

[1] R. J. Theil, *Combining Old and New*, Naturopathy for the 21st Century (Warsaw, IN: Whitman).
[2] Ibid.
[3] Ibid.
[4] Ibid.
[5] Ibid.
[6] Ibid.

something that provides an alternative to traditional medicine by practice and definition. It is an oxymoron for a naturopath to perform surgery.

Naturopathy, according to Benedict Lust[7], is a distinct school of healing, employing the beneficial agency of Nature's forces of water, air, sunlight, earth power, electricity, magnetism, exercise, rest, proper diet, various kinds of mechanical treatment, and mental and moral science. Furthermore, because none of the aforementioned agents of rejuvenation can cure every disease by itself, the naturopath employs the combination that is best adapted to each individual case. The objective of naturopathy is to remove foreign or poisonous matter from the system, allowing the restoration of nerve and blood vitality, the invigoration of organs and tissues, and the regeneration of the entire organism. Examples of some therapies that fall under the purview of naturopathy are iridology, kinesiology, reflexology, acupressure, and the like.

What most people have forgotten or do not know is that the original naturopaths were medical doctors[8] dissatisfied with the medical options available to them, and others were straight naturopaths, using only natural modalities, and naturopaths who were medical doctors. There are still medical doctors who incorporate some form of naturopathy in their recommendations to their patients, especially in the area of stress management and nutrition. A medical degree, however, is not a prerequisite to being a naturopath and should not be.

What follows is an overview of water, air, iridology, kinesiology, and two kinds of naturopathic manipulation: reflexology and acupressure.

Water is the most ancient of all remedial agents for disease.[9] Among the Spartans of ancient Greece, cold bathing was made obligatory by law.[10] Hippocrates directed that cold baths should be of short duration and should be preceded and followed by friction—that after a cold bath, the body quickly recuperates its heat and remains warm, while a hot bath produces the opposite effect.[11] Hippocrates employed both hot and cold water in the treatment of fevers, ulcers, and hemorrhages and for a variety of maladies, both medical and surgical.[12]

Well, most people agree that polluted air is dangerous. It is through the medium of the air, with its life-giving oxygen, that the blood is purified.[13] It therefore follows logically that air, pure air, is necessary to health.[14] Four minutes is the limit of time that most people can be deprived of oxygen and live.[15]

---

[7] Ibid.

[8] Ibid.

[9] R. Dextiet and M. Abehsera, *Health Handbook* (Provo, UT: Woodlands, 1993)

[10] Ibid.

[11] Ibid.

[12] Ibid.

[13] Theil, "Combining Old and New."

[14] Ibid.

[15] Ibid.

Correct breathing supplies more oxygen to the blood, circulates it properly, and purifies it, which can be clearly observed by a clear and bright complexion, while the blood of those who breathe imperfectly is bluish, darkish, and lacking in oxygen, which can be observed by a livid or pale complexion.[16]

According to Thiel, iridology was defined by Dr. J. Haskell Kritzer as follows: "Iridology is a science revealing pathological and functional disturbances in the human body by means of abnormal spots, lines, and discolorations of the eye."[17] Dr. Jensen adds that toxemias and, where located, the activity of each organ, glandular conditions, and drug poisonings can be accurately identified through the observation of the iris of the eye.[18]

A form of kinesiology is reflex nutrition assessment (RNA), which is an ancillary form of nutrition assessment.[19] It is a technique used to assess nutrition status by observing the response of muscles under externally provided human force.[20]

Many naturopaths use forms of acupressure.[21] In acupressure, fingertips are applied to acupuncture points. The fact that it is finger pressure that is applied to Oriental acupuncture points suggests a relationship to reflexology (actually, reflexology should be considered a form of acupressure).[22] There are too many points to list here, but there is one acupressure point used against anxiety or nervousness where one applies slight pressure to the indentation at the point. Holding four fingers over the area opens up breathing and relieves tension.[23]

I hope your interest is piqued and that you will pursue more knowledge and experience a journey through the natural world of healing and preventive medicine.

Be well.

About the Author

Parthenia S. Izzard, CNHP, is a psychologist and president and founder of Alternative Medicine Therapies. In addition to being a certified natural healthcare practitioner (CNHP) and Pennsylvania State Certified Psychologist, she is in the dissertation phase of her PhD in Clinical and Health Psychology. You can listen to her radio program, Wellness, Wholeness, and Wisdom, on Delaware Valley's WWDB, 860 AM at 9:00 a.m. every Saturday. The program is simulcast on VoiceAmerica Radio's 7th Wave Network (the link is on her site). To contact her, send e-mails to consult@amtherapies.com, and visit her Web site, http://www.amtherapies.com.

---

[16] Ibid.

[17] Ibid, 83.

[18] Ibid.

[19] Ibid.

[20] Ibid.

[21] Ibid.

[22] Ibid.

[23] Ibid.

64

Control Autoimmune Diseases with Stomach Acid?

Marcus Laux, ND

I believe proper digestion is vital to addressing the epidemic of autoimmune diseases in this country. Digestion is the ability to take what isn't you and turn it into you by breaking it down, assimilating the useful components, and disposing of the rest. It's a complicated sequence of secretions, hormones, enzymes, and bacteria, and the proper balance of these substances is important.

A key part of the process is hydrochloric acid (HCl), or stomach acid. The complete absence of HCl in the stomach is called achlorhydria, and an insufficient amount is called hypochlorhydria. If HCl is not present at the proper levels, the digestive process is disrupted from beginning to end—with one or more autoimmune diseases as a possible outcome.

Essentially, HCl sterilizes your stomach and food by killing most pathogens on contact, which means it prevents the overgrowth of yeast, fungi, and bacteria in your upper GI tract (an exception appears to be *H. pylori* bacteria). When you have enough HCl, pathogens and parasites just become part of a meal for your body. But when you have insufficient HCl, your body can become the meal.

In addition to sterilizing, HCl denatures proteins so that the digestive enzyme pepsin can break them down further. In fact, without enough HCl, the enzyme pepsinogen that is secreted in the stomach can't be converted into pepsin, leading to poor protein absorption and impaired metabolism that then affects the body's other enzymes, hormones, neurotransmitters, and so on.

Additionally, proper HCl levels signal the release of secretin, a hormone that then aids in the proper functioning of enzymes from the pancreas that are needed for the digestion of fat and carbohydrates. In other words, a person with low HCl isn't able to digest any foods adequately and so has difficulty absorbing minerals, vitamins, and other nutrients from those foods.

It's easy to see how the scenario of little or no HCl can start a whole cascade of health compromises that can lead to severe health problems. I believe that the majority of people in their sixties and older who have multiple health complaints (particularly autoimmune diseases) should have their doctors consider hypochlorhydria as a contributing factor.

Because it hasn't been well researched, most doctors don't realize how common hypochlorhydria is in their patients. We do know, though, that over 30 percent of people over sixty have atrophic gastritis (which means that little to no HCl is being made), and that's just one reason for low HCl levels.

The Purple Pill and Other Autoimmune Perpetrators

They used to call it "heartburn" and treat it with antacids such as Rolaids, Pepto-Bismol, Tums, and so on. Then they started calling it "GERD" (for gastroesophageal reflux disease) because the pharmaceutical companies developed prescription drugs that didn't just neutralize stomach acid, but inhibited its production. Now it's been shortened to "acid reflux"—I guess because people weren't considering GERD a problem that they recognized and weren't buying the drugs.

Whatever we want to call the condition that is the result of stomach acid entering the esophagus, the current fashion is to use either over-the-counter or prescription drugs to address it. Along with antacids, the expensive methods preferred by conventional medicine include proton pump inhibitors (such as Nexium, Prevacid, and Prilosec) and H_2 blockers (such as Pepcid and Zantac).

While these drugs may be appropriate for a few people who need to get some temporary relief, they are actually a setup for disease for nearly everyone. Even if they help with the discomfort of heartburn or acid reflux, they are the wrong treatments because it's rare for the stomach to actually produce too much acid on a long-term basis. When you think of all that HCl does for you, it makes no sense to try to limit its production or neutralize its effects.

Even worse is the fact that the symptoms of low HCl levels are strikingly similar to the symptoms of high HCl levels. That's right, you can have the same symptoms with either too little or too much stomach acid, which means that low acid is often diagnosed as either high acid or an ulcer, unless the doctor runs a test to confirm which end of the acid spectrum the symptoms are coming from.[1]

---

[1] The Heidelberg Gastric Analysis Test is an accurate way of measuring HCl levels. The test involves swallowing a capsule that contains a hi-tech pH meter connected to a radio transmitter. After swallowing it when the stomach is empty of food, you drink a mixture of water and bicarbonate that stimulates a rebound release of HCl. The pH information is then transmitted back to a receiver that is located close to the stomach. The normal pH in a healthy stomach when it is empty of food is about 2.1 in men and 2.7 in women. However, with low to no HCl, the pH is around 7.4–7.6. Other lab tests can document the absence of HCl by extremely low serum level measurements of pepsinogen A and high serum gastrin levels.

By following the drug companies, most doctors just diagnose too much acid after a patient reports one or more of the following complaints: indigestion, heartburn, chest pain, diarrhea, flatulence, abdominal pain, or cramps. The tests that truly reflect acid levels are rarely ordered, unless the doctor actually suspects hypochlorhydria.

A diagnosis of high acid is almost always made based solely on the symptoms and the influence of the slick drug ads. However, proton pump inhibitors can lead to headaches and lung infections, and H_2 blockers can cause confusion, diarrhea, and erectile dysfunction—and these adverse effects are from drugs that may have been incorrectly prescribed in the first place.

Suppress Stress for More Slime

Another possibility when it comes to a diagnosis of too much acid could actually be a faulty mucus barrier. Mucus is the slime that covers many tissue surfaces to keep them moist and to protect them from harm. Two of the jobs of the stomach's mucosal barrier are to prevent HCl from eating the stomach and to provide another barrier to pathogens.

A gastric ulcer can develop if this barrier breaks down. Forty years ago, a patient with an ulcer was told that stress was the likely cause. Lately, conventional doctors and researchers have been saying that stress is no longer a culprit. Instead, they believe that most peptic ulcers (of which gastric ulcers are one type) are thought to be caused by an infection of *H. pylori* in the gastrointestinal tract. However, most people with *H. pylori* never develop ulcers, so there is clearly more going on, including reactions to nonsteroidal anti-inflammatory drugs (NSAIDs) and food allergens.

Despite the current emphasis on *H. pylori*, stress can indeed contribute to the formation of peptic ulcers. Stress overworks the sympathetic nervous system that, in turn, affects the production of mucus, causing a breakdown of the barrier that allows HCl and *H. pylori* to attack weak spots. Supporting the parasympathetic system can help keep your gut sublimely slimy.

For rebuilding the barrier and easing the pain, I've had great success with licorice in a deglycyrrhizinated form known as DGL. It has been shown to promote mucin production and protect your stomach lining while soothing irritated tissues. However, it appears that DGL must be chewed for it to work, which means you should make sure you can handle it since the flavor is intense.

However, my top recommendation for supporting your mucosal barrier is Ulcinex. It's based on a traditional Chinese formula of nine herbs, and it's designed to relieve heartburn and indigestion, quiet dyspepsia, relax reflux symptoms, and support healthy flora and digestion. I recommend taking two tablets thirty minutes before each meal. For additional support, you can also take one tablet between meals.

Low Stomach Acid Causes the Body to Attack Itself

As I mentioned earlier, it's rare to actually have too much stomach acid. If your mucosal barrier is strong, there really shouldn't be a problem. However, low stomach acid is a real possibility, and it will alter your body's metabolism and cause you to be functionally malnourished, which in turn means increased oxidative damage, inflammation, waste buildup with increased toxin absorption, and altered immune response (such as autoimmune diseases). There is no complete explanation for why we get autoimmune diseases. However, we know that bacterial and microbial overgrowth in the gut and intestinal barrier can leak into the bloodstream and cause immune sensitivity and hyperreactivity.

If improperly digested foods, pathogens, or even cells from your own intestinal wall enter your bloodstream, your immune system has to attack and eliminate them. In the case of food, your immune system is literally finishing the job that should have been done by the digestive system. One of the problems with the immune system disposing of foods is that the cellular structures of some foods are similar to some of the cellular structures in your body. Similarly, perceived pathogens may actually be some of your own cells that shouldn't be in the bloodstream. Either way, your immune system will be programmed to think of some of your own cells as invaders that it will attack more vigorously the next time it encounters them. The consequences can be dire since autoimmunity, allergies, and inflammation are all potential outcomes.

Additionally, some of our microflora share antigenic determinants with our healthy, normal tissues. Even intestinal yeast overgrowth can have systemic effects and play a role in autoimmunity due to yeast antigens translocating to other parts of the body. We know, for instance, that autoimmune arthritis can be activated by intestinal infections of *Yersinia*, *Salmonella*, and other enterobacteria, with further evidence showing bacterial antigens discovered in the synovial cells of joints.

This evidence has led to the theory that the immune system is attacking cells that are hiding bacteria or other pathogens. For instance, some people may have infections that are hiding in their own cells. As the body attempts to eliminate the infection, it attacks its own cells and is then programmed to see them as invaders as well. The process may differ from that for other forms of autoimmunity, but the effects are the same.

We have been conditioned to think of stomach acid as a bad thing. However, based on my own clinical experience, I can assuredly state that many patients with a variety of autoimmune diseases can markedly improve their condition by improving their HCl, which means either getting off the antacids, proton pump inhibitors, and other acid reflux drugs or addressing hypochlorhydria if the body really isn't making enough stomach acid.

Increasing Your HCl Levels

For anyone with an autoimmune disease (or anyone who suspects that they might have low stomach acid), I recommend supplementing with betaine hydrochloride. It's listed under different names, depending on the manufacturer. The Vitamin Shoppe (http://www.VitaminShoppe.com) calls their version "Betaine HCl with Pepsin," while TwinLab calls it "Betaine HCl Caps" and Solaray simply calls theirs "HCl with Pepsin."

The treatment strategy is to gradually increase the amount of betaine HCl you take until you truly have too much acid in your stomach, then back down slightly to the correct maintenance dose. Betaine HCl has been used safely for over one hundred years, and it's often combined with pepsin—which I recommend as well. All three of the brands I mentioned above contain pepsin, even though TwinLab doesn't say so in the name of their product.

If you currently have a peptic ulcer, *do not* supplement with betaine HCl or pepsin. You need to heal your peptic ulcer first by taking plant digestive enzymes (without protease) and by rebuilding the mucosal barrier in the way I discussed earlier. After the peptic ulcer problem is cleared up, then consider the betaine HCl program.

People with a history of ulcers, gastritis, stomach pain, or heartburn must be closely supervised when taking betaine HCl. Also, people taking NSAIDs, cortisone-like drugs, or other drugs that may cause a peptic ulcer should not use betaine HCl.

Finally, if you've been taking antacids, proton pump inhibitors, or other acid blockers for a while, wean off them slowly before following the betaine HCl supplementation program since the possible rebound effect can be significant and painful.

Getting with the Program

I recommend this simple and straightforward protocol for taking betaine HCl. Take one capsule (500–700 mg of HCl with 100–175 mg of pepsin) at the beginning of your first complex meal that contains protein and fat (not with a simple meal of mostly carbohydrates, such as salad, soup, or fruit). Take two capsules at the beginning of your second complex meal, three capsules at the beginning of your third complex meal, and so on. Keep adding an additional capsule with each meal until you get heartburn or irritation.

On your next meal after irritation was achieved, take one capsule less than the amount that caused the irritation—this will be your maintenance dose. Whenever you have a meal of mostly carbohydrates, take only one-third to half of your full dose.

Most people with low acid will have symptoms that they should notice an improvement in as they take betaine over several days or weeks.[2] The symptoms may not go away immediately, but they should not get any worse. If the symptoms do get worse, then you either have an ulcer that needs to be addressed, or you might be one of the rare people who truly has too much HCl. If supplementing with betaine HCl is right for you, you should experience better digestion, health, energy, and the gradual relief of many complaints.

Also be aware that as your body's normal acid production resumes, you will again experience the irritation that helped you identify the proper dose. When this irritation recurs, reduce your dose by one capsule with each meal until the irritation is no longer recurring—which means that you may eventually end up not taking any betaine at all. Later, if the low acid symptoms or digestive problems come back, start the betaine HCl program again from the beginning.

One final note for those people who have acid reflux because of a malfunctioning sphincter: improving your HCl and avoiding food allergens should help as well.

About the Author

Marcus Laux, ND, is a licensed naturopathic physician who earned his doctorate at the National College of Naturopathic Medicine in Portland, Oregon. He has been clinically trained in acupuncture, homeopathy, and physical medicine, among other healing modalities. He also writes a monthly newsletter, *Naturally Well Today*, which brings his readers the best of new healing methods and traditional healing wisdom. For more information, visit http://www.DrMarcusLaux.com.

---

[2] Rather than waiting for serious health problems to arise (such as an autoimmune disease), the following symptoms may be an indication of insufficient HCl levels: bloating, burping, and belching; flatulence after meals; foul-smelling flatulence; indigestion, lasting fullness, or feeling full too easily; diarrhea or constipation; soreness, burning, or dryness of the mouth; heartburn or acid reflux; multiple food allergies that get worse over time; frequently nauseous after eating or taking supplements; adult acne, rosacea, or dermatitis, especially on the cheeks and nose; hair loss in women; undigested food in the stools; rectal itching; chronic yeast infections; and hunger all the time or the desire to eat when not hungry.

65

How to Treat Your Colds and Viral Sore Throats

Dr. Joseph Mercola

How Do I Catch a Cold?

The humble cold is the most common infectious disease in the United States. It accounts for more absences from school and work than any other illness. It is the leading cause of patient visits to physicians.

It is not easy to catch a cold. Your body's natural defenses usually fight off these viruses. There is a direct relation between your risk of catching a cold and the amount of time spent in contact with an infected person. That is why families tend to get sick together.

The most common route of infection is not from coughing or sneezing, or walking barefoot in the rain, but from hand-to-hand contact. That is why when you have a cold, washing your hands frequently is so important. The likelihood of you becoming a victim of the cold virus increases, however, if you are overtired or physically exhausted.

Children under two generally get ten to twelve colds a year, especially if they are in day care. Older children and young adults get about six colds per year. After the age of thirty, the number starts to decrease to about two per year.

How Long Will It Last?

Most uncomplicated colds last between eight and nine days, but about 25 percent last two weeks, and 5 to 10 percent last three weeks.

What Should I Do for Treatment?

1. As long as your temperature remains below 102°F, there is no need to lower it. Cold viruses do not reproduce at higher body temperatures. A slight fever should help you get rid of the virus quicker and feel better much sooner.

2. A study in *Journal of Infectious Disease* showed that people who take aspirin and Tylenol (acetaminophen) suppress the body's ability to produce antibodies to destroy the cold virus. You should only use these medications if you have a temperature greater than 105°F, severe muscle aches, or weakness.

3. Chicken soup does help the symptoms. Chicken contains a natural amino acid called cysteine. Cysteine can thin the mucus in the lungs and make it less sticky so that you can expel it more easily. Campbell's soup won't work as well as the homemade version. Make the soup hot and spicy, with plenty of pepper. The spices will trigger a sudden release of watery fluids in the mouth, throat, and lungs. This will help thin down the respiratory mucus so that it's easier to cough up and expel.

4. Rest. It is important to rest and take it easy throughout the time you are ill. The time you are ill may be longer if you do not allow yourself to recuperate and recover completely. If you exercise regularly, you need not stop. However, you should definitely cut back on the intensity until you feel better.

5. Wash your hands frequently, and try to keep them away from your nose and eyes. Use disposable tissues as opposed to cloth handkerchiefs. If you are caring for a child with a cold, *please wash your hands* every time you have to wipe his or her nose. This will protect you from being infected. Dove soap is the mildest soap that you can use for this purpose.

6. Drink plenty of fluids. Water is the best. Try to drink at least eight to ten glasses a day. This will help the stuffiness and help the secretions loosen. Avoid using tap water; use bottled or filtered water to limit your exposure to chlorine. You can put lemon juice in your water or also try green tea as a water alternative.

7. If you are congested and can't breathe very well because your nose is plugged up, we recommend the decongestant Sudafed (pseudoephedrine). We can give you a twelve-hour preparation that also has guaifenesin to help you breath better. You must be careful and make sure the medicine is out of your system before bedtime. Most people will not sleep well on Sudafed, and sleep is what will make you better. You can use AFRIN (or generic equivalent) at night. This spray will open up your nose without interfering with your sleep.

8. However, if you are not congested and drowning in nasal discharge, an antihistamine will help dry up the secretions. Please note that there are two problems with nonprescription antihistamines (such as Chlor-Trimeton (chlorphenairamine) and Benadryl). (1) They can put you to sleep. This isn't a difficulty at night but might be in the day. (2) We encourage you to minimize their use because they can also increase your risk of developing a secondary sinus infection by thickening the nasal secretions and impairing drainage.

9. It will be very important to stop all milk products. This includes not only milk, but ice cream, all yogurt except plain, and especially cheese. Lactaid milk is *not* acceptable. This step is helpful to decrease the extra mucous that dairy products can cause you to produce.

10. Eating refined sugars weakens your immune system and promotes yeast overgrowth. This includes *all* nondiet pops that have eight teaspoons of sugar per can. Honey, molasses, maple syrup, date sugar, cane sugar, corn sugar, beet sugar, corn syrup, fructose, lactose, and other refined carbohydrates are known promoters of yeast growth. Reducing or eliminating these in your diet will help your immune system. However, you need not become obsessive about the sugar. If it is the fourth or fifth ingredient in a food, that would probably be acceptable.

11. Many people will start to drink large amounts of orange juice when they are sick. All the simple sugars (fructose) in the juice will actually make you worse. If you feel the need to take extra vitamin C, please read tip 13. Try to avoid *all* juices, including organic juices or ones with no sugar added; Gatorade-type sports drinks also need to be avoided. If you must have a juice, use diluted organic apple juice; do *not* use orange juice as it is the most allergic fruit.

12. Researchers have shown that zinc lozenges reduce the severity and duration of cold symptoms, particularly a sore throat. They believe the zinc is directly toxic to the virus and stimulates your body to produce antibodies to destroy the virus. They seem to work for about three out of four colds. You can suck on *one-quarter* of a zinc lozenge every thirty minutes. Do not chew the tablets and swallow them directly as they won't work. If you get nauseous, you should stop the zinc immediately as it is a sign of toxicity.

13. Extra vitamin C is also helpful. You can take 500–2,000 mg every one to two hours. The only side effect you may have are loose stools at higher doses. If this happens, decreasing the dose will quickly clear up the symptoms.

14. Vitamin A in large doses may be helpful: 200,000 units twice a day for five days (eight of the 25,000 unit capsules twice a day). Children can take half the dose. Even though vitamin A is oil-soluble, this dose is very safe if not taken for long periods. However, if you are pregnant, you should not use it.

15. Garlic is an excellent natural antibiotic. Kyolic is one of the best brands. You might use six capsules four times a day for several days. Echinacea is the most widely used herbal medication in Europe for colds and infections. It contains insulin, which enhances the production of immunoglobulins. Astralgalas and goldenseal also enhance the immune system and are widely used in Europe and China for infections.

16. Essential fatty acids like flax oil should also be taken regularly. This will help your immune system build the proper antibodies.

Why Should I Avoid an Antibiotic?

More than three hundred different viruses can cause colds. Each time you have a cold, it is caused by a distinct virus (i.e., adenovirus, rhinovirus, parainfluenza virus, coronavirus). A virus is much smaller than a bacteria. It is a tiny cluster of genetic material surrounded by a protein wrapper.

Medical science currently does not have any drugs that can kill these viruses. Antibiotics, including penicillin, *do not* have any effect on viruses. We only use them to treat the secondary bacterial infections that can complicate a cold.

When Should I Call the Office?

Sinus, ear, and lung infections (bronchitis and pneumonia) are examples of bacterial infections that do respond to antibiotics. If you develop any of the following symptoms, you should call your doctor's office:

- fever over 102°
- ear pain
- pain around your eyes, especially with a green nasal discharge
- shortness of breath or a persistent, uncontrollable cough
- green and yellow sputum persistently coughed up.

You should also call if you have any questions.

About the Author

Dr. Joseph Mercola is the founder and director of the Optimal Wellness Center in Schaumburg, Illinois. His Web site, Mercola.com, is the most popular natural health Web site in the world, with over 1 million subscribers to his free health e-newsletter and ten million page views per month. You can take a free test to learn what foods your unique biochemistry suggests you eat at http://www.mercola.com.

66

Qualifying Natural Health

Susanne Morrone, CNC

When the topic of natural health is brought up in conversation, some individuals have preconceived notions and associate it with what they know about modern medicine. Thus they consider it to be the taking of a supplement instead of a drug. Others immediately think of vegetarianism with hippie food faddists nibbling on nuts, berries, and birdseed. Still others acknowledge alternative practitioners such as herbalists, naturopaths, chiropractors, and acupuncturists.

To qualify natural health, it is important to understand from the onset that natural health and modern medicine are very different systems of health and healing. The medical system is concerned with symptom suppression, naming or finding a disease and then effecting a cure through the intervention of drugs and/or surgery. Natural health, on the other hand, recognizes that the body heals itself by wondrous design. Rather than immediate surgical removal of a diseased organ, the body is allowed to use its innate intelligence to bring about a cure. To assist this process, nature-provided raw materials and proven therapies are incorporated that do not interfere with or overtake the healing. This healing concept is easily understood by looking individually at the two words in its name.

Natural means derived from nature, in harmony with nature, or occurring in nature. Perhaps Thomas Edison best captured the essence of nature when he said, "Until man duplicates a blade of grass, nature can laugh at his so-called scientific knowledge. It's obvious we don't know one millionth of one percent about anything." Owing to its beauty, evidence of supreme intelligence, divine order, and creative genius, nature is the place where we can become grounded in thoughts and heart. Nature gives us a glimpse of the following foundational precepts:

1. Universal laws exist to which we must adhere.
2. One senses an awesome Designer when looking into the expansive universe or within the human body itself.
3. The human body is continually trying to heal itself.
4. Mankind benefits by practicing healthy living principles.
5. Nature provides therapeutic complements to the healing capacity within.

6. To see positive changes, causes of imbalances must be addressed; these may exist on a physical, emotional, and spiritual level.
7. Natural healing is long lasting since the body must do the work.
8. Health must encompass a holistic view, respecting the biodiversity, ecosystems, and harmonious balance within the human body itself.
9. Health requires stewardship of this planet.
10. We have an obligation to enlighten others of these precepts.

Health, the second word, means the absence of disease, possessing vitality or wellness. Since there is no disease in health, disease management is not a health-building process. Natural health requires one to work on building and achieving optimal health. The individual must make appropriate lifestyle changes to address the causes of imbalances such as poor diet, toxic exposures, lack of sleep, poor elimination, and so on.

The concept of natural health has been more common to cultures embracing Ayurveda or Chinese medicine, where empirical knowledge has been gathered over the millenniums using herbs and foods as medicines, along with body work, to support the healing processes. In the Western world, there were empiric herbalists, homeopaths, traditional naturopaths, and other practitioners who lost their familiarity to the general populace as allopathic medicine emerged in a changing political climate. Medical societies were restructured to embrace pharmaceuticals at the close of the nineteenth and in the early twentieth centuries.

Divergent thoughts have brought about changing systems of health care throughout history. Each time period has given birth to individuals who break free from the common mold of thinking of their day. For example, during the Renaissance in the fifteenth century, Paracelsus disagreed with the accepted Galen and Aristotle teachings. He wrote, "All that man needs for health and healing has been provided by God in nature; the challenge of science is to find it." Three hundred years later, Samuel Hahnemann, the "Father of Homeopathy," rejected the common use of toxic substances in the treatment of maladies. His contemporaries were using arsenic, opium, and mercury. Hahnemann set himself apart and delivered a kinder, gentler medicine. Interestingly enough, those physicians of medicine using mercury, or quicksilver as it was also called, were labeled "quacksilvers" by the herbalists of their day.

Within the realm of natural health, many modalities have emerged to enhance one's quality of life and health. No single modality is the end all, for each of us has unique biochemical needs, health histories, genetics, patterns of living, and exposures to a variety of toxic substances. As time goes on, life presents each of us with new and different health challenges. Of greatest benefit would be a program that does not neglect any of the basic principles of healthy living:

a. nutrient-dense organic foods and quality supplementation
b. regular exercise
c. exposure to sunshine and fresh air
d. pure water
e. satisfying work
f. adequate rest and relaxation
g. proper sleep
h. effective management of stress
i. effective healing from emotional traumas
j. humor and laughter
k. feeding the spirit
l. periodic cleansing

A natural health approach is true prevention. It's about not needing to rent space in the doctor's waiting room. Instead, it makes us aware that responsibility rests with each of us individually to take excellent care of ourselves—yes, each and every day. Awareness acquired through an education and understanding of natural healing along with enthusiastic follow-through is a major part of a life of health, happiness, and real purpose.

Skilled direction goes a long way to bring about improvement where these areas of life need some tweaking. As in nature, balance is important. Our approach to health and healing must be balanced, taking into consideration all the aforesaid aspects. Leaving any one out would probably have us miss our goal of good health.

Natural health, qualified, should make good sense. After all, it is in harmony with life itself and all that seeks to perpetuate it. All we need do to begin is have the desire for better health and start asking questions of professionals in the natural health field.

About the Author

Susanne Morrone, CNC, grew up on a small farm in rural Pennsylvania amid a menagerie of domestic and wild animals. These early years were character building as they helped cultivate a deep appreciation for nature. She was later lured to the big city with a promising career in advertising and public relations. Creative writing became a passion, and she enjoyed publishing newsletters and working as assistant editor of a nationally distributed company magazine. Her career soon shifted to the medical field, and her experience helped her refocus on the importance of good health and serving others. Susanne graduated from Clayton College of Natural Health with a degree in holistic nutrition. She is the author of *The Best Little Health Book Ever* (Llumina Press, 2004). She can be reached by e-mail at naturalhealthchat@yahoo.com. For more information, visit her Web site at http://www.naturalhealthchat.com.

67

How to Control and Manage Stress and Stress-Related Conditions

D. Andrew Neville, ND

There is no denying that many of the chronic ailments people suffer from today are worsened by (or even directly caused by) stress. This has been demonstrated in doctors' offices for decades as well as being discussed in the media and in medical conferences and confirmed by medical research. Illnesses such as anxiety, depression, heart disease, cancer, multiple sclerosis, chronic fatigue syndrome, and fibromyalgia all have connections to stressors we are exposed to in our lives. If we know this to be true, why then don't more doctors (and their patients) pay more attention to stress itself?

Although many physicians tell patients that stress is merely in their heads, true stress and our response to it is a full-body phenomenon, from the immune system to digestion to hormones to neurological function and all points in between. In particular, people who are more sensitive to stress generally need only some type of added stimulus (the straw that breaks the camel's back, if you will) to finally trigger the symptoms (a normal biological response) of whatever their particular chronic illness may be. This stress can be of any nature, not just emotional, and is certainly not just "all in our heads." Some examples include the physical stress of an automobile accident, a physical trauma, a virus, the energy expenditure of caring for an ailing parent, the mental stress of an exam or large project at work, or a true emotional stressor like a death in the family, divorce, or abuse of some kind. No matter what the cause, the response to all these stressors has one thing in common: the adrenal glands.

The adrenals are small glands that sit on top of your kidneys and function as part of your hormone system. These relatively unheard of glands have the incredible job, in conjunction with the hypothalamus and pituitary gland in the brain, of determining how we handle any stress in our lives. When presented with a stressor, whether concrete or perceived, the adrenals are automatically stimulated by the nervous system to release the stress hormones cortisol, epinephrine, and norepinephrine. These hormones have a global effect on the organs and tissues of the body, resulting in modulation of our blood sugar, inflammation and the immune response, cardiovascular tone, digestive function, and even the construction and breakdown of our muscles and connective tissue.

To get an idea of what it's like when the adrenals are vigorously stimulated, picture your immediate response to speaking in public or getting cut off in traffic. Feel the blood rushing to your muscles and heart as your eyes dilate, your pores open with sweat, and your breathing and heart rate quicken—you are now experiencing fight or flight. This is the stress response. At this point you are, in effect, set either to run away from or to try to kill the proverbial tiger. The problem is that there are far too many "tigers" (stresses and demands) in society today—our jobs and bosses, families, schedules, children's schedules, gas prices, politics, and what kind of protein, fat, and carbohydrate (if any at all) is okay for dinner. It is precisely this combination of an inability to adapt to constant overstimulation of the adrenal glands and the adrenals far-reaching influence over the body's systems that make them the common denominator in the various illnesses experienced by so many patients.

Signs and symptoms of weakened adrenal glands include (but are in no way limited to) fatigue, pain, frequent colds, allergy, headaches, irritable bowel, low (or high) blood pressure, lightheadedness, anxiety, panic attacks, insomnia, poor blood sugar control, "brain fog," and a multitude of other hormone-related imbalances such as PMS, menopausal complaints, low libido, hypothyroidism . . . and the list goes on. Any of this sound like anyone you know? If so, then he needs to be evaluated for adrenal dysfunction and will more than likely need to find ways to both reduce and better cope with his stress. A simple salivary hormone test, available online, that can be done at home has been shown to provide an accurate assessment of adrenal hormone status.

The bottom line is that too much stress weakens adrenal function, which may lead to a myriad of symptoms. Can we as doctors and patients do something about this? The answer is a resounding *yes!*

The first and foremost way to strengthen adrenal function is to reduce stress. The bottom line is that we have choices in life, and the trouble is that we are choosing to make our lives more stressful than they need to be. The reduction of stress starts with the recognition of the various stressors in our world; it is only then that we can begin to deal with them. This requires work and effort, but the fruits of this labor include a greater sense of health, balance, energy, love, satisfaction, and well-being.

One of the major stressors that we have in society today is a poor diet. Proper diet and nutrition starts with proper prenatal nutrition, which is currently inadequate; continues through breast-feeding, which we've been told is not all that important because it can be replaced by formula; and continues on throughout life with the often appalling choices of what we call food. The quality of our current food supply and eating habits is, to put it quite simply, abysmal and beyond the scope of this article.

One of the major tenets in naturopathic medicine is that we must follow the laws of nature. These laws are undeniable—if you don't believe this, put down this article, decide not to be subjected to the law of gravity, and see how you fare. Nature provides us with high-quality, nutrient-dense, nourishing foods from the earth. This is what is required to truly build our bodies, our minds, and our spirits. What we don't need is so-called food created in a chemist's lab from genetically modified seed, farmed in nutritionally deplete soils laden with so-called safe pesticides and chemicals—food that has been stripped down (i.e., "enriched") to make it last longer on the shelf or food that has been manipulated to be "low-fat," "low-carb," or "sugar-free." Sounds not only delicious, but nutritious, right?

We need to shift from blindly accepting that everything in the supermarket is good for us and from eating for purposes other than nutrition to eating to nourish our entire beings. Specific to adrenal patients is the necessity for a blood sugar–balancing diet, the principles of which are relatively simple. Eat small, frequent meals of whole foods, eat protein and fiber with each meal, eat only whole grains, and avoid refined carbohydrates such as most breads, pastas, and potatoes as well as sugar-laden foods like cakes, cookies, and most processed foods. This may be easy to say but can be a lot less easy to put into daily practice. However, if *we* control our blood sugar (and nutritional status) with our diets, then our adrenals have just one less thing to do. And in a world of constant, unavoidable stress, we have to pick our battles by focusing on those stressors that we *can* control.

Another crucial aspect of stress reduction is balance—in all things. Our lives are too hectic and busy and often too overscheduled and demanding. We work too much and play too little. To survive this life, we must make time for ourselves and our families, we must find quiet and peace, and we must find balance. There are many ways for us to bring about this balance: from deep breathing and prayer, to meditation and massage, to walking and exercise. This is essential if we are to heal ourselves for the long term. Balance is possible if we prioritize it and focus on it.

In addition to lifestyle modification and dietary changes, there are certainly nutritional supplements, vitamins, and herbs that can be utilized to supplement these core changes in our lives, but these things must only be used *in addition to* these other very fundamental changes if we want to avoid the ongoing cycle of transient improvements followed by relapses when the next stressor presents itself.

About the Author

D. Andrew Neville, ND, trained as a naturopathic physician at Bastyr University in Seattle, Washington, prior to undertaking a residency with Dr. Gerald Poesnecker, a pioneer in the treatment of chronic fatigue syndrome and adrenal weakness. He now focuses his entire practice on helping people with this debilitating yet largely unrecognized condition. He practices at Clymer Healing Center in beautiful Bucks County, Pennsylvania, in an integrated medical setting. He is a member of the International Association of Chronic Fatigue Syndrome, the CFIDS Association of America, and the Weston A. Price Foundation. As a board member of the Pennsylvania Association of Naturopathic Physicians, he is active in pursuing state licensing efforts for trained naturopathic physicians to ensure freedom of choice to all qualified health care providers.

68

The Mouth-Body Connection:
Oral Health Equals Body Health

Ellie Phillips, DDS

Oral Health Impacts General Health

Bacteria in plaque around teeth are related to the plaque in blood vessels that can cause high blood pressure, heart disease, and risk for stroke. Pregnant women with gum infections may be seven times more likely to have a baby born prematurely, and there is a well-recognized link between diabetes and gum disease. Every dentist knows the association of chronic ear infections with gastric reflux and how stomach acids will destroy teeth, both young and old.

Studies show that over one third of working Americans having long-term relationships with their dentists, yet the surgeon general's report of 2001 indicates that almost all American adults have dental disease. Despite insurance coverage and regular visits, one out of five people rate their oral health as fair or poor.

Oral Care Products

Unfortunately, many oral care products contain harsh chemicals that damage teeth, even though they may claim to help you. Plaque control or whitening ingredients often make teeth porous and sensitive. Sorbitol, an artificial sweetener in many sugar-free products, may actually thicken plaque bacteria. A recent study shows that almost a quarter of young people aged eighteen to thirty-four have gum disease and say that their teeth hurt when they drink hot or cold beverages.

Patients are blamed for poor flossing or missed dental visits and mistakenly assume that teeth automatically become sensitive, that fillings need repair, or that problems are inherited. None of these are true facts. Sensitivity and soft or weak teeth are always associated with either or both of the following factors: a dry or acidic mouth.

Dental Disease: A Progressive, Destructive Disease

Women in their forties frequently experience hormonal changes that make their mouths drier and more acidic. A dry mouth is like an engine motor without oil, and in an acidic mouth, teeth become vulnerable to wear and breakage. Without the cleansing action of healthy saliva, food and drinks can create conditions that encourage harmful bacteria to flourish.

Mouth acidity dissolves minerals from tooth enamel, making it more porous, more likely to stain, and sensitive to hot and cold. Weak enamel easily flakes away, forming a groove at the gum line or around the edges of fillings. Damaged enamel allows liquids to leak underneath fillings, irritating the nerves inside teeth and setting up infection. Sensitivity, broken fillings, and bad breath are the symptoms of these problems that can lead to root canals, crowns, and gum surgery.

Men with dry or acidic mouths will find that their teeth become brittle and start to wear away. Even after complicated repairs, their gum disease, tartar buildup, and bad breath will continue, and no amount of flossing or dental cleanings will prevent it.

The solution to these painful and expensive problems is twofold: we must (1) stimulate natural tooth repair and (2) protect teeth from dryness and mouth acidity.

Stimulating Natural Tooth Repair

In a moist and healthy mouth, natural tooth repair and healing occur rapidly. Minerals deposit into teeth to keep them strong, supple, and resilient. Even damaged teeth and early cavities can repair themselves if they are bathed in alkaline and mineral-rich saliva.

I suggest finishing meals and snacks with an alkaline or mineral-rich food such as celery, fresh apples, nuts, or dairy products. Evian and Fiji mineral waters create healthy alkaline conditions for tooth repair, as do dairy products and carrot or vegetable juices.

Possibly the easiest way to promote natural tooth repair and protect teeth is to eat a few xylitol mints or gum after every meal, snack, or drink.

Xylitol

Xylitol has been recognized for decades as a safe, delicious, diabetic-friendly sweetener and sugar substitute. Xylitol is found naturally in fruits and vegetables and notably the woody fibers of birch trees. The dental benefit of xylitol is that it stimulates a flow of healthy alkaline saliva into the mouth and also progressively eliminates harmful bacteria to prevent the formation of plaque.

Regular consumption of about six grams of xylitol a day gives dental benefits. Xylitol mints and gum are available on the Internet and in health stores. Unfortunately, some commercial gums, such as Trident, advertise xylitol on the package but contain such small amounts they would be inadequate for tooth healing. Look for xylitol as a main ingredient, and ideally choose 100 percent xylitol products.

Following is a calendar of expected events when you eat xylitol regularly. In four weeks,

- your teeth will feel smoother
- less plaque will build on and around your teeth
- your teeth will feel more comfortable and less sensitive.

In six months,

- most harmful bacteria will have vanished from your saliva and mouth
- people may notice that your teeth are shinier
- your dentist may congratulate you on your oral health.

In one year,

- you may need fewer dental cleanings.

Complete Oral Health

Besides eating xylitol, it is important to select your oral care products carefully and ensure that their chemistry is in harmony with natural healing. Remember that acidic foods and drinks soften teeth, especially if consumed before tooth brushing. An alkaline or balanced prerinse removes mouth acidity to help protect teeth from toothbrush wear or abrasion.

I recommend a sequence of three rinses, used in this specific order:

- a pH-balanced prerinse called Closys, which prepares teeth for brushing
- a simple toothpaste used with a clean, well-designed tooth brush
- an effective antiseptic formulated with essential oils such as Listerine, which prevents early gum disease
- a protective finishing rinse such as ACT fluoride, which gives teeth strength and shine. For those who refuse all fluoride products, I would substitute a xylitol rinse for ACT.

This three-rinse system should be used every night before sleeping and again during the day, if possible. It should be combined with xylitol after all meals and snacks.

This balanced oral care program will allow natural protection and repair to give you the oral health you have dreamed of. No matter what your age or your past experiences with dental disease, try this easy system and enjoy clean, bright, and healthy teeth.

Bibliography

Featherstone, J. D., "The Caries Balance: The Basis for Caries Management by Risk Assessment," *Oral Health and Preventive Dentistry* 2 (2004): 259–64.

Geerts S. O., M. Nys, P. De Mol, J. Charpentier, A. Albert, V. Legrand, and E. H. Rompen, "Systemic Release of Endotoxins Induced by Gentle Mastication: Association with Periodontitis Severity," *Journal of Periodontology* 73 (2002): 73–78.

Hogg, S. D., and A. J. Rugg-Gunn, "Can the Oral Flora Adapt to Sorbitol?" *Journal of Dentistry* 19 (1991): 263–71.

Jeffcoat, M. K., J. C. Hauth, and N. C. Geurs, "Periodontal Disease and Pre-term Birth: Results of a Pilot Intervention Study." *Journal of Dental Research* 82 (2003): 1214–18.

Mealey, B. L., and T. W. Oates, "Diabetes Mellitus and Periodontal Disease," *Journal of Periodontology* 77 (2006): 1289–1303.

Milgrom, P., K. A. Ly, M. C. Roberts, M. Rothern, G. Mueller, and D. K. Yamaguchi, "Mutans Streptococci Dose Response to Xylitol Chewing Gum." *Journal of Dental Research* 85 (2006): 177–81.

Nieuw Amerongen, A. V., and E. C. I. Veerman. "Saliva—The Defender of the Oral Cavity." *Oral Diseases* 8 (2002): 12–22.

Tweetman, S., L. G. Petersson, and S. Axelsson, "Caries-Preventive Effect of Sodium Fluoride Mouth Rinses: A Systematic Review of Controlled Clinical Trials." *Acta Odontologica Scandinavica* 62 (2004): 230–33.

About the Author

Ellie Phillips, DDS, is a member of the American Dental Association, American Academy of Pediatric Dentistry and Honorary Member of the Eastman Institute London, England. She has graduate specialties in General and Pediatric Dentistry from Eastman Dental Center, Rochester New York. She has been in Private Practice and a Faculty member of the University of Rochester and Outpatient Clinic Director of the Eastman Dental Center.

Dr. Ellie has worked in the United Kingdom, Switzerland, and the United States. Dr. Ellie lectures to the public and has helped mothers, schoolchildren, and health professionals see dentistry in a new light and tooth decay as a preventable disease. Dr. Ellie has been an outspoken advocate for xylitol in an otherwise quiet dental community. Her book *The Power of Xylitol* and her children's book *My Friend Zellie* are some of the first written on the subject of xylitol for dental prevention. Online or telephone consultations about dental prevention may be scheduled through her Web site http://www.CleanWhiteTeeth.com. For more information about xylitol, please visit http://www.Zellies.com.

69

Referred Pain and Trigger Point Therapy

Paul Svacina, PE, LMT

Human Physiology versus Modern Living

Human bodies have not changed much in the past 10,000 years; however, during the last 150 years, we have greatly changed our lifestyles. Our bodies deal with new chemicals, sleep habits, physical tasks, indoor lighting, noise, and other unnatural stimulation. The increase of psychological stress, repetitive tasks, and decrease of physical activity in modern lives has contributed to chronic pain.

It is difficult to change a lifestyle, but trigger point therapy can be used to reduce or eliminate the source of various types of pain, without drugs or surgery.

Pain Can Be Tricky

The Centers for Disease Control and Prevention reported in 2006 that over 25 percent of Americans aged twenty and older report pain lasting over twenty-four hours. The *Annals of Internal Medicine* reported that twenty-five billion dollars per year was spent in search of low back pain relief in 2003.

Typical allopathic treatments for pain are medications, cortisone, and surgery. For many patients, surgery provides welcome relief, at least temporarily, from sciatica, carpal tunnel syndrome, and other mechanical and pathophysiologic problems. However, symptoms mimicking such problems can be caused by trigger points, which surgery does not improve.

In general, trigger points frequently remain overlooked, unrecognized, and untreated. After a back injury, medication was prescribed for me for a year with little relief. Then I visited another medical doctor who, in one session, removed my pain using manual therapy. He explained that my pain was referred from the actual problem areas.

Referred Pain

Referred pain is sensed in an area away from the actual pain source. Examples of referred pain are headaches, phantom limb pain in amputated limbs, pain down the left arm during a heart attack, and the infamous so-called brain freeze caused by drinking cold liquid, which cools the vagus nerve running along the throat. During a brain freeze, one may feel it in the head, when the cause may be down the throat.

Pain referral is also common in myofascial pain syndromes, which are caused by trigger points in muscle, fascia (fibrous tissue that connects, separates, and supports muscles, bones, skin, and other organs), tendon, and ligament tissue. These trigger points are among the most common causes of chronic pain.

Trigger Points

A trigger point can be thought of as a muscle protection mechanism, which stiffens the muscle in order to limit range of motion, triggered by injury, overuse, and adrenaline—all phenomena in which modern humans excel. Resultant stiffening or spasms of muscles cause blood stagnation, nutrient loss, and buildup of toxins. Such protection can become chronic and painful and can activate other trigger points, spreading pain and disability like an infection.

Postural muscles, as in the neck, shoulders, back, and pelvic girdle, and others, such as forearms, hands, calves, and face, that are used in repetitive actions are most vulnerable to trigger points. Trigger points may cause headaches (tension and migraine), temporomandibular joint pain, sciatica, and apparent carpal tunnel syndrome and can be associated with burning, numbness, weakness, temperature, sweating, dryness, dizziness, nausea, tinnitus, vision, decreased range of motion, and other problems. Since trigger point syndromes are unfamiliar to many physicians, these familiar symptoms can make diagnosis difficult.

Sedentary people and those, such as computer operators, dentists, drivers, and specialized athletes, who hold unnatural positions or perform repetitive tasks are at high risk of developing active trigger points. After sitting at a desk, running or a gym workout may seem to make up for the sedentary time, but it actually may promote the pain and dysfunction. Rigid use then overuse is not the best.

Most trigger points are reduced or deactivated by acupuncture, electric stimulation, or injections. Fortunately, trigger points also respond to manual therapy.

Trigger Point History

Some researchers think that many trigger points and acupuncture points overlap. Hence trigger point therapy was accomplished by acupuncture thousands of years ago in China and other parts of the world. In the seventh-century book *A Thousand Golden Remedies*, Sun Su-Miao (Si miao) described "ah-shi" tender points—most probably trigger points.

In the 1940s, trigger points were first clearly described and mapped by Janet G. Travell, MD, who eased John F. Kennedy's pain in 1955, allowing him to run for president. Dr. Travell then served as the personal physician for both presidents Kennedy and Johnson. Drs. Travell and David Simons later wrote the seminal text on Trigger Point Therapy: *Myofascial Pain and Dysfunction: The Trigger Point Manual.*

Although sixty years of medical research has shown that trigger point therapy relieves pain, the medical community has been slow to promote this therapy. Doctors who do treat trigger points inject steroids, local anesthetics, carbon dioxide, dextrose, Botox®, Myox™, and even muscle relaxants to disarm trigger points, and such injections have been covered by U.S. medical insurance since 2005.

Manual Trigger Point Therapy

In Europe, manual approaches are used by myoskeletal medical doctors and practitioners. In the United States, physical therapists use spray and stretch techniques, which numb the skin, interfering with pain conduction, allowing stretching to release trigger points. Also, massage therapists use direct pressure by hand, foot, or tool.

The simplest and least invasive method of trigger point therapy involves manually locating the trigger point, which may feel like a pea or knot, and pressing or holding firmly, using thumb and finger, for fifteen seconds or more. Elbows and feet may also be used, as in barefoot deep tissue therapy. Best of all, this modality can be incorporated into a Swedish, barefoot, deep tissue, or other type of massage, whether the client is clothed or not.

Trigger point referral patterns in muscles have been thoroughly mapped; for example, temple headaches are most often caused by trigger points in the temporalis or upper trapezius. So when a patient complains of a temple headache, the therapist knows, or looks up, which points on which muscles harbor this referred pain. When manual pressure is applied to the correct point, the pain will temporarily increase, and then fade.

Many massage schools now teach manual trigger point therapy, and popular lay books have been written that can prove extremely useful for self-help.

Self-Massage

For self-treatment, a tennis ball may be placed inside a sock and dropped over the shoulder between the shoulder blades and pressed against a wall into tender spots for fifteen seconds or so, whether or not "good" pain decreases. This can be done several times a day. For more force, or for gluteal areas, one can lie on the floor or use a harder ball. Several tools are available to aid self-treatment.

Not all pain is caused by trigger points, so if one to three therapy visits do not produce relief, then referral to a licensed health specialist is recommended.

Conclusion

Over the last hundred years, Western medicine has been straying from manual therapies to drugs, surgery, and other invasive treatments.

Manual trigger point therapy is a noninvasive method for relieving many types of pain. It may be used by doctors as well as massage therapists, and even by patients themselves, to help reach the goal of a pain-free body.

To find a trigger point therapist near you, ask your doctor, physical therapist, or local massage school.

About the Author

Paul Svacina, BS, PE, LMT, has a BS in aerospace engineering from Texas A&M University and learned bodywork and health sciences in Europe and the United States, most recently at the Santa Barbara Body Therapy Institute, and with John Harris, Olympic therapist and coauthor of *Fix Pain – Bodywork Protocols for Myofascial Pain Syndromes,* explaining treatments for trigger points and sports injuries. Paul specializes in trigger point therapy, barefoot deep tissue massage, and myofascial release. For more information and resources about trigger point therapy, visit Paul Svacina's websites at http://trisoma.com or http://santabarbarabodytherapy.com.

70

Deep Cleaning:
Letting Go and Becoming New with Colon Hydrotherapy

Dr. Carlos M. Viana

Modern Living versus Human Physiology

W e clean our clothes, skin, houses, and cars, but what about our insides? Natural physicians will tell you, "Old age starts in the colon." And certainly, colon toxicity underlies many commonly reported health problems—not only constipation, diarrhea, gas, bloating, and irritable bowel syndrome, but also back pain, PMS, skin conditions, weight gain, insomnia, hypertension, headaches, arthritis, bad breath, asthma, allergies, fatigue, and depression. Americans spend more than four hundred million dollars on laxatives each year, treating symptoms rather than the underlying cause. In 2006 alone, 130,000 new cases of colon and rectal cancer were diagnosed in the United States, making it the fourth most common form of cancer among Americans.

As a treatment and preventative measure, we introduced colon hydrotherapy in our clinic in the Caribbean nation of Aruba, where for the past decade, this natural procedure has effected small miracles. Patients once ill and despondent excitedly report, in addition to relief from the symptoms that plagued them, renewed vigor and vitality, softer and more radiant skin, increased sex drive, mental clarity, and even a sense of emotional and spiritual well-being.

What Does the Colon Do?

The physical purpose of the colon is to separate the pure from the not pure. A major organ of elimination, along with the lungs and skin, the colon absorbs water, electrolytes, and nutrients from digested matter passing through the small intestine; it then expels the waste. Traditional Chinese medicine recognizes that each organ of the body also has an *emotional* purpose, and the colon's is, not surprisingly, letting go of old stuff. Never have I treated someone with an unhealthy colon who was not also grappling with old, obstructing patterns. Colon hydrotherapy works deeply to heal not only physical ailments, but emotional and even spiritual blockages, too.

What Is Colon Hydrotherapy?

Also known as colon irrigation or colonics, colon hydrotherapy was first recorded in 1550 b.c.e. in the Ebers Papyrus, an ancient Egyptian medical text. A popular form of treatment in the 1930s and 1940s, it is making a comeback among natural physicians today.

Colon hydrotherapy cleanses the large intestine above the rectum all the way to the cecum, on the lower right side of the abdomen. The client lies comfortably on his or her back or side while the therapist gently infuses warm, filtered water into the rectum through a tube attached to the colonics machine. As the water flows through the colon, it removes excess gas, mucus, and hardened fecal matter. Free of chemicals, the procedure is safe, clean, and comfortable. A typical session takes about forty-five minutes, during which clients often become so deeply relaxed that they "let it all go" and "start anew." Multiple sessions over several weeks are often recommended to rebuild optimal colon health.

Is Colon Hydrotherapy Safe and Effective?

The medical term for this procedure is *colon lavage*, which literally means a washing out of the colon with infusions of water or a medicated solution, a practice researchers worldwide[1] have found to be both safe and effective. British researchers report that "on-table lavage of the colon" is "an effective method" enabling surgeons to perform operations "with reasonable safety."[2] A team of Italian surgeons have deemed colon lavage safer than operating on the colon in the event of obstruction.[3] Physicians in Germany using saline solutions to expand the colon for sonography as well as physicians in Japan using saline irrigation pumped through an endotracheal tube to clear impacted feces have determined that the technique is

---

[1] As of this writing, a search of PubMed alone reveals 905 citations on various aspects of colon lavage.

[2] N. M. Koruth Z., H. Krukowski, G. G. Youngson, W. S. Hendry, J. R. C. Logie, P. F. Jones, and A. Munro, "Intra-operative Colonic Irrigation in the Management of Left-Sided Large Bowel Emergencies," *British Journal of Surgery* 72 (September 1985): 708–11.

[3] P. Fabiani and F. Maghetti, "Intraoperative Anterograde Lavage of the Occluded Left Colon," *Annali Italiani di Chirurgia* 67 (1996): 171–75.

useful and effective.[4] This past year, in the United States, federal health agencies (the National Institutes of Health, the National Cancer Institute, and the Food and Drug Administration) concluded that coffee enemas, found previously to be 20 percent as effective as colon hydrotherapy in ensuring colon health,[5] are "harmless."[6]

How Does the Colon Become Unhealthy?

An unclean, weak, or impaired colon is a breeding ground for disease. The culprits are mainly a combination of poor diet, dehydration, limited exercise, and accumulated toxins. The standard American/Aruban diet (SAD) of refined, processed foods high in saturated fats, sugar, flour, and preservatives and low in fiber kills healthy bacteria in the bowels, paving the way for intestinal parasites. What's more, highly refined foods are difficult to digest, and undigested as well as partially chewed food, along with environmental toxins such as heavy metals, stagnate in the colon. Over time, the accumulation of old, hardened feces sticks to the walls of the colon, inhibiting its ability to absorb nutrients. At this point, it is forced instead to absorb toxins from the fecal buildup and fight off the parasites that have been feeding on it.

But the problem doesn't stop there. The toxins and parasites soon pass into the circulatory system, which then distributes them throughout the body. When these poisons accumulate in the nervous system, we feel irritable and depressed. When they back up into the heart, we feel weak, and when they reach the stomach, bloated. If they contact the lungs, our breath will turn foul. If they try to escape through the skin, rashes, blotches, or acne may develop, or our skin might turn pale and wrinkly, adding years to our appearance. Should the toxins and parasites make it to the glands, we will feel fatigued and lethargic, so much so that our sex drive may cease.

What Are the Signs of an Unhealthy Colon?

The colon signals its distress through many easily identifiable symptoms. The most common symptom is chronic constipation. Contrary to accepted medical

---

[4] Franklin Greif, Alexander Belenky, David Aranovich, Igal Yampolski, and Nisim Hannanel, "Intraoperative Ultrasonography: A Tool for Localizing Small Colonic Polyps," *International Journal of Colorectal Disease* 20 (2005): 502–6; and M. Shimotsuma, T. Takahashi, T. Yamane, A. Noguchi, and T. Sakakibara, "Intraoperative Cleansing of the Impacted Colon Using an Endotracheal Tube," *Diseases of the Colon and Rectum* 33 (1990): 241–42.

[5] Gar Hildenbrand, "A Bottoms-Up Summary of Past and Recent Impressions Regarding Coffee Enemas," *Townsend Letter* (August/September 2006): 78–82.

[6] Ibid.

standards, a bowel movement every few days is not normal; the digestive system is designed to eliminate waste daily, with no straining. Other telltale signs are excessive gas, bloating, burping, and an uncomfortable fullness after eating. Physical appearance, too, can give clues such as poor skin tone or blemishes; dry, drab hair; or a distended belly. Additional indicators include mood swings, fatigue, depression, irritability, low energy, PMS, and insomnia. Another outcome is congestion. The malodorous chemicals the compromised colon produces, aptly named cadaverine and putrescine, stimulate mucus production in the sinuses, which can result in headaches, frequent colds, sinus infections, allergies, or food intolerances—all of which signal an unhealthy colon.

How Can I Keep My Colon Healthy?

In addition to getting regular colonic treatments, following are some easy ways to rebuild and maintain colon health:

1. Drink plenty of filtered water every day, preferably half your body weight in ounces.
2. Eat brown rice daily, a food rich in B vitamins.
3. Take a magnesium capsule to hydrate the intestinal tract and liberate oxygen, which encourages the growth of healthy (aerobic) bacteria, while inhibiting the proliferation of unhealthy (anaerobic) bacteria and fungi.
4. Take probiotics, friendly microscopic organisms that enhance digestion and aid the absorption of nutrients.
5. Control Candida—a yeast-like parasitic fungus that can cause thrush in the mouth, vagina, or intestinal tract—through diet and supplements. Ask your health practitioner for recommendations.
6. Exercise to the level of your ability.
7. Practice releasing old patterns and embracing new ones.

Think of colon hydrotherapy as a deep cleaning of the house (some would say temple) that is your body. It flushes away bowel toxicities, reducing the burden on the liver. Simultaneously, it hydrates the body, cooling the fire of inflammation. It also removes excess yeast and rids the intestines of dangerous parasites. Ultimately, it helps you eliminate old stuff, both physical and emotional. More than a highly effective treatment for a variety of ailments, colon hydrotherapy is a pathway to vibrant health.

About the Author

Dr. Carlos M. Viana, known internationally as the barefoot doctor of Aruba, founded and directs the Viana Natural Healing Center, the island's only medical provider outside the socialized health care system. An Oriental Medical Doctor, Certified Clinical Nutritionist, certified addiction professional, and age management specialist as well as a colon therapist and colon therapy instructor, Viana views chronic inflammation due to long-standing acidity as the foundation of all degenerative illness. His comprehensive treatment modality, biocompatible medicine, combines the best of alternative and conventional care to guide people back to health. This integrative approach to healing is described in his book *Introduction to Biocompatible Medicine: A Holistic Protocol for Today's World* (Healing Spirit Press, 2008). Visit his Web site at http://www.viananaturalhealing.com.

PART SEVEN

Physical or Mental Disorders & Problems

Life always brings new challenges.
It's our response to these challenges
that enables us to thrive.

-- Dr. Joseph Cilea

71

Seven Ways I Fought My Daughter's Arthritis and Won

Amy Butler

At the tender age of seven years old, my daughter Cassandra was given the devastating news that she was suffering from a severe case of juvenile rheumatoid arthritis. I was shocked and unaware that arthritis afflicts 300,000 American children.[1]

Following more than a year of medical doctors, anti-inflammatory medications, and procedures without any significant improvement, I'd had enough. I immersed myself in finding answers. I've spent hundreds of hours researching medical and alternative therapies as well as the impact of diet and exercise.

To my delight, Cassandra has defied the odds! Just six months after beginning the steps I will outline below, her blood tests came back negative for arthritis! Considering that I was told she could potentially suffer from this disease for the rest of her life while experiencing stunted growth and possible deformity, I am ecstatic!

There are seven major steps I took through our journey. I did not find one Web site or person who detailed this plan for me, but through research and using my mother's intuition, these are the things that I chose to use. Although I cannot say which step or steps are the reason Cassandra is free from arthritis today, I can share with you what we did. I hope this will guide you in your journey to finding freedom for yourself or loved ones from ill health.

Research, Research, Research

Research is the first crucial step. If you asked me two years ago what the words *rheumatologist, JRA, hydrogenated oils,* and *homeopathy* meant, I would have answered "I'm not sure" for all of them. Cassandra's illness changed all of that, including my outlook on nutrition, health, and doctors.

After being told by her rheumatologist that she needed to be given an adult rheumatoid arthritis medication, Methotrexate, I began my quest for alternatives.

---

[1] Donald W. Miller Jr., "A user-friendly vaccination schedule," 2004, http://www.mercola.com/2004/dec/29/vaccination_schedule.htm.

The thought of giving my daughter's fifty-pound body a chemotherapy drug that, according to the clinical trials, may potentially cause liver damage and affect the reproductive system made me cringe.

Learning about autoimmune disease, proper nutrition, and alternative medicine online became my part-time job. I began simply by typing in arthritis and autoimmune diseases into a search engine. After months and months of reading, it became apparent to me that I wanted to heal Cassandra's autoimmune system, not just treat her arthritic symptoms. This led me to alternative medicine because treating the cause, not the symptoms, seemed to make more sense to me. Some reputable sites I found very helpful include Mercola.com, NaturalHealthWeb.com, and HealingWithNutrition.com.

Although a large percentage of my research was done via the Internet, it did not stop there. I asked anyone—family members, friends, and hairdresser—really, anyone I came in contact with, if they had ever tried something for an illness that had worked. I would take any information I received and research it.

Nutrition

Nutrition is, in my opinion, the most important for a lifetime of good health. Although I am a college graduate and a dedicated mother, I was very uneducated when it came to nutrition and its effects on one's health. I fed Cassandra vegetables and fruit regularly and limited the amount of candy and junk food she ate, or so I thought. I learned that this was not nearly enough.

Most likely, you are unaware of the unhealthy ingredients you are consuming—I sure was. My education on nutrition began when a friend, who was studying to become a research scientist, had a child. She had a book sitting in her kitchen called *Super Baby Food* by Ruth Yaron. In light of Cassandra's health, my friend urged me to read it.

Although the book is intended for new mothers wanting to provide proper nutrition to infants, I found it enlightening for people of all ages. Ms. Yaron thoroughly covers every aspect of eating properly, from shopping for food, to reading labels, to knowing what ingredients to look for (and which to avoid, and why), to kid-friendly recipes.

My first trip to the grocery store after reading the book took two hours, and I left without buying a thing. When I read the ingredients on every loaf of bread I picked up, I found that only a few, if any, contained whole grains, but rather, they were filled with toxic substances such as high-fructose corn syrup, sugar, hydrogenated oils, and so on. This also applies to just about every snack food that children typically eat, for example, Goldfish, pretzels, peanut butter, milk, and so on. Now I only shop at health food stores, and I still read labels even there.

To my surprise, one evening, after eating lentil pasta with organic spaghetti sauce and broccoli, Cassandra turned to me and said, "Mommy, I feel better when I eat organic." From the mouth of babes!

It was like learning how to shop and cook all over again. Throwing out a whole dish of macaroni and cheese because it tasted awful, a box of sesame sticks because she didn't like them, and doubling the amount of time and money on food took patience. However, I believe that this was the most important part of Cassandra's success. By the way, don't try to use lentil pasta to make your own baked macaroni and cheese—it's awful!

Supplements

Supplements are also an essential part of a healthy diet. Pesticides, overworked soil, and extended time from harvest to consumption are a few of the reasons to supplement. The most important factor in determining what products to choose is bioavailability. This is your body's ability to absorb what you are taking. When you consume supplements from a whole food source that is free of fillers and flowing agents, this can happen.

Again, I learned all of this information from reading alternative health magazines and online articles as well as by asking people about their personal experiences. After learning about all of the awful ingredients in the food I had been consuming, I assumed that all supplements were not created equal. It was daunting at times sifting through promotional jargon to figure out which products were the best. Following what I had learned about food, I chose supplements that were from a whole food source, organic, and free of preservatives.

Some of the essential products that I used to improve Cassandra's health included probiotics, digestive enzymes, green foods, minerals, and omega-3 fatty acids. All of these supplements help the body function properly; therefore it is able to maintain balanced pH levels and in turn reduce inflammation.

Chiropractic Care

Chiropractic goes far beyond simply alleviating back and neck pain, which was a surprise to me. I had sought out a chiropractor prior to Cassandra's illness for back pain from multiple car accidents earlier in life. After trying two others, we were lucky to find a chiropractor, Dr. Janet McGaurn of West Chester, Pennsylvania, who adapts her approach to each client's needs. I personally felt more comfortable with her soft touch approach that did not involve any jerking or snapping of the neck. Cassandra looked forward to her appointments because she felt immediate relief from some of her pain.

Chiropractic care is an essential part of maintaining optimal health. Aside from direct trauma, science has discovered a major interference to our system of nerves called *vertebral subluxation*. This is a mechanical problem in the spine that reduces a person's ability to heal, regulate, and express well-being.[2] Chiropractors are the only professionals trained in the detection and correction of this problem.

In addition to the care she provided, Dr. McGaurn offered her knowledge of disease and treating it naturally. When I spoke with her about my quest to treat Cassandra's illness without pharmaceutical drugs, she referred me to a homeopathic doctor that she had personally seen for over twenty years. Trusting her, I was able to try more confidently another alternative approach I knew nothing about.

Homeopathy

Homeopathy is an alternative medical approach that believes in stimulating the body's own innate healing mechanisms. We had to wait a month in between remedies, the name given to their medicines, which are natural forms of an extremely diluted amount of substances that would cause illness in a healthy person.

The first three times we went, we saw little to no results; however, we continued on. After the fourth visit, she had a breakthrough within three days. She attended physical therapy on a Friday afternoon, and her affected shoulder had not improved. Saturday morning, she saw the homeopath. Tuesday afternoon, at her physical therapy appointment, her therapist was shocked that she had full mobility back in her shoulder. All the muscular tension and knots were gone. It sold us both on homeopathy instantly!

Exercise

Exercise is one of the most important aspects of good health, and even more so if you have arthritis. This was advice that was consistently given to me from all medical and alternative medical professionals as well as being detailed in most online and health magazines.

The more active you are, the better you will probably feel. Non-impact workouts are best as to not put any undue stress on joints.

Cassandra swims and thoroughly enjoys it. It doesn't seem like exercise because it's fun. I found a yoga DVD for children that provides her with fun stretching and strengthening exercises that are very important. Also, she is in a karate class, which she resisted at first but has come to love.

---

[2] Christopher Kent, "Beyond bad backs: What chiropractic is and how it can help you," 2003, http://www.mercola.com/2003/nov/12/beyond_bad_backs.htm.

Reiki

Reiki is a Japanese term that is translated as "universal life-force energy." I had heard the word *reiki* before, but I found it hard to believe that without being touched, you could experience any relief from pain. As with all the methods I employed to help my daughter heal from arthritis, I tried them first. *Amazing* is the one word I would use to describe reiki. Cassandra agreed, and after one session would ask to go back because she felt so much better.

During a reiki session, a certified practitioner will place his or her hands over you at different points, depending on your needs. The practitioner channels healing energy to you. This can help facilitate healing from physical and emotional trauma.[3]

Cassandra is now a happy and healthy ten-year-old. When we first learned of her illness, I was distraught, questioning why this happened to her. Now we look at it as a blessing because we learned so much through this journey. Our whole family is healthier and happier than we've ever been. It has also given me a new passion, and I am planning to return to school to obtain a naturopathic medical degree. I hope to be able to help many more people heal.

So, know that you can cure illness naturally. It won't happen by itself; you'll need to give it your all, but I believe unequivocally that anything is possible. I've seen it with my own eyes. Best wishes to living a happy and healthy life!

About the Author

Amy Butler is a devoted mother and freelance writer. She is the co-owner of GreenLifeSaver.net, an online store where you can now purchase many of the supplements that she used to help aid in Cassandra's recovery from juvenile rheumatoid arthritis. Amy is dedicated to creating awareness about the potential life-altering benefits of natural living. If you have any questions about the supplements or any of the methods she spoke about, you can ask at ricamy@greenlifesaver.net.

---

[3] Learn more about reiki at http://www.heatherreiki.com.

72

Backpack Safety to Protect Spinal Health

Noah De Koyer, DC

Your daughter rolls out of bed to the sound of a blaring alarm and heads for the shower. She brushes her teeth, washes her face, dresses herself with the outfit you left out the night before, and heads downstairs for a piping hot bowl of oatmeal that her father just prepared for her. After breakfast, she grabs her backpack and jams her science and math textbooks inside, followed by her spelling workbook, lunch bag, and the makeup she is hiding from you. She slings the bag loosely over one shoulder, and off to school she goes. She has become accustomed to filling her bag with all the books she needs for the entire school day so as to avoid making several trips back to her locker. At the end of the day, she makes the trek back home with her backpack loosely slung over the same shoulder as it was for the morning commute.

Let's look at the above scenario in terms of this fictitious young girl's spine and nervous system. The straps pull down on her shoulders, placing a downward compression force on the spinal column. Depending on how heavy the bag is and how many straps are used, the bag will cause a slumped posture, a head that is jutting forward, and shoulder muscles that are working overtime to maintain some semblance of proper biomechanics. In our scenario, a bag worn on one shoulder consistently can cause a head tilt or rotation, unbalanced shoulders and hips, a winging of the shoulder blades, and/or rucksack palsy, which, in the most severe cases, can lead to permanent nerve damage. Early-onset spinal degeneration, disc herniations, vertebral subluxations or misalignments, abnormal curvatures of the spine, muscle imbalances, fatigue, and a decrease in health potential are more than a possibility. What can complicate this even further is if this child has an underlying neurologic or orthopedic condition such as a scoliosis, or the student is an athlete playing full-contact sports. I challenge you to look at your children, how heavy their backpacks are, their posture, and how these factors are affecting their performance in school and, more importantly, their health.

Current research points to the health of your spine and nervous system leading to long-term wellness. Let's examine how we can avoid any problems from improperly worn backpacks.

Backpack safety can be broken down into a few easy steps, with many of these ideas and recommendations coming from Dr. Marvin Arnsdorff, cofounder of Backpack Safety America/International. First and foremost, your child needs to choose the proper size bag. The proper size is approximately the space between your child's shoulder blades and waist. A disproportionately large bag will result in carrying too many unnecessary books, toys, and so on, while a too small bag will result in your son or daughter carrying too many objects in his or her hands, thus causing even greater balance and postural problems. Remember, nature abhors a vacuum, and it is likely that your student will fill his or her bag to capacity, whatever the size, so it is critical to have the right-sized bag.

Packing the bag is also very important and has two distinct areas of concern. First, a loaded backpack should not exceed 15 percent of your child's body weight. To accomplish this, your son or daughter may find it necessary to make a list of what is needed throughout each day to limit the amount of unnecessary cargo. If a backpack is too heavy, the wearer often has to lean forward to carry the bag or balance himself. Below is a 15 percent chart.

User's weight (lbs.)	Backpack weight (lbs.)
50	7.5
75	11.25
100	15
125	18.75

In addition, your child needs to be taught how to pack his or her bag, rather than simply shove belongings inside without any regard for safety. You should always pack the heaviest books nearest your back and the lightest books farthest away from your back. This will help avoid an excessive lean backward and help prevent tipping over. Also of concern are sharp objects such as scissors. These items should be kept in a special place, such as a small box or bag, designed to avoid harming the wearer or any passersby.

If parents and educators model proper lifting habits and teach children backpack safety at an early age, many childhood injuries and spinal conditions can be avoided. The first lesson students should be taught is to gently check the weight of their bags. The weight can certainly be deceiving simply by observing the bag, so your child should pick up the backpack slowly and cautiously, as he or she may be surprised with the weight of the contents. Your son or daughter should be facing the bag and use both hands to lift the bag up using his or her leg muscles. It is important to have your children realize that their leg muscles are infinitely stronger and less prone to injury than the lower back muscles, which most people erroneously use to lift objects. Any quick turning or twisting should also always be avoided when lifting anything.

The last step to proper backpack safety is wearing the bag in a manner that distributes its weight equally. Primarily, this means always using well-cushioned arm straps—all the time and without exception. While it may be more fashionable for your daughter to wear her bag hanging off one shoulder, this practice should always be avoided. I also suggest that parents look for bags that include a waist strap to provide the wearer with even more support. If your child has a bag with only one strap, make sure it is worn fully across the chest to evenly distribute the weight of the bag as much as possible. I typically do not recommend suitcase-style backpacks that are on rollers. These bags become very cumbersome when anyone has to carry them up flights of stairs, and a child is made to twist and torque the spine to pull the bag along. The only benefit of this type of bag is that on flat surfaces, the wheels cause the weight of the bag to become almost negligent.

Simple education and demonstrating the proper way to use and wear backpacks can have a huge impact on the health and vitality of your school-aged children. Not only is it important to teach our children the content in the books they carry, but also how to safely transport their materials between school and home each day.

If you suspect that your son or daughter may have some underlying condition, such as a scoliosis, or his or her posture has been getting progressively worse, first look to your child's backpack-wearing habits. The next step should be a visit to your chiropractor for a full evaluation. He or she will be able to determine whether conservative chiropractic care with some lifestyle changes will be able to correct the problems uncovered or if more aggressive steps need to be taken. Chiropractically maintained scoliosis or postural problems can save a young child a lifetime of pain, discomfort, lack of self-esteem, and ill health.

About the Author

Dr. Noah De Koyer graduated magna cum laude from Montclair State University in 1997 with a BS in biology and summa cum laude from Life University Chiropractic College in 2000, obtaining his DC degree. Dr. Noah has been practicing passionately in Bayonne, New Jersey, for the past six years. He is a certified Toastmaster and a member of the Association of New Jersey Chiropractors. Dr. Noah can be reached at (201) 437-0033 or at http://www.familychiropracticcenters.info for speaking engagements, consultations, or patient care.

73

Postpartum Emotional Health

Cheryl Jazzar, MHR

The period surrounding the birth of a child is a joy, but for many families, it can also be a time of concern. Changing roles and physical changes can leave both mothers and fathers feeling irritable, depressed, or unable to cope. Mood changes are the most common complications of pregnancy. Most new mothers will experience a disruption in their mood. In addition, it is estimated that 20 percent of pregnant women experience clinical depression.

Perinatal (occurring before and after birth) mood changes can fall within several distinct categories:

- *Prenatal depression.* Symptoms of depression interfere with the ability to perform life tasks such as working or caring for oneself or older children. This is a biochemical reaction to the increased demands for proper nutrition.

- *Baby blues.* Up to 80 percent of new mothers experience so-called baby blues within the first week of delivery. This condition *is not* a psychiatric disorder, and it passes within a few weeks. Mothers can become weepy, nervous, or dependent. Baby blues have been described as "normal crazy"—part of a reaction to rapid lifestyle and hormonal changes.

- *Postpartum anxiety reactions.* Postpartum anxiety is much more common than depression. Occurring any time during the first eighteen months, anxiety reactions can range from mild feelings of nervousness to panic attacks involving physical symptoms such as a racing heart, hot flashes, or sleep troubles. Emotional components may include feelings of loss of control, wanting to run away, extreme irritability or nervousness, or excessive worry. Postpartum posttraumatic stress disorder is an anxiety reaction that can occur due to past trauma or a negative birth experience.

- *Postpartum obsessive-compulsive disorder.* Intrusive, recurrent thoughts or behaviors characterize this disorder. In new mothers, this can include extreme worry over the baby's safety. Mothers may continually count or check things, hide or get rid of dangerous objects, or stay away from situations where they perceive threats.

The mother may imagine harm coming to the baby—sometimes at her own hand. In the case of postpartum obsessive-compulsive disorder, the mother is horrified at these thoughts, and so far, there has never been a report of actual harm taking place toward a baby. To the contrary, these mothers are typically overprotective.

- *Postpartum depression.* Depression can be experienced as a lack of energy, a loss of interest in life in general, or a lack of interest in the baby. New mothers can cry uncontrollably, lose or gain weight excessively, and lose the ability to concentrate or make simple decisions. Occurring any time in the first eighteen months postpartum, mothers may feel guilty or overwhelmed or fear that they are unworthy of their new role.

- *Postpartum psychosis.* Psychosis is a medical emergency requiring hospitalization. Five percent of new mothers experiencing psychosis commit suicide, and nearly as many commit infanticide. Women experiencing postpartum psychosis have lost touch with reality, and they should not be left to care for their children, even for a moment. These mothers may be profoundly confused and afraid, seeing things or hearing voices that are not there. This disorder is rare, occurring in only 1–2 percent of births.

- *Postpartum bipolar disorder.* Mood can rapidly shift from profound depression to mania, characterized by a flight of grand ideas, little need for sleep, excessive energy, or paranoid thoughts.

What Are Risk Factors for Postpartum Mood Changes?

Any stressful situation during the perinatal period increases the incidence of mood reactions. Stress reduces the body's ability to cope with drastic change. Typical stressors include the following:

- financial demands
- marital discord
- moving to a new home within several months of delivery
- previous emotional instability of either parent *or* their families
- changes in employment status or the lack of support of the new parents' employers
- lack of social support
- the mother's attitude toward motherhood
- thyroid imbalances
- multiple births
- real or perceived defect with the infant

- a traumatic birth experience
- some types of birth control, especially Depo Provera.

Biochemical Issues Affecting Mood

- *Low B-complex vitamin levels.* These are the so-called stress vitamins—they are crucial to proper brain function. Being under stress makes the body use more B vitamins and also leach more of them.
- *Low levels of minerals,* especially calcium and magnesium. Many new mothers have found relief by supplementing these nutrients. The bioavailability of these minerals can be increased by adding vitamin D or spending time in the sunshine.
- *Inadequate hormone production,* especially progesterone. Typically, women who are more depressed, lethargic, and fatigued are low in estrogen, and women who are more irritable, anxious, and edgy are lower in progesterone.
- *General toxicity in the body,* especially of the colon. It is true that proper colon function is the basis for optimal health. An unhealthy colon may be unable to absorb adequate nutrients into the bloodstream; the brain may not have the tools needed to function properly.
- *Low levels of healthy fats.* The brain is made up of 60 percent fat. Fats are needed to encourage proper nerve function.

What Can Be Done to Treat or Prevent Mood Issues?

1. Protect the mother's general health by ensuring adequate nutrition. Ideally, a woman should strive for optimal health *before* pregnancy. This way, the body is prepared for the physical demands of growing a fetus, and nutrient stores are not exhausted by the pregnancy itself. Today's inferior food supply warrants supplementation of vitamins, minerals, omega-3 fatty acids, and amino acids.
2. Seek guidance in choosing a safe, healthy internal body cleansing system. Although deep cellular cleanses are not appropriate during pregnancy and lactation, certain daily cleanses are excellent for promoting brain chemistry health. Mood issues can be a direct result of a yeast imbalance, heavy metal or chemical toxicity, or even an electromagnetic disruption. Go to http://www.PostpartumDepressionHelp.com to find an excellent cleansing and nutrition program for pregnancy and postpartum.
3. Call the Postpartum Depression Helpline staffed by trained volunteers at Postpartum Support International at (800) 944-4PPD (http://www.postpartum.net).

4. Find time to sleep. This may be the hardest bit of advice to follow, but remember, prisoners of war are tortured by sleep deprivation!

5. Exercise can be a wonderful prevention and treatment of mood issues for many reasons. Exercise helps flush toxins from the body via the lymph system and releases endorphins in the body.

6. Hire a doula. While an obstetrician or midwife is there for the baby, a doula is there for the mother and father. Doulas can work to ensure that the mother's needs are met during delivery and are typically very valuable in addressing the various surprises of delivery. Postpartum doulas can be invaluable in the early months of parenthood.

7. Join a mother's group. Many mothers feel isolated and unable to share in the wisdom of our society regarding how best to raise their babies. Increasing discussions of the rigors of motherhood can help women to adjust.

8. If seeking counseling, be sure that the therapist uses cognitive-behavioral therapy. Postpartum is not the time for intensive psychoanalysis.

9. Check hormone balance using a saliva test from a qualified alternative health care practitioner. Refrain from starting a birth control prescription until several months after mood symptoms have passed.

It is my hope that through this article, I have provided women and their families with the knowledge they need to confront—and, with proper nutrition, battle against—mood disorders during and after pregnancy. The transition to motherhood is the most fragile time in a woman's life. Childbirth affects women emotionally, biochemically, financially, and socially. A pregnant woman is entering into the most important position of authority in the world: that of shaping the next generation. New mothers deserve all the support available to encourage them during this time. If a woman happens to experience a mood disorder, she is not alone, she is not to blame, and she will get better.

About the Author

Cheryl Jazzar, MHR, is a volunteer counselor trained in the diagnosis and treatment of postpartum mood disorders. She is Postpartum Support International's coordinator for the state of Oklahoma (http://www.postpartum.net). Her interests in holistic health care combined with experiences in supporting new mothers have led her to realize that most postpartum mood disturbances have a nutritional etiology. Mrs. Jazzar is a home schooling mother to two of her four children. Her role is to listen, support, value, and pamper women through their various life stages, especially in their transition to motherhood.

74

Man vs. Paper Clip

Dr. Michael J. Kaye

My patient Bob told me his story: "Look, Doc, all I did was bend over to pick up a paper clip. Wham! I was down on the floor, sucking wind. The pain in my lower back was so intense, it brought tears to my eyes. Just breathing caused excruciating pain. I don't even want to remember what happened when I tried to move. I have had treatment, but I still have some level of pain every day."

Bob initially had an acute (new) injury—a sprain/strain of his lower back. Now his condition is chronic (ongoing). According to the International Association for the Study of Pain, *pain* is defined as "an unpleasant sensory and emotional experience associated with actual or potential tissue damage, or described in terms of such damage." Chronic pain is pain that lasts more than six weeks and is resistant to treatment. It can be physical and/or emotional. Chronic pain can occur in conditions such as colitis, multiple sclerosis, burn injuries, anxiety disorders, arthritis, and diabetes.

Quite often, the patient who comes to my office with chronic pain has seen his or her primary care physician, a physical therapist, a chiropractor, an orthopedist, a massage therapist, and/or an acupuncturist. The patient may be on medications for pain, depression, sleep difficulties, and stomach discomfort (most likely caused by all the other medications). The usual presentation of a chronic pain patient in my office is fifteen to twenty weeks after the initial injury. By this time, the patient is wondering, "What in the world has happened to me? Four months ago, I was in control of my life. Now, I wake up in pain, and I go to sleep in pain."

Many questions and thoughts run through the mind of someone suffering from chronic pain: Does anyone believe I am in pain? Does anyone even care? No one understands the pain I have. Simple movement kills me. The heat bothers me. The cold bothers me. The rain bothers me. Why doesn't my spouse understand? Sneezing bothers me. Coughing bothers me. I am depressed. I easily get headaches. I can't pick up my kids. I can't toss a ball with my kids. I don't want to drive or ride in a car. I am tired of taking these medications. My stomach hurts. I have reflux. I get pains in my chest. It hurts to do the laundry, cook, and wash the dishes. I'll probably be like this for the rest of my life.

Everyone wonders how a small injury can become a chronic injury. Was the condition or injury incorrectly diagnosed? Was the wrong medication prescribed? Did the patient receive improper therapy? Are secondary issues (lawsuits, addiction to medication, etc.) a concern? What did the patient do wrong? What did the doctors or therapists do wrong? The answer is nothing. Everyone did his or her best. The most important question now is, What can a chronic pain patient do to achieve a pain-free life? The patient must take responsibility for his or her own care.

Step 1

Research your problem, and educate yourself on your specific condition. This is not to act as a doctor or to impress the doctor, but to make sure you understand what the doctor is explaining. It is your responsibility to educate yourself.

Step 2

Learn about the traditional branches of medicine such as internal medicine, family medicine, orthopedics, neurology, psychiatry, psychology, osteopathy, physical therapy, and pain management. Learn about alternative or holistic health fields such as chiropractic, acupuncture, massage, homeopathy, and naturopathy. All disciplines and all practitioners are not created equal.

Step 3

Find a multidisciplinary facility. These facilities may combine treatments such as alternative with traditional, traditional with traditional, or alternative with alternative. Usually, the best type of facility provides a cross between traditional and alternative treatments.

Step 4

If you choose a multidisciplinary facility, ask if you can be afforded the opportunity to learn more about the types of care and patient management before you agree to treatment. You want to find out if the doctors truly communicate with each other. Doctors who work together in the same facility don't necessarily speak with each other. Remember that you want a true team approach. You also want to find out if the facility has treated problems like yours and what the specific outcomes have been. Often, by the time a patient reaches this type of facility, insurance benefits have been exhausted. Therefore it is important to learn all the costs that will be associated with your care at the facility of your choice. Always ask about payment plans.

Step 5

Have all your previous medical records mailed to your new medical team prior to your first visit. This will allow your new doctors ample time to review the records.

Step 6

Keep a typed chronological history of your injury and treatments. Note the doctors' names, types and durations of treatment, what helped you and what didn't help. Keep track of all your medications (current and past). Don't forget to include any vitamins or supplements you may be taking as well. Always share any allergies or sensitivities to medicines. Obtain copies of any special reports such as blood work, MRI scans, CAT scans, ultrasounds, and so on.

Step 7

During your first appointment, tell the doctor *everything*. Include all your past medical history and current complaints, even those you think do not matter. What seems trivial to you might be very important to your doctor.

Conclusion

Remember, the goal of treatment should be to determine the cause of your pain, then to set out a specific regimen combining the best of both worlds of traditional medicine and alternative treatment to address your individual needs.

In today's society of failing health insurance and mismanagement of care, you must become responsible for your own health. Health and time are our most precious gifts.

In the words of Johann Wolfgang von Goethe, "Take care of your body with steadfast fidelity. The soul must see through these eyes alone, and if they are dim, the whole world is clouded."

About the Author

Michael J. Kaye is a chiropractic physician practicing in Bucks County, Pennsylvania. He is a member of the American Chiropractic Association, the Pennsylvania Chiropractic Association, and the American Chiropractic Rehabilitation Board. He has a subspecialty in chiropractic rehabilitation. He is the director of the Rehab Group of Bucks/Montgomery County—a multidisciplinary clinic with an emphasis on chronic pain and wellness. He has published two papers on rehabilitation of chronic injuries. Dr. Kaye also developed a Web site dedicated to health, wealth, and happiness (http://www.frompaintopersonalgain.com). He authored an e-book titled *The Living Triad*—a book about building a foundation for a well-lived life.

75

Seven Simple Steps to Beat Your Depression and Take Back Control of Your Life[1]

Connie Maranca

Depression affects many of us at various stages of our lives. If it hasn't affected us personally, we know someone who has been affected by it. We can feel sad and depressed for a variety of reasons such as relationship difficulties or being rejected by a lover, losing a job, divorce, workplace conflict, financial difficulties, or the death of a loved one.

However, depression is more than just feeling sad. It is usually longer lasting and can have life-altering consequences that can destroy your self-esteem, health, and well-being. It can also affect your job and personal relationships. It is commonly characterized by melancholic moods that typically last longer than two weeks. Many people describe it like a dark cloud of desperation descending on their lives.

Symptoms of depression may include some or all of the following:

- lack of concentration, impaired decision making ability
- constant feelings of stress, anxiety, sadness, emptiness, or melancholy
- feelings of guilt, worthlessness, helplessness
- feelings of hopelessness and negativity
- fatigue or lack of energy
- reduced libido, sex drive
- insomnia, oversleeping, or waking early in the morning

---

[1] This article, Web site, and its authors, affiliates, and associated companies are not promoting any cures, medical advice, or diagnoses. Content is not intended to be a substitute for professional medical diagnosis, advice, or treatment. Never self-diagnose. Please consult a qualified professional or GP for medical advice and the applicability of any recommendations, opinions, or suggestions with respect to your symptoms or medical condition. All material is provided for informational or educational purposes only.

- overeating, loss of appetite
- recurrent thoughts of death or suicide
- physical symptoms such as headaches, muscle or nerve tension/spasm, digestive issues, and generalized pain
- unable to feel good and enjoy things like you used to, withdrawal from friends.

These symptoms can be experienced in varied combinations and for different durations of time, depending on the individual circumstances.

Sometimes there may be no obvious or clear cause for depression. However, in many cases, there are triggers or causes for depression, and some of these include genetic factors, personality types, major life stressors such as job loss or relationship breakdown, family conflict, abuse, rape, and death.

Another common cause are biochemical changes in the brain. In people with depression, specific neurotransmitters (brain cell chemical messengers) do not function as normal. These are the mood-regulating neurotransmitters that are responsible for our emotional states. Depression occurs when these neurotransmitters do not deliver the chemical messages effectively between brain cells, thus disrupting brain cell communication.

For this type of depression, it is best to see a medical professional for treatment. They will usually recommend some form of psychotherapy and most commonly prescribe an antidepressant or a treatment program that consists of a combination of both.

For some of the other causes of depression, cognitive behavioral therapy may be recommended to address dysfunctional personality traits, stress, anxiety, and negative thinking patterns. This is a form of psychological treatment carried out over several sessions aimed at changing behavior or managing mental and emotional responses to depression triggers.

Apart from the professional treatments available through various medical professionals such as counselors, psychologists, doctors, and psychiatrists, there are various self-help methods you can try to help alleviate your depressive moods and minimize the impact of depression on your life.

Following are some simple strategies that can make a big difference to how quickly you can overcome depression and get the most joy out of your daily activities.

1. Eat Right and Exercise Regularly
Never underestimate the power of diet and exercise on your ability to function at your best and its effects on your brain's ability to function healthily. Avoid foods that contain artificial preservatives, additives, colors, and flavors (when possible), and also avoid or minimize consumption of caffeine, alcohol, and sugar. Caffeine and sugar are popular pick-me-ups and short-term energy boosters; however, they deplete your body

of hydration, and after the quick fix wears off, they contribute to anxiety, to tension, and to digestive and nervous system problems.

So many people drink alcohol to forget about their problems and stressors without realizing that alcohol can exacerbate depressive moods and thus have the reverse effect.

Instead of consuming alcohol or other substances to facilitate relaxation and stress release, exercising regularly causes your body to produce more feel-good chemicals called endorphins, which can have a similar feel-good and relaxing effect to the consumption of alcohol. These endorphins are known to help alleviate stress and induce states of happiness. You also produce endorphins when you fall in love and make love.

2. Go Outdoors and Get an Hour of Sunshine or Daylight

Lack of sunlight exposure can cause your body to be depleted of vitamin D, which is known for its mood-enhancing properties. It also encourages the secretion of the hormone melatonin, which plays an important role in your sleep-wake cycles or circadian rhythms. Excessive melatonin production can trigger melancholy and encourage fatigue.

Melatonin is produced in darkness and lowers your body temperature and creates lethargy. So, although you may feel like staying in bed keeping the covers drawn over your head and the curtains shut, this is actually counterproductive, and you would be better off getting up and walking outside in the morning light.

This is one of the primary reasons why so many more people suffer from depression during winter than in any other season. It is due to the reduced daylight hours and longer nights.

Make the effort to get enough sunlight during the day as often as you can by having lunch in the park, going for a walk during your lunch break, or riding your bike to work if it's safe and your trip to work entails minimal traffic and smog.

3. Find Inspiration or a Purposeful Activity, and Get Busy

Find something that is meaningful to you and that you are passionate about. Actively pursue this activity, whether it be spiritual, career related, a hobby, or a project you are working on. Find inspiration in what you do. If you are really busy pursuing a worthwhile goal or activity, you won't even have the time to notice the depression and will be more likely to conquer any feelings of depression or mood conditions.

Alternatively, find a simple activity that you love. It doesn't need to be an expensive pastime or hobby. It could be as simple as reading your favorite books, watching comedy movies, playing sports, or spending time in nature. Nature can be very soothing and can also provide the perfect environment for reflection and introspection.

4. Take Time Out to Rest and Relax

This is very important. Take time out for yourself. Go for a walk in the park. Have a massage, or jump into a hot bubble bath with your favorite book and some soothing music. Take a day off where you do not check your diary or e-mail and just have fun, completely removed from your work. Meditation and light physical activities, such as yoga or Tai Chi, are extremely beneficial and are also effective at alleviating mild depression.

5. Create a Healthy Social Life

Spend time developing friendships. Your friends are there for moral support, love, and fun. Participate in quality activities with them such as dancing, sports, book clubs, or a discussion group. There is nothing like the feeling of knowing that your friends are there supporting you.

6. Develop Intimate Relationships

Form close bonds with your friends and family. All humans have an innate need for touch. The love and warmth we feel when we give and receive hugs, kisses, massages, and embraces from people we care about nourishes the body, mind, heart, and soul. It feels so good to be openly loved and cared for and to express the same in return. Perhaps this is one reason why feeling loved has been shown to reduce heart disease and recovery time in heart disease patients, with scientists documenting the benefits of loving relationships on heart health and general well-being.

7. Remain Positive and Keep an Open Mind

Finally, stay as positive as you can, and keep a firm belief that you can achieve what you set out to do. Do an analysis of your achievements, strengths, and weaknesses, then set some realistic short-term goals and get to work on them. If you do this, despite any difficulties or challenges that may arise, you will see it through with a joyous attitude and happy disposition, and you should effectively come out to conquer your depression.

About the Author

Connie Maranca is a qualified massage therapist, currently pursuing studies in psychology and counseling. To find out more about her books and articles and information relating to health, well-being, and her personal experiences with depression, please visit http://www.beatingyourdepression.com and sign up for a *free* e-mini-course Beating Depression and Loving the Life You Live. To contact Connie directly, please e-mail her at beatdepression@gmail.com.

76

Eye Disease and Nutrition: Has the Fringe Become the Cutting Edge?

Edward Paul, OD, PhD

Imagine not being able to see the face of a grandchild, watch television, or be able to tell what time it is. Age-related macular degeneration (AMD) is the leading cause of blindness for Americans over the age of sixty-five and affects as many as fifteen million people in the United States alone. That number is projected to grow in epidemic proportions to a staggering thirty million by 2010. Individuals over the age of sixty-five have a one-in-four chance of developing the disease, and in those over seventy-five years of age, the chances increase to one-in-three.

The majority of well-meaning eye doctors in practice today were trained to believe that AMD is an untreatable and incurable disease. Subsequently, you, a family member, or a friend has probably been told that nothing can be done for this blinding condition. Well, there is good news. AMD can not only be prevented, but in many cases, it can be safely treated and even reversed.

Getting old and going blind is not the only recourse for people diagnosed with AMD. In this article, we will cover the latest nutritional breakthroughs and treatments in conquering AMD. There is now hope, where previously, there was none.

The Nutrition Connection

For years, eye doctors have been recommending antioxidant vitamins for AMD patients. Up until recently, the AREDS formula was considered to be the standard of care in treating AMD. While the AREDS study fell short in terms of evaluating many of the possible nutrients that can help AMD, it did come out with findings that 25 percent of patients with *advanced* AMD could slow the progression of their vision loss by taking antioxidants plus zinc.

In 2007, the landmark TOZAL study was published, which evaluated lutein and omega-3 fatty acids in addition to the antioxidants studied in AREDS. Remarkably, the results of the TOZAL study revealed that more than half (57 percent) of the subjects had improved vision at six months. In contrast to the well-known natural course of AMD that demonstrates deterioration, nearly 77 percent of those treated with the TOZAL nutritional supplement improved or stayed the same. This is the first study to show both statistical and clinical significance with respect to vision improvement in patients with dry AMD.

Antioxidants that protect your retina—such as beta-carotene and vitamins A, C, and E—in combination with omega-3 fatty acids may also *prevent* the development of this serious eye disorder. Two particular carotenoids, lutein and zeaxanthin, may be particularly beneficial. Antioxidants can be obtained from foods or supplements. Vegetables rich in carotene include orange and yellow squash and dark, leafy greens such as kale, collards, spinach, and watercress.

If you have AMD, the following are some suggested amounts of key nutrients found in the TOZAL formula:

- the carotinoid beta-carotene,[1] 15,000–25,000 international units (IU) a day
- the carotenoid lutein, 6–10 milligrams (mg) a day
- zinc, 60–70 mg a day
- taurine, 400–500 mg a day
- vitamin A, 5,000–10,000 IU a day
- vitamin C, 400–500 mg a day
- vitamin E, 200 IU a day.

As mentioned previously, omega-3 fatty acids also offer protection against AMD. In a study of more than three thousand people over the age of forty-nine, those who consumed more fish in their diets were less likely to have AMD than those who consumed less fish (most types of fish are rich in omega-3 fatty acids). Similarly, a study comparing 350 people with macular degeneration to 500 without found that those with a proper ratio of omega-3 to omega-6 fatty acids and higher intake of fish in their diets were less likely to have this particular eye disorder. Another larger study found that consuming docosahexaenoic acid and eicosapentaenoic acid, two types of omega-3 fatty acids found in fish, four or more times per week may reduce the risk of developing macular degeneration.

Flavonoids (such as quercetin, rutin, and resveritrol) may also play a role in preventing AMD. A study of 3,072 adults with macular changes showed that moderate red wine consumption may offer some protection against the development or progression of AMD. Red wine is high in certain flavonoids

---

[1] If you smoke or have smoked in the past, you should consult your doctor before taking beta-carotene supplements.

(including quercetin, rutin, and resveritrol) that have antioxidant activity; damage from oxidative stress is thought to contribute to the development of AMD. Dark berries, such as blueberries, blackberries, and dark cherries, are high in flavonoids as well.

Here is a summary of preventive and therapeutic measures that a person should follow:

1. Take a nutritional supplement based on the TOZAL study.
2. Exercise—walking is an excellent source of exercise and improves circulation.
3. Limit caffeine intake from coffee, tea, and soft drinks.
4. Quit smoking—smoking increases your risk of AMD by 350 percent.
5. Drink eight 8-ounce glasses of water daily.
6. Avoid aspirin and ibuprofen.
7. Wear sunglasses or brimmed hats outside.
8. Develop a PMA—positive mental attitude!

About the Author

Edward Paul, OD, PhD, is widely regarded as one of the world's leading authorities on eye disease and nutrition. Dr. Paul has been in private practice for more than twenty years, with offices located in Wilmington, North Carolina. Dr. Paul graduated from the Southern College of Optometry in Memphis, Tennessee, and completed his internship training at Womack Army Hospital at Fort Bragg in Fayetteville, North Carolina, and St. Luke's Eye Institute in Tarpon Springs, Florida. In addition to his doctorate in optometry, he also holds a PhD in nutrition. He has authored and coauthored four books and serves as a consultant to Rodale, publishers of *PREVENTION* magazine. Visit his Web site at http://www.DrEdwardPaul.com.

77

Chiropractic and Spinal Health

Dr. Aaron Peters

The healing art of chiropractic was discovered in 1895 by D. D. Palmer and since that time has become the largest nondrug natural healing art in the United States. On average, each year, over two hundred million visits are made to the sixty thousand plus practicing chiropractors. By 2008, it is estimated that nearly 50 percent of all visits to complementary and alternative practitioners will be to chiropractic doctors.[1]

In its 112-year history, chiropractic has come a long way in its development and practice. Initially, skeptics considered chiropractic to be quackery. However, as chiropractic science and practice evolved, chiropractic itself has become one of the most accepted and widely used forms of health care.

For many people, when they think of chiropractic, a vision of bad backs or necks comes to mind. Although many people first go to see a chiropractor because of back pain or a neck problem, patients often find many other aspects of their health improving for the better.

One common question most people have regarding chiropractic care is, What conditions do chiropractors treat? This is a misleading question since chiropractic is not a specific treatment for any condition. Instead, rather than treating a specific disease or condition, chiropractic focuses on the inherent ability of the human body to heal itself.

Many people are surprised to learn that their bodies have the ability to heal themselves. In fact, your miraculous human body is constantly changing and adapting. Throughout your life, virtually all the cells of the body are in a continual state of growth. When old cells are worn away, they die and are replaced by brand new ones.

Chiropractors respect the factual knowledge that it is the body that does the healing and that the job of the doctor is to help the patient by removing barriers to healing. The specific focus of the chiropractor is on the spine and nervous system. The nervous system is the control, communication, and coordination system of your

---

[1] American Chiropractic Association Web site, http://www.amerchiro.org.

body. The job of the brain is to monitor, run, and control the functions in your body, and it uses the spinal cord and nerves of the body as its communication lines.

As long as the brain and nervous system are able to communicate with the body without any interference, then the body can function at a higher level. When someone has a nerve or spinal cord injury, often they have numbness, paralysis, or lose the ability to breathe on their own. More severe injuries to the nervous system can result in loss of life. This is why the most vulnerable parts of the nervous system are protected by bone.

Your brain is protected by your skull, and the spinal cord is protected by your spine. The spine is truly an engineering masterpiece. It is structured primarily for protecting the nervous system but is also the main support system for the human body. The spine is composed of twenty-four moving bones called vertebrae, and each vertebra contributes to the overall support, stability, and protection of the spinal cord. When a vertebra loses its ability to move properly, or its alignment relative to the other vertebrae is altered, it places abnormal stress on the spinal joints, ligaments, muscles, and discs (cushions between vertebrae). This changes a person's overall posture. If you have ever seen someone with bad posture, it is likely they have a spinal problem. In addition, when a vertebra loses motion or alignment, it creates abnormal stress and irritation on the nervous system. Between each vertebra, a pair of nerves branches off the spinal cord. These nerves go directly to the muscles in the spine, arms, and legs. The spinal nerves also connect to a major part of the nervous system that controls the function of the internal organs, blood vessels, and glands of the body.

The chiropractic term for this condition is *vertebral subluxation*. Subluxations of vertebrae can negatively affect nerve function. When nerve function is disturbed by a spinal subluxation, any body part connected to that nerve pathway can also be affected. Dr. Chung Ha Suh of the University of Colorado showed that even a small pressure (about the weight of a dime) on a nerve can reduce the function of the nerve by 60 percent and that the nerve will start to degenerate if the pressure is sustained for three hours.[2] Most of my patients have had a health challenge for longer than three hours!

Many people are taught that if they do not have a symptom, they are healthy. The majority of the time, the body can be malfunctioning without any signs or symptoms. Perhaps one of the most common symptoms associated with a subluxation is pain. Pain, however, is only one of many different signs that can show up. Some of the other common problems people have are lack of energy, poor immune function, loss of sleep, muscle aches, digestive problems, headaches, menstrual difficulty, infertility, weight problems, allergies, and asthma. Children who have spinal subluxations often

---

[2] C. H. Suh, "Researching the Fundamentals of Chiropractic," *Journal of the Biomechanical Conference of the Spine* 5 (1974): 1–52.

have frequent illnesses; are more likely to have ear, nose, and throat infections; and are more likely to develop a condition of the spine called a "scoliosis." A scoliosis is an abnormal sideways bend in the spine that usually begins early in life. If left untreated, it has the potential to create many problems with the spine but also with the overall health of the child.

The cause of spinal subluxations usually comes from three areas. First and most common are physical injuries to the body. One of the initial injuries to the spine can occur during the birth process. If the mother experiences a difficult delivery, then injuries can happen in the upper neck region. Noted researcher Abraham Towbin of Harvard University found that damage to the upper spinal cord and the first several vertebrae can negatively affect the function of the nervous system and the development of the spine.[3]

As a person moves through childhood, thousands of falls, accidents, sports injuries, and other traumas can have a negative cumulative effect on the continuing growth of the spine. This is often when a scoliosis will develop. Add car accidents, work injuries, repeated stressful movements from jobs or housework, and the spine can be subjected to a great deal of physical trauma. Often, many of the problems adults suffer with their spines have their origins in childhood.

Another cause of subluxations are emotional and mental stresses. Chronic exposure to mental and emotional stresses create long-standing muscle tension in the spine and body. Over time, the body must adapt to these changes as the abnormal muscle tension becomes a pattern. These muscle imbalances further weaken the spine.

The last main cause of subluxations are biochemical stresses. For example, when a person has a poor diet, does not exercise the body, or is exposed to toxins in the environment, it can create inflammation throughout the body. The increase in inflammation causes pain and dysfunction of the joints in the body, particularly those in the spine.

Spinal subluxations not only have the potential to cause dysfunction in the nervous system and body, but also have a degenerative effect on spine itself. Because of the vertebrae being out of position, an abnormal stress is placed on the bones. The spinal joints, the spinal discs, muscles, and ligaments are overloaded. As the force of gravity works on the vertebrae that are misaligned, it creates a wear-and-tear effect on the spine. Areas where there are subluxations frequently have an accelerated rate of arthritis, bone spurs, and disc degeneration.[4] This is most commonly observed on patient X rays.

---

[3] Abraham Towbin, "Latent Spinal Cord and Brain Stem Injury in Newborn Infants," *Developmental Medicine and Child Neurology* 11 (1969): 54–78.
[4] O. J. Ressel, "Disc Regeneration: Reversibility Is Possible in Spinal Osteoarthritis," *ICA Journal*, March/April 1989, 39–61.

The good news is that spinal degeneration can be halted and, in some cases, reversed, depending on how severe it is. Noted researcher, author, and chiropractic pediatrician Dr. Ogi Ressel conducted a landmark study that showed evidence supporting the reversal of spinal deterioration with chiropractic care.[4]

Chiropractic can be an excellent way to improve the health and well-being of you and your family. In the age of preventative care, the spine is unfortunately often most overlooked but is one of the most important parts of the body to take care of. The doctor of chiropractic is extensively trained to be able to detect and help correct spinal problems.

There are many types of chiropractic healing techniques. Some of the chiropractic approaches focus on the spine only. Other chiropractors utilize care for the spine and other parts of the body such as the arms, legs, and muscles. Also, many chiropractors focus on specialties such as rehabilitation, nutrition, weight loss, and family care.

Many people have been told that chiropractic is unsafe or harmful. As compared to other forms of health care, chiropractic is one of the safest methods of care available. Many chiropractors now offer a low-force care approach for those who do not prefer the traditional hands-on style of adjusting. It is also useful to know that some chiropractors only work with patients until they are out of pain, while other chiropractors offer their patients additional options for the overall holistic improvement of health. If you are unsure of the type of care a chiropractor offers, always ask ahead of time, and find the one who is right for you.

If you are concerned about the health and well-being of your spine and the impact the spine can have on your overall health and well-being, I would highly recommend seeing a chiropractor. Today's chiropractic has advanced considerably—as millions of people find each year, chiropractic can make a tremendous difference in your life.

About the Author

Dr. Aaron Peters graduated with honors from the New York Chiropractic College in 2000. Prior to chiropractic school, Dr. Peters attended the Pennsylvania State University and majored in electrical engineering. In 2002, he opened a chiropractic practice with his wife, Dr. Jennifer Peters, at their current location in DuBois, Pennsylvania. Since 2005, Dr Peters has been the host of the weekly health show he created called The Healthy for Life Show. The program can be heard every Wednesday morning on 1420 WCED. For more information on chiropractic, visit Dr. Peters on the Web at http://www.advancedchiro.org. Dr. Peters can also be contacted via e-mail at docaaron@earthlink.net.

78

Your Best Defense Is a Progressive Offense
The Lymphatic System—The Heart of It All

Mary Jo Ruggieri, PhD

The foundation of all good health lies within the function and operation of an individual's lymphatic system. Those pesky nodes, when stressed out, will swell in your neck, especially behind the ear, and will make it impossible to swallow.

The lymphatic system, according to the *Microbiology Coloring Book*,[1] is a series of vessels, structures, and organs that collect fluid throughout the body and return it to the main circulation for distribution. The lymphocytes function in the immune process; the fluid draining through the lymphatic system is lymph. The clusters of lymph nodes, almost like a bunch of grapes, are located throughout the lymphatic vessels.

These nodes provide a filtration system for the body. They contain the all-important T-cells that eventually will fight for your life. It's a well-known fact that a highly functioning lymphatic system can handle even the toughest invader of your body—cancer!

It is important to remember that the immune system is your main defense for healing and long-term immunity to diseases. The immune process and your entire body's defense mechanism is located in the lymphatic system, a system we hardly pay attention to until it's in a state of trauma or stops functioning properly.

When bacteria, viruses, foreign chemicals, and environmental pollutants enter the body, the lymphocytes—the body's little soldiers—begin preparing for war. But this type of war doesn't depend on large defense spending. It is a natural part of our everyday internal health care—the physician within. When these soldiers are activated, they secrete large quantities of antibodies. These antibodies move into the sites of the virus or bacteria or even cancer cells and begin to engulf and destroy the disease or abnormal cells.

It doesn't take much to understand who runs the show in our human biological house. The lymphatic system is a sure bet. It is the only thing that really lets us

---

[1] E. Alcamo, *Microbiology Coloring Book* (Princeton, NJ: Princeton Review, 1998).

function and live a normal life in a germ-infested world.

The body houses hundreds and hundreds of lymph nodes, which are located everywhere imaginable. If we are to keep our lymphatic system functioning, we must be aware of their locations:

- *Head and neck.* Under the jaw, behind the ears, in the back of neck, at the base of skull, around the eyes, on the side of the cheek, and on the floor of the mouth.
- *Chest.* Shoulder area, under the armpits, in the breast or mammary glands, at the clavicle or collar bone area, along the upper arm extending into the elbow, and all along the sternum.
- *Stomach.* Nodes sit on the stomach, the colon, and all major organs such as liver and kidneys.
- *Lower body.* Groin area, pelvic girdle, and all through the inner thighs. They even go along the spine in many areas.
- The lymphatic system functions only as well as it is kept in good working order. Surprisingly, the lymphs are easy to care for, especially if you become aware of how they function.

Exercise is a key factor:

- Walking, biking, or any cardiovascular work. Both the cardiovascular and the respiratory systems are tied into the lymphatic system.
- Get a mini trampoline and jump on it for five to ten minutes daily. Great for pumping leg lymphs.
- Sit-ups and push-ups.

Self-help techniques include the following:

- Constantly do self massage or polarity acupressure points—your jawbone, under your eyes, behind your ears, squeeze the muscles under your armpit and along the side of your neck.
- If a node is swollen or hard to touch, work around the area, not on it.
- Skin brush. It is good to use a dry vegetable brush daily on your entire body, stroking toward the heart.
- Meditate. Stress suppresses immune function.

Bodywork options include the following:

- Lymphatic massage manually drains the lymphs and helps promote positive movement.

- Lymphodema, especially after surgery, should be attended to immediately through bodywork.
- Polarity lymphatic balance uses key acupressure points to help the body move fluids and create a good energy flow.
- Foot reflexology will stimulate certain lymphatic reflexes.

Personal cleansing is also important:

- Fast regularly—drink green juices or fresh carrot juice, which flush the lymphs.
- Do a colon cleanse. Work with a holistic health practitioner to set up a system to help cleanse your digestive system.
- Sweat. Soaking in hot tubs helps release fluids in lymphs.
- Eat good fats—avocados, olive oil, and almond oil, for example.
- Drink water every hour on the hour.

Specific herbs for immunity include Echinacea, goldenseal, and garlic for surface immunity, and ginseng, liquorices, and astragali for deep immunity.

The health care of the lymphatic system is truly the heart of it all. I remember a yoga teacher once saying, "You have everything you need to do what you want; you have everything you want to do what you need."

It's simple: your best defense is a progressive offense.

About the Author

Mary Jo has a doctorate degree from the University of Cincinnati and was a former professor of twenty-five years at the Ohio State University. She has a background in all facets of education with a focus in health science, physiology of exercise, and Ayurvedic health care. Mary Jo is the founder and director of Columbus Polarity, Center for Integrative Health and Wellness and the Ohio Institute of Energetic Studies, which trains professional practitioners in energy medicine, polarity therapy, and holistic health education. She also teaches complementary and alternative therapies in several medical schools and has numerous articles, books, and manuals published. For further contact, go to http://www.ohioinstitute.com or e-mail satnam170@aol.com.

79

Heal Brain Chemistry Disorders without Drugs.
You Can. I Swear. I Did.

MJ Sawyer

It is my belief that brain chemistry disorders come to be when a brain functions at different energetic frequencies than the so-called normal brain. The names assigned to each type of frequency—*attention-deficit/hyperactivity disorder, obsessive-compulsive disorder, bipolar, autism*—are simply nomenclature. I contend that it is important to go past the labels and work toward healing by embracing the idea that the brain is a physical entity that can be healed in the same way any other part of the body can be healed. I know this is possible because I used my own body as a laboratory to discover the way to end my battle with several brain chemistry disorders that are considered by most to be incurable.

In the past, I endured thirty-six years of relentless, treatment-resistant rapid cycling bipolar disorder, obsessive-compulsive disorder, panic disorder, and social anxiety disorder. Occasionally, autistic behaviors would surface when I felt severely threatened. The bipolar disorder manifested when I was about thirteen years old. I was finally diagnosed about a decade later, in the early 1970s. This was the time when lithium and psychotropic drugs came far more fully into play. I was a willing guinea pig in those days. I was desperate to find relief from the turbulent violent mood swings that usurped my days. For seven years, I lived in and out of mental hospitals. I underwent several series of electroconvulsive therapy (shock treatments). Every variety and combination of mood elevator, MAO inhibitor, hypnotic, and mood stabilizer was administered by my psychiatrists. I only worsened with each chemical assist. I was often lost and unable to find my home, hallucinating and violently physically ill from lithium-induced toxic poisoning. I was prone to repeated suicide attempts, which were always conducted in an incoherent daze.

Despite an exhaustive search for the appropriate medications, all drugs consistently failed. So I did my absolute best to function in the world without them while I sought out every variety of alternative healing to help ease other aspects of my life that required assistance. Ultimately, the nightmare-like years finally culminated in my last mental, emotional, physical, and spiritual breakdown, which was of spectacular proportions. This event was a gift. It forced me to commit to do whatever was necessary to heal my mental illness.

I can tell you that since I have healed, the world is a new and remarkable place. I'm amazed at how simple life is without faulty brain chemistry determining my reactions and perceptions. Things are so easy now. I can work, play, laugh, sleep, and tend to the day-to-day without having to fight through every moment to stay present and calm. And mercifully, I now have the ability to choose thoughts that nurture and support me. I can finally change my mind.

Several Necessities for Healing Brain Chemistry

- Discern the way(s) the imbalance is serving you. (*Example:* What does it protect you from having to do or be?)
- Recognize and give up your attachment to keeping your illness. (*Example:* It may be so familiar that it's like a home that you are afraid to leave.)
- Commit to complete healing and to living your life in a way you never have before.
- Ask whatever you consider a Higher Power to be to help you heal completely.
- Trust that healing is possible; never give up hope.
- Research alternative healing modalities; learn to trust that you can intuit those which are right for you.
- Be mindful that the physical, emotional, mental, and spiritual bodies are interconnected; they must all be addressed and healed.

Suggestions for Healing Brain Chemistry

1. You can improve your condition through diet and nutrition because the brain is a physical entity. Foods have great impact on the brain. The brain manufactures neurotransmitters, which carry impulses between nerve cells and regulate our behavior. Nutrient concentrations affect them. They are controlled by what we eat. (*Example:* When ingested, sugar increases serotonin levels, which elevate the mood. This sugar-induced boost is usually followed by fatigue and depression.) It is advisable to avoid sugar, chocolate, caffeine, alcohol, and drugs. If you can tolerate carbohydrates, stick with small amounts of the high-complex variety. Also avoid foods high in saturated fats.

2. Check for food allergies. Certain foods can produce inflammatory compounds that manifest as psychological disorders once they have traveled to the brain. The gluten in wheat and the casein in dairy are especially prominent in causing brain allergies.

3. Be sure that your *Candida* yeast is in balance. If you crave sugar, carbohydrates, and other yeast or fermented foods, chances are you have candidiasis, an overgrowth of yeast that releases large amounts of toxins into the body. This condition can wreak havoc with the brain, often manifesting as anxiety, fear, and/or depression.

4. Check for heavy metal poisonings. They often manifest symptoms that resemble those of brain chemistry imbalances. Homeopathic remedies can eradicate these debilitating intruders.

5. Hormones strongly affect brain chemistry. The more balanced the hormones, the better brain chemistries fare. Naturopaths, Chinese medicine practitioners, and homeopaths can be helpful with glands and hormone balance.

6. Rectify vitamin and mineral deficiencies with the guidance of an alternative medicine practitioner, if necessary.

7. There are homeopathies that cleanse and heal the physical, emotional, mental, and spiritual bodies thoroughly. If you are not a professional homeopath, I strongly suggest you find one to help you determine which remedies are appropriate for you. There are a number of remedies available for balancing brain chemistry such as *Argentum nitricum* for attention-deficit disorder and/or panic disorder; *Tarentula hispana* for attention-deficit disorder and/or mania; medorrhimum, *Hepar sulphuris*, phosphoros, and *Cyclamen europaeum* for depression; and *Plumbum metallicum* and *Lycopodium clavatum* for anxiety.

8. Vibrational sound healing is an extremely valuable tool for realigning brain chemistry. The principle of entrainment, which helps explain how sound heals, states that high-frequency energies from one source (particular vibrational sounds) will affect a lower-frequency source (the imbalanced energy in each atom, cell, gland, organ), bringing it into alignment with the vibration of the first higher-frequency source. This is possible because nature always seeks the path of least resistance. Sound healing can produce brain entrainment and heal the cells in brain structures, rectify faulty chemical responses, and realign the electrical circuitry of the brain.

9. Brain chemistry healings require enormous faith that a Higher Power can assist you and complete trust that you have an ability to intuit your Higher Wisdom, which can guide you to wellness.

For those of you wrestling with so-called incurable brain chemistry disorders, take heart. Know that I suffered severe unremitting mental illness for more than three decades, and I am completely healed today. My prayers for my own amelioration have been answered. I pray now that you, too, will find your path to the peace, relief, and freedom that complete healing brings.

Please note: If you are on medications, do not discontinue them. They can help you stay focused while you take control of your healing process. You and your doctor will know if and when alternative methods alone will suffice. If you do not have a doctor who is open to holistic modalities, find one who is.

Bibliography

Balch, J., and P. Balch. *Prescription for Nutritional Healing.* Garden City Park, NY: Avery, 1990.

Leonard, G. *The Silent Pulse: A Search for the Perfect Rhythm That Exists in Each of Us.* Layton, UT: Gibbs Smith, 2006.

Null, G. *The Complete Encyclopedia of Natural Healing.* Stanford, CT: Bottom Line Books, 1998.

Perlmutter, D. *The Better Brain Book.* New York: Penguin Group, 2004.

About the Author

MJ Sawyer, a vibrational sound healer who facilitates multidimensional energies and guidance, is a pioneer and highly acclaimed expert in transmuting brain imbalances through the use of sound and energy infusions. MJ has healed herself of bipolar disorder as well as liver disease and the ramifications of abuse. Her private practice is based in New York City, where she continues to succeed in assisting individual clients as they conquer disease and find joy. For more information, visit http://www.mjsawyer.com. MJ's new book, *Choosing Sanity: An Unprecedented Guide to Healing Brain Chemistry Disorders without Medications,* will be available in 2008.

80

End Chronic Pain

Julian Whitaker, MD

Kathy Stevens, who has been training my dogs for the past three years, is a battle-scarred veteran of the war against chronic pain. Kathy injured her back when she fell from a ladder in 1996. As a result of her injury, she lost the feeling in her legs for four weeks. When sensation did return, she almost wished it hadn't—she suffered intense pain that deprived her of sleep and interfered with her ability to do her job. Her legs were so weak that at times, they would simply give out from under her.

Kathy went through the usual merry-go-round of treatments with painkillers, physical therapy, and even a high-tech procedure called thermocoagulation, in which a hot needle was inserted into her lumbar spine to shrink a swollen disc. But none of these relieved her pain, so after living with it for a year, she consulted an orthopedic surgeon, who advised her to have the damaged disc removed. When she mentioned to me that she was contemplating surgery, I urged her to try prolotherapy first, a nonsurgical intervention that eliminates pain by addressing the underlying cause: weakened ligaments and tendons.

Kathy's Pain Is History

Kathy came to the Whitaker Wellness Institute for her first prolotherapy treatment in September. Once a month for four months, she received several strategically placed injections of a mildly irritating solution containing dextrose or a cod liver oil extract. By the third month, her pain had lessened considerably, and after her fourth treatment, she had regained much of the strength in her legs. Today, she exercises on a treadmill, sits through movies without suffering pain, and has no trouble keeping up with her dogs.

This patient's experience is not unique. George Hackett, MD, the father of prolotherapy, treated thousands of patients and achieved a success rate of about 90 percent. Contemporary research, including double-blind placebo-controlled studies, shows similar results for a wide range of musculoskeletal conditions. The procedure is safe—much safer than aspirin, ibuprofen, and other nonsteroidal anti-inflammatory drugs (NSAIDs), which result in more than 16,000 deaths from gastrointestinal complications every year—and much less costly and traumatic than surgery. Most important, it works.

Loose Ligaments Cause Pain

To understand how prolotherapy works, you need to know a little about joint anatomy. Synovial joints, the free-moving joints that give us our remarkable flexibility, consist of bones covered with cartilage, held in place by thick fibers called ligaments that attach bone to bone. Ligaments are normally taut, strong bands of connective tissue, but when they are injured, they become weak and lax, making it difficult for them to do their job of holding a joint in place. As a result, nerve fibers within the ligament are activated and cause local pain and inflammation. Injury to tendons, which connect bones to muscles, can similarly cause pain and inflammation.

NSAIDs relieve joint pain by countering inflammation. Unfortunately, because inflammation is the first stage of your body's healing process, these drugs also hinder recovery. In addition, they damage the stomach lining and destroy cartilage, the cushioning material that protects joints. Finally, NSAIDs do nothing to address the underlying laxity of ligaments and tendons that is the source of chronic pain. This is where prolotherapy comes in.

Prolotherapy Stimulates Healing

Prolotherapy (also called sclerotherapy or reconstructive therapy) is a nonsurgical intervention that causes a proliferation and shortening of collagen fibers in connective tissue. It involves the injection of a mildly irritating solution, such as dextrose or sodium morrhuate (from cod liver oil), into the area where ligaments or tendons attach to bone. Just as a fire alarm triggered in a burning building calls fire fighters to the site, the injection of an irritant provokes inflammation and draws specialized immune cells to the area. These cells go to work engulfing and removing cellular debris and foreign material in preparation for phase two of the healing process.

A day or two after this, rebuilding begins. The workhorses of this phase are the fibroblasts that form new collagen tissue, the basic building blocks of ligaments and tendons. Over the next few weeks, tissue growth continues, resulting in thicker, stronger ligaments and tendons that regain their ability to stabilize the joint and take the pressure off sensitive nerve endings. Sometimes one treatment is enough to achieve complete pain relief, but it usually takes about four treatments, administered at three- to four-week intervals, to produce sufficient collagen growth to relieve pain and restore normal function.

Results Are Miraculous

For patients with chronic pain who have tried everything from drugs and surgery to physical therapy and chiropractic manipulation, prolotherapy can be a miracle. These patients may have suffered for years with chronic pain that sapped their energy, deprived them of sleep, and left them unable to do the things that they enjoy. Yet within four to six months, they are free of pain and feel normal for the first time in years.

If you haven't heard of prolotherapy until now, you're not alone. This simple and effective therapy has been around for at least half a century, but due to the bias toward drugs and surgery that pervades the medical profession, it has never gotten the attention it deserves. That's why I've brought prolotherapy to the Whitaker Wellness Institute, and that's why I'm writing about it here. No one who suffers from chronic pain should have to learn to live with it. Patients like Kathy who have come to the Whitaker Wellness Institute for prolotherapy are living proof that permanent pain relief is possible.

Recommendations

- Prolotherapy is useful for many chronic, painful conditions, including back pain, arthritis pain, migraines, sciatica, TMJ, tendinitis, and sports-related injuries. To find a doctor who administers this procedure, please contact the American Association of Orthopaedic Medicine (AAOM) via their Web site at http://www.aaomed.org. Once on the Web site, go to "Find a Doctor." Type in your state. The Web site will then list the various doctors in your area. The ones that perform prolotherapy will be coded with an *A* under the "Therapies" section in the listing. Because of the high volume of calls they receive, the AAOM prefers you use this Web site. They may not be able to refer you to a specific doctor by phone.

- Another source for referrals is the American College of Osteopathic Pain Management and Sclerotherapy at (302) 996-0300.

- If you're interested in receiving treatment at the Whitaker Wellness Institute, call (800) 488-1500.

Bibliography

Hauser, R. A., *Prolo Your Pain Away!* Oak Park, IL: Beulah Land Press, 1998.
Ko, G., "Prolotherapy: A New 'Old' Treatment for Chronic Back Pain," *Natural Medicine Journal* 1 (1998): 12–17.

About the Author

Julian Whitaker, MD, is director of the Whitaker Wellness Institute and editor of the "Health and Healing" newsletter, which provides important health advice for more than 500,000 people nationwide. Dr. Whitaker graduated from Dartmouth College in 1966 and received his MD degree in 1970 from Emory University Medical School. He completed his surgical internship at Grady Memorial Hospital in 1971 and continued at the University of California in San Francisco in orthopedic surgery. In 1974, Dr. Whitaker founded the California Orthomolecular Medical Society, along with four other physicians and the Nobel Prize–winning scientist Dr. Linus Pauling. Dr. Whitaker is the author of several books, including the best-selling *Shed 10 Years in 10 Weeks*. For more information, visit http://www.DrWhitaker.com.

PART EIGHT

Stress & Mental Health

The life of inner peace, being harmonious
and without stress, is the easiest type of existence.

-- Norman Vincent Peale

81

Let Your Mind Heal Your Body

Shayn Cutino

Hypnotherapy uses the techniques of suggestion and trance-like states to access the deepest levels of an individual's mind to achieve positive changes in his or her physical and mental health. Furthermore, people have come to accept hypnotherapy's value since its formal sanction by the American Medical Association in 1958. Hypnosis, a technique used in hypnotherapy, is the most powerful nonpharmacological relaxing agent known to science and can best be described as a state of focused attention that facilitates access to the subconscious mind.

There are two methods used by hypnotherapists to initiate hypnosis: (1) passivity of mind with distraction and (2) active participation with attention. The passivity of mind with distraction approach is to engage in some kind of mental activity to occupy your mind and remove your focus from induction into hypnosis. This allows the subconscious to be more accessible because the distraction will produce sensory fatigue.

Active participation with attention is the opposite. This method encourages you to pay strict attention to what is being verbalized and what is taking place around you, including all feelings and sensory awareness. Hypnosis is a two-person process, and a hypnotherapist can aid you in determining which method will work best for you. It is important to remember that motivation is the most important factor affecting your ability to be hypnotized by a hypnotist or yourself.

Hypnosis will enable you to make productive changes to your inner self by working with your subconscious. The main objective for induction into hypnosis is to quiet the conscious mind and make the unconscious mind more accessible. The reason this is so effective is because the unconscious mind is noncritical, and suggestions have a better chance of being more effectual than they would if given during a waking state.

Even though the changes you have not been able to make in the past but want to make are in your best interest and would greatly improve your quality of life and personal health, they still elude you. Five years ago, Mary Wilson[1] suffered a neck

---

[1] Name changed to protect real identity.

injury on the job. Her life became a chronic neck pain nightmare inundated with migraines, depression, and an excessive weight gain of sixty pounds. Mary began to define herself by her pain, which had taken over her life. It became increasingly difficult for Mary to create any positive thoughts for her well-being and personal health as long as these traumatic experiences dominated her subconscious.

The wonderful thing about the subconscious is that while it can work against us, as in Mary Wilson's case, it can also be used as our most powerful ally to effect positive changes in our lives. The subconscious contains all of your memories from the past, your belief system, and sensory information from all five senses. There are things stored from the most traumatic experiences of our lives and from repetitive negative thoughts we have had about ourselves or been told to us by others. Unfortunately, our subconscious does not have a sense of humor or a sense of time, and therefore everything from the gentle jibes we may get from a coworker about having love handles to teasing from a classmate about not being cool enough are stored there as serious, real, and current realities. These negative imprints, also called blocks or obstacles, get in the way of our more positive thoughts and ideas, which can produce physical symptoms.

Mary Wilson embraced hypnotherapy to help her overcome her chronic neck pain and migraines. Through the process of hypnotherapy, Mary was able to remove the negative imprints that had impacted her daily life. Moreover, hypnotherapy enabled her to reclaim her self-confidence and inner strength, allowing her to become the adventurous, spontaneous, loving, and passionate person that she was before her injury.

Whatever path you are considering taking to improve your health, it is highly likely that you have made the same agreement with yourself in the past, and after a few months, you are faced with old behaviors and unhealthy symptoms once again. In fact, it seems like the more we want something and the harder we try to obtain it, the worse our problem becomes. Why exactly does it work this way? Why is it so hard for us to keep our promises to ourselves?

The reason is surprisingly simple. While you are obviously aware of and can control your conscious thoughts (for example, "I will exercise more," "I will give up chocolate"), your unconscious thoughts are not within your awareness or control and may be telling you the exact opposite ("You cannot succeed," "You are ill"). The unconscious or subconscious thoughts win this battle most of the time because they are more powerful, making up as much as 95 percent of our mental potential. You are what your conscious mind tells your subconscious. Subconsciously, you are still accepting and living by negative thoughts and ideas that you have had for a long time. It is these negative ideas or thoughts at the subconscious level that keep you doing the very things that you consciously no longer want to do.

Research has demonstrated that a person's body chemistry actually changes during a hypnotic state. For instance, a lowering of blood pressure and stress reduction are common. However, not only does hypnotherapy provide these therapeutic benefits, it has been shown to serve as an effective adjunct therapy for medical procedures such as chemotherapy and orthopedics.

Some medical conditions may appear to be beyond one's ability to control and are frequently the most distressing aspects of being ill. Learning how to relax will give you a sense of confidence in your ability to focus your mind and influence your body. Additionally, conditions caused or aggravated by stress often respond to relaxation techniques used in hypnotherapy. Remember that relaxation is a learned skill, and you can practice techniques through self-hypnosis at home.

Self-hypnosis is a one-person process where you take on a dual role. You can become your own hypnotist. This is not difficult to accomplish because the mind is used to doing two things at once. With self-hypnosis, you are multitasking as you do in your daily life while in a waking state. For example, when you go shopping and are looking for a parking place at the mall, you are able to find a parking place while your mind is also thinking about what you are going to purchase at the store.

There are few ways to give yourself suggestions to induce a self-hypnosis state of mind. Record suggestions on a cassette tape and relax quietly with your hands in your lap as you play the tape back. Memorize suggestions and repeat them back to yourself after hypnosis has been induced, or you can write the suggestions out and read them a number of times prior to inducing the hypnotic state in yourself. This produces an autosuggestion sequence that you can visualize floating across the screen in your mind.

All ethical hypnotherapists should teach self-hypnosis. This discourages dependency on the clinician and encourages empowerment on your part. In addition, a trained hypnotherapist should never require recreational drugs, especially hallucinogenic agents, under any circumstances. The purpose of hypnotherapy is to bring one's energy into balance and raise its quality. No drug can do that for you.

So before you decide to make better choices in your life, consider making this one first: explore the idea that the key to good health lies within your own mind. Understanding this and deciding how to use it to your highest potential is one of the greatest gifts you can give yourself. Reclaim your desire for good health and a great life.

About the Author

Shayn Cutino, a holistic health practitioner and certified clinical hypnotherapist, is the owner of Anja Alternative Health Center in Brentwood, California. Shayn has been in the medical field for over twenty-five years, and through hypnotherapy, she empowers and inspires individuals to achieve improved personal health and become the best they can be on a daily basis. More information can be obtained by visiting her Web site: http://www.anjahealthcenter.com.

82

Energy Psychology

Jef Gazley, MS, LMFT, DCC

The term *energy psychology* refers to a number of related energy therapies that are based on the Chinese meridian system of medicine. Energy psychology quickly and thoroughly relieves mental health problems by eliminating emotional traumas or blockages from the mind-body continuum by touching or tapping key points on the body. Some of the more popular forms of energy psychology are Neuro Emotional Technique (NET™), Thought Field Therapy (TFT), and Emotional Freedom Technique (EFT).

All these energy psychology techniques were developed in the mid-1980s to mid-1990s but are still rather unknown by the general public. These energy psychologies have been dubbed "power therapies" because they work so quickly compared to traditional talk therapy. This appears to be in part because they target the more primitive parts of the brain. These include the limbic system, the medulla oblongata, and the enkephalin system, which is in every cell of the body. Eye movement desensitization and reprocessing and hypnosis are often included as power therapies, although they do not directly utilize the meridian system.

EFT, TFT, and NET™ all work by accessing the mind-body matrix, or the meridian system in Chinese medicine. Chinese medicine addresses the body's need for balance or homeostasis. If the Chi or energy of the body is in balance, then it is assumed that the body will be able to cure itself and run at top efficiency. Practitioners assess the body's balance by testing acupressure or acupuncture points in the body, which are divided into twelve main meridian systems. These meridian systems are named for the main organs of the body such as the lung meridian or the liver meridian. Each of these systems corresponds with particular emotions. For example, the lung meridian is associated with grief and sorrow and the liver meridian with anger and resentment. Through a process of tapping acupuncture points on the body, trauma is relieved, and homeostasis is reestablished.

Applied kinesiology tests the Chi or energy by taking a strong indicator muscle, almost any major muscle, and asking the client or patient to lock that muscle while the practitioner tries to challenge the strength of the muscle to see if it will hold its position. The practitioner might ask a client to hold his arm straight out in front of him and lock it, while the clinician, with an open hand, firmly pushes down on the arm right above the wrist.

The body consists of water and electricity. It is believed that muscle testing checks to see if the muscle has enough electrical activity in it to hold. It appears that Chi is essentially the same as this electricity. Dr. Goodheart, the father of applied kinesiology, first demonstrated therapy localization. Therapy localization occurs when the therapist tests a strong muscle alone or in the clear. Then either the client or the therapist touches another part of the client's body to test if a change of muscle strength occurs. If it does, then dysfunction is assumed to be present in the localized area.

Chiropractors who practice applied kinesiology routinely test or challenge a vertebra in the neck or the back, and if the muscle goes weak, then they can assume that the vertebra is misaligned. They then put the vertebra back in and retest. When the muscle is strong, it is assumed that the vertebra is back in alignment. The client routinely reports feeling much better.

Although there are great similarities among these three main forms of energy therapy in that they are all based in Eastern medicine, there are also many salient differences, at least between TFT and NET™. Robert Callahan is the formulator of TFT. He developed his system after being introduced to Chinese medicine from a chiropractor who was practicing applied kinesiology, which is the same way that I became aware of these principles in 1990.

The energy therapies adapted and built on Dr. Goodheart's work by applying applied kinesiology to the emotional arena. Emotions are energy, and therefore emotions can be muscle tested through the electrical system of the body. TFT differs from traditional applied kinesiology, however, because most of Dr. Callahan's techniques do not utilize muscle testing, except minimally. Instead, he developed several algorithms of tapping certain acupressure points while thinking of a problem, such as an addiction or a phobia. This method often allows the body to return to homeostasis, and therefore the craving is reduced or the fear alleviated. Not only is it a highly effective system for many problems, but recent studies have shown that it is quicker and more effective than cognitive behavioral therapy. However, many repetitions of the treatment are often necessary with this particular type of energy therapy.

EFT is an offshoot of TFT. It was developed by Gary Craig, a minister and personal trainer, who, in this book, has written an article describing the details of EFT. Most of the following systems, which are offshoots of TFT, also differ mostly in slight variations of tapping and/or affirmations and were developed later than TFT: Be Set Free Fast, Energy Diagnostic and Treatment Methods, Emotional Self-Management, Evolving Thought Field Therapy, Freedom from Fear Forever,

Healing from the Body Level Up, Human Software Engineering, Psycho Energetic Auro Technology, Seemorg Matrix Work, TAAP, Tapas Acupressure Technique, Thought Energy Synchronization Therapies, and Three-in-One Concepts.

Dr. Scott Walker, a chiropractor and applied kinesiologist, developed NET™ in the early 1980s. He developed his system independently from Dr. Callahan and within the same time frame. Both men were influenced by Dr. John Diamond, who worked with meridian systems in the late 1970s and early 1980s and developed behavioral kinesiology. Dr. Diamond stressed the use of positive verbal affirmations to change meridian systems.

All of the energy systems have great merit and are quite effective. What makes NET™ vastly superior and versatile is the tailored muscle testing that is the standard in this technique. Individual muscle testing makes pinpoint diagnosis of a problem possible.

Dr. Callahan was a cognitive behavioral therapist before becoming an energy therapist. Possibly because of this, practitioners of TFT often stress the theoretical importance of operant and classical conditioning or stimulus and response learning to explain why energy therapy is effective. Conditioning is certainly one of the main ways through which energy therapies work, but it is not the only component.

The essential reason that I believe NET™ is so much more effective than any of the other energy therapies is that part of the muscle testing protocol involves assessing for the earliest event where a feeling or problem originated. Because of this component, the energy balance is more complete, and as a clinician, there usually isn't a need to repeat the corrections multiple times, which is often the case with the other energy therapies.

The theoretical basis behind NET™ is not only behavioral in nature, but psychodynamic. Freud's concept of repetition compulsion is one of the central tenets of NET™. Freud believed that when a trauma is not fully processed or relieved, an individual will develop a maladaptive symptom or behavior pattern in a fruitless attempt to resolve the original problem. A present stressor is more likely to become a trauma if it is similar to an event that was traumatic to an individual in his past. When the earliest trauma is relieved at the basic energy level, most present traumas collapse in response. Not addressing this earliest pain is the most common reason for psychological reversal, which shows up with much greater frequency in the other systems for energy rebalancing. Therefore NET™ seems to be more thorough in its approach, although it is still relatively unknown by mental health practitioners and the general public compared to knowledge of TFT or EFT.

The world continues to shrink dramatically due to the amazing advances in technology and communication. In the past, knowledge was often encapsulated by individual cultures. The brilliance of Eastern and Western thought is now beginning to mingle. The scientific method of the West is now being applied to some of the techniques of the East. There have been several studies in Florida universities and South America wherein TFT has been proved effective, and NET™ is now under extensive study at Oxford University. It will not be long until these recently discovered energy systems will take their place as accepted and respected treatment modalities. I believe that NET™ will become the gold standard of these mind-energy therapies.

About the Author

Jef Gazley, MS, LMFT, DCC, has practiced psychotherapy for over thirty years and has been the owner-operator of http://www.AskTheInternetTherapist.com and http://www.HypnosisTapes4Health.com since 1998. He is the author of eight mental health educational videos and DVDs and is currently writing a book on distance counseling. Jef is state licensed in general, marriage/family, and substance abuse counseling in Arizona and is a certified hypnotherapist. He is dedicated to guiding individuals to achieving a lifelong commitment to mental health and relationship mastery. In his private practice in Scottsdale, Arizona, Jef specializes in ADD, love addiction, hypnotherapy, dysfunctional families, codependency, and trauma. He is a trained counselor in EMDR, NET™, TFT, hypnosis, and applied kinesiology. Jef received his BA in psychology, history, and teaching from the University of Washington and his master's in counseling from the University of Oregon.

83

The Single Cause and Cure for Any Health Challenge[1]

Ray Gebauer, PhD

What if there was a *single cause* of all health problems? What if there was something you could do about it *daily*?

Unresolved stress is the root cause of *all* health problems—it can kill you. However, stress itself is not harmful—it can be good for you, as long as you recover from it. For example, without stress from gravity, bones demineralize and muscles become too weak to walk. Because stress can cause us to become stronger, it can be appreciated as a valuable gift, just as fire can, *if* it is properly controlled. If not, it will, like fire, kill you.

Mice and the Electric Grid Experiment

Did you know that unresolved stress accelerates the aging process?

When mice were placed on an electric grid with very mild shocks, they were unaffected as long as they were given enough time to recover from the stress of the shocks. But if these mild shocks were too frequent, the mice were not able to recover from this harmless stress, and they died from old age within a few short days.

Even though each shock itself was harmless, the accumulative effect of frequent stress without enough recovery time causes the body to just give up and die. When you don't have enough time to recover from a particular stress before the next one comes, your reserves ("account balance") in your "health checking account" are depleted, putting you on the slippery slope toward degenerative disease, such as heart disease, diabetes, cancer, and so on, which takes out over 90 percent of all Americans. Where does stress come from?

---

[1] Article based on *How to Cure and Prevent Any Disease* and *Healing in Your Pocket* by Ray Gebauer (http://www.RayGebauer.net).

Five Different Sources of Stress

- *Physical stress.* Stress can be physical, as in lifting or falling down stairs, a car accident, getting cut, or from being sedentary (not moving enough).
- *Chemical stress.* Stress can be chemically based. One hundred percent of us are exposed daily to chemical stress from the environment and/or prescriptions. The chemical/pollutant load in the average American home is five times that of outdoors! Many scientists believe that stress (and damage) from chemicals is the primary cause of cancer and many other diseases.
- *Electromagnetic stress.* Stress can be electromagnetic, for example, from cell phones and computers. You may not feel this stress, but it adds up, moving you toward disease.
- *Deficiency-based stress.* Stress can be deficiency based; for example, insufficient oxygen, food, water, or sunlight creates stress. Deficiency-based stress can be nutritional. It's easy to get too many calories, but no one gets enough nutrients, which creates a deficiency-based stress that handicaps your cells and organs from doing their job, which is a setup for disease. The key principle is that the most critical nutrient is the one that is most missing, which will cause the greatest stress and thus serious problems. Among the most common missing nutrients are glyconutrients. There is an abundance of two of the eight essential glyconutrients, but virtually everyone is deficient in six of the eight, which causes a tremendous stress in the body that can lead to virtually any disease.
- *Psychological stress.* Most psychological stress is *not* based on what actually happens to you. It is based on your interpretation of events. Once you accept this fact, you no longer feel like a helpless victim to stress because you realize that stress is self-induced. Because we create our own emotional stress by how we respond to our circumstances, we also have the power to alter our perception so as to *not* create stress or recover quickly from it.

What can you do about stress from these five sources? The short answer, in a word, is *lifestyle.* Live your life in a way that minimizes all five sources of stress. One of the key ways to do this is through movement, as described below.

SHALOM WISH

Here are ten antistress and energy-releasing movements I do twice every day. Each takes less than one minute. To make it easy to remember, I created the acronym SHALOM WISH (*shalom* is a Hebrew word that means "health," "happiness," "well-being," and "peace").

Each movement is like making a one-thousand-dollar deposit into your health account! Maximize your benefit by doing these with the goal of curing your specific challenge or enhancing your health in a specific way.

- *Stretching.* Stretch your body in the morning, doing it slowly, with deep breathing and feeling appreciation. Stretch your spine by squatting, holding yourself up for ten seconds on a bathroom or kitchen counter or on the arms of a chair. Install a bar in a doorway and hang (stretch) for ten seconds three times a day. Try to stretch *all* your muscles daily.

- *Humming.* Humming increases nitric oxide, which is very good for your arteries and healing in general. Do this hourly, as much as possible.

- *Activation/acupuncture points.* Activate the flow of your energy by stimulating key acupuncture points with either firm pressure for twenty to thirty seconds each or for ten seconds with a pointer laser on these points: Kidney 27, Pericardium 6, Large Intestines 4, and CV-8. Do *not* use pressure on the navel (CV-8)—use only a laser, but laser this very important point twice a day.

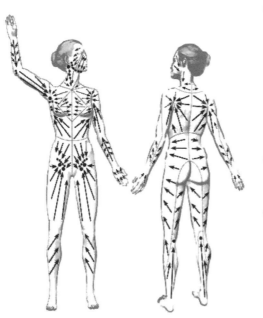

- *Lymphatic drainage* (See Fig. 1). Lymphatic massage is extremely valuable and gives you benefits that you can feel instantly (alertness, energy, strength, pain reduction). Do this in sixty seconds first thing in the morning (even in bed) and last thing at night.

- *Oxygenate.* Oxygenate your blood by deep abdominal breathing hourly.

- *Massage/mobility.* Massage your ears, neck, hands, feet, arms, and anywhere you feel tight or stiff for ten to thirty seconds. Increase your joint mobility by moving or rotating every joint in your body, including your jaw joint, your arms (wide circles), your ankles, your

Figure 1 -- Lymphatic Drainage
Flow Line Diagram

wrists, and your neck. Suck your stomach in (exhale first); bend side to side, backward and forward, slowly, breathing deeply.

- *Walk and wiggle/bounce.* Walk for at least thirty seconds each hour, and ideally for thirty minutes continuously during the day. Wiggle your entire body by bouncing or jumping in place for ten to thirty seconds several times a day. The vibration is very healthy for every cell, organ, and muscle.
- *Isometric contraction.* Isometric contraction is the most effective way to build strength. Exert one muscle against another for five seconds, *exhaling*, using 100 percent of your strength. For example, (1) push your palms together at full intensity (five seconds), (2) grip your hands and pull apart, and (3) tighten your abdomen for five seconds. Figure out how to do this with all your muscles. Maximize your benefits by *also* contracting every other muscle in your body at the same time, from your nose to your toes, as *intensely* as you can for five seconds.
- *Stimulating organs: tapping/slapping.* Stimulate your organs by tapping or slapping over them for five to ten seconds each, including your thymus, heart, lungs, liver, intestines, kidneys, lower spine, neck, and the back of your head.
- *Holding your breath.* Hold your breath for thirty seconds or longer every half hour. This can permanently dilate your carotid arteries so that you get more oxygen to your brain, which can improve your memory.

Even though these stress reduction movements are easy to do, they are easy *not* to do. Knowing about them will not help you if you don't use them. So do yourself, your family, and your future a huge favor by doing them every day. I can't guarantee that if you do, you will live one hundred years, but what if you lived an extra ten or twenty healthy years?

If you are not *proactively* making deposits into your health checking account (healing yourself), you are *passively* making withdrawals (killing yourself).

I say, choose life by making large, frequent deposits!

About the Author

Ray Gebauer is the director of Empower Enterprises. With a PhD in Energy Health Care and thirty years in health research and training from "out the box thinking" doctors, he is retired from a holistic health care practice in which he used numerous energy-based modalities along with nutrition. As the author of several workshops, a dozen books, and hundreds of articles, Ray's mission is to educate and empower people to be more self-sufficient and proactive in their health recovery or enhancement in multiple ways. With a worldwide network of over one million associates, he invites you to join in spreading the truth that anyone can experience vibrant health and longevity. For more valuable free articles on health, visit www.RaysHealthPage.com and www.CureAnyDisease.com. This short chapter is an extremely condensed version of the free full version e-booklet at my web site under free e-booklets. Contact Ray at (425) 957-1851.

84

Looking Back into the Future!

Tom Goode, ND, DD

Imagine living in a future world where people are not taught how to breathe. What if, instead of teaching citizens about this vital subject, the government ignored the matter? What if there were no schools teaching breathing as part of their health instruction? What if there were no Say Yes to Breath™ program to correct the stress breathing that otherwise begins robbing people of life, even as children? What would happen if people were left, abandoned, to let nature take its course and became habitual shallow breathers?

What if there were no Breathers Anonymous to help overcome the resistance to deep, full breathing and the addiction to stress chemistry? What would be the consequence of such a planned or even innocent ignorance regarding a natural process affecting 85 percent of individual biochemistry and responsible for the elimination of 70 percent of bodily toxic waste?

The future result would reveal a nation with a generally unhealthy population experiencing high levels of obesity and sluggishness, lowered metabolic rates, and decreased energy and activity. There would be a general dullness of mind as well that would spill over to their offspring. This is because the brain doesn't work well without ample supplies of oxygen. The normally small amount available through shallow breathing is shunted off for survival purposes instead of cognitive or creative ones. The emotions shut down, and the muscles tense, producing fatigue.

Since their breathing would be impaired, we could expect the general population to suffer from tension headaches and poor digestive and eliminative processes. Their "plumbing" systems could expect to decline as well. They would become a nation reliant on over-the-counter pain killers and stomach remedies, liniments, and laxatives. In addition, to deal with mood swings, the general public would become reliant on stimulants to energize their bodies and depressants to calm them. Their drugs of choice would become caffeine and alcohol, which, used excessively, would undermine their health and peace of mind.

Corporations, schools, and institutions would have personnel and performance problems. Their workers, shallow breathers, would be more anxious and impulsive, displaying unbalanced emotions and, often, high blood pressure. They'd operate in a perpetual panic mode, as if life were a fight or flight situation. They wouldn't sleep very well either or live as long as those with greater vital capacity. They would make mistakes that affect the quality of their work and lower the company profits while increasing health care costs.

Can you imagine a world where only a few, plus some athletes and singers, have incorporated deep breathing into their lives? Wouldn't it be strange to live in a society where the average sixty-year-old had half the vital capacity remaining of the amount that was present at age thirty—when the lungs themselves don't shrink?

The citizenry would also notice their immune function declining as aging took place. Even more insidious would be the growth of a chronic stress syndrome that characterizes the life of the shallow breather. Shallow breathing produces stress, which causes shallow breathing—and, unless interrupted and corrected, leads to discomfort and disability. Eventually, the entire mind-body system would become debilitated, and the body's natural tendency toward self-healing would be compromised.

You can do your part to prevent this future from occurring by learning to breathe in ways that uplift you, rather than drain you. It is a simple thing to do. You have read popular articles in magazines and on the Web telling you to manage your stress with deep breathing. What is left untold, however, is how to do it, how to avoid habitual shallow breathing, and how to *make deeper breathing a habit.*

The process requires only moderate focus and minimal effort. The muscles of the diaphragm, left unused by "normal" chest breathing, become flaccid and ineffective over time. You can recondition them in as little as a month. The exercise to restore them and increase vital capacity is simple in its mechanics, yet highly significant in the benefits it provides.

By practicing as outlined below, you can begin to retrain your normally shallow— and life draining—breathing to that of habitual, deep, life-enriching breathing. It is a simple thing to understand, although more difficult to create as a habit with its profound benefits to mind and body. Practice this breathing exercise for thirty days, and you will transform the way you feel—and your life!

Set aside one-half hour daily—six days a week—to complete the process. This period is broken up into activity and stillness. Find a place that is quiet and where you won't be interrupted. Adjust your surroundings for comfort. Begin with five to fifteen minutes daily, progressing toward a goal of one hundred continuous cycles of inhalations and exhalations during one exercise session. Meditate and rest before resuming activities.

- Sit, recline, or lie down face-up in a relaxed position.
- After pursing your lips and blowing out any stale air by drawing the abdomen back toward the spine with the initial exhalation, inhale and distend the lower abdomen as if filling a balloon. The diaphragm flexes, and the lungs fill naturally.
- When the lungs are filled, relax and allow the exhalation to take place with no effort.
- Next, without a pause between the exhalation and inhalation, inhale once more.

- Repeat this process up to a count of one hundred breaths at a slow and full pace of six breaths per minute to balance brain hemispheres.

The active part of the exercise takes less than seventeen minutes. Most of us will breathe faster than six breaths each minute, and the actual time to reach one hundred breaths will vary with the individual. Out of the thirty minutes allocated, any time remaining after the active breathing is for you to rest.

Allow your breathing to return to normal and rest, watching your breathing. You will know when you are through resting when you feel energized and relaxed, ready to resume your activity.

You can breathe through the nostrils or the mouth for the purpose of the exercise. Normal breathing should be performed by breathing through the nostrils. I prefer to have beginners breathe through the mouth because it almost doubles the intake of oxygen for detoxification and energization. Any resulting dizziness experienced is a result of the brain adapting to accommodate an increase in oxygen and usually passes within a few days. Consider any discomfort as a signal to slow the rate of breathing and rest. Conclude the exercise by resting for a few minutes afterward and before returning to your normal activities.

Now that you know how to reverse the otherwise inevitable decline of breathing function that results in impaired oxygenation and function, it is a basic matter. Either you want to live to your fullest, or you don't. You will either be a victim of aging, or you won't. You will either allow yourself to slowly fade away, dependent on drugs and medicines, or not. Which choice would an intelligent person make who desired to be at his best? With all the lifestyle choices you get to make about your diet and exercise habits, remember the importance of oxygen and breathing to your life and Say Yes to Breath.

About the Author

Tom Goode, ND, DD, developer of Full Wave Breathing, is the author of several books, including *The Holistic Guide to Weight Loss, Anti-Aging and Fat Prevention*, and *Help Kids Cope with Stress and Trauma*. His latest e-book, *Fully Alive!*, is available on his Web site at http://www.internationalbreathinstitute.com. He provides a free newsletter on holistic and alternative health. His other Web sites are http://www.inspiredparenting.net, providing holistic parenting information and a free newsletter, and http://www.acpi.biz, providing information about owning your own business as a parent coach. His speaker's Web site is http://www.drtomgoode.com. He and his wife, Dr. Caron Goode, live in Fort Worth, Texas.

85

Stress . . . Big Deal!
Ten Thoughts about Your Stress

Randall J. Hammett, DC

Stress is a normal reaction to life. In fact, we all need a certain amount of stress to be healthy. What is not healthy for us is the small day in, day out stresses that accumulate over time. These cause our body to deplete the stores of vital chemicals and energy necessary for health. Stress does kill; stress does shorten life. Remember, the stress is your own and no one else's.

Some Thoughts about Stress and Your Life

1. *Quit controlling.* Let's face facts. You can't even control your own bladder for one day, and yet you expect yourself to control everything that's around you? Get real. Control only what you can, and let the rest handle itself. Keep the big things big and the small things small, and let me give you a hint: it's all small. Life is not a five-alarm fire.

2. *Worry?* Worry is based on fear! Fear of loss and even fear of gain. Worry is about people or things we care about. Here are the facts: 80 percent of what you worry about will never come to pass. The 10 percent that does happen will never be as bad as you thought it would be. The last 10 percent will be bad, painful, and irritating. But the truth about the last 10 percent is that you probably will not remember it accurately in ten years. So any time you have worries, remember the 80-10-10 rule.

And especially remember this: the brightest future in your life will always be based on a forgotten past. You cannot go forward until you let go of the past. Practice living in the now.

3. *Passion and goals.* Have you ever noticed that a person with passion for goals or a dream that he has committed himself to doesn't seem to worry as much? It's true. Find out what your passion in life is and focus on that, rather than on the millions of negative things that happen. Focus on your goals and what you love. When you're busy working toward your goals, you're generally too busy to worry or stress.

4. *Present time consciousness.* Present time consciousness means living right now in the moment, in the zone. The past is gone; leave it where it is. The future is guaranteed to no one. Plan for the future, but keep your body and mind in the same place at the same time—it's all that you have. If you find your mind wandering, as it will, ask yourself the following questions: What's next? What's important? What's not? Will this matter in five years?

5. *Fifty thousand thoughts a day.* That's what the average person's brain thinks every day. Most of these thoughts are negative. Typically, they're about fears, losses, or weakness and low self-esteem. Some remember the great boxer Mohammed Ali saying frequently that he was "the greatest," and he was because that is what he told himself many times a day. What are you telling yourself about you? We become what we think about. Self-esteem and self-image are all-important and not what others think. Put reminders around your home and office of the past successes you've enjoyed. When you find yourself busy thinking negatively, focus on these reminders, and know that nothing in our lives stays the same and that everything changes.

6. *Get organized.* We come to our lives naked, with nothing, and we will leave that way. Are you a pack rat? A collector junky? If you are, you are slowing down your life by carrying too much. Every year, note on your calendar a day for cleaning out and getting organized. The rule is very simple: if you haven't used it in a year, donate it or throw it out. Lighten your load in life. Never let your possessions possess you. After all, you're not taking it with you.

7. *Avoid toxic people, places, or things.* There are people, places, and things that emotionally drain our energy. We call them energy vampires—they suck your good energy away from you. You must divorce yourself from anyone or anything that sucks the good and positive from you. Let's face facts: you only have 90–150 years to live. Choose wisely how and who you'll spend your energy and time with.

   How do you know you've come up against a toxic person or place? Simply ask yourself how you feel after your exposure to these people or places. Typically, when you feel confused, depressed, low in energy, or physically ill, you have exposed yourself to a toxic situation. The best advice is to avoid or minimalize your exposure, and at all costs, do not try to change the toxic person or place, or you'll find it's a waste of time. Hot stoves are always hot; toxic things are always toxic.

8. *Rest, dream, and awaken charged.* Sleeping allows our bodies to heal and our brains to relax and refocus. You must guard your sleep as if your life depended on it, for it does. We need six to eight hours of sleep every night to cope with the world. Never let anyone or anything keep you from a good night's rest. It's critical for stress management.

9. *Exercise.* Research has shown that exercising over a period of time creates a wide variety of brain chemicals that inhibit the day's stress effects. Rigorous exercise

twenty to thirty minutes a day is necessary to allow these brain chemicals to function correctly. Rowing or vigorous walking are key exercises that you should do every day.

One of the best overall exercises everyone should do twice a week is called the slow burn exercise. These exercises are done with free weights or machines, and your muscles are taxed with heavy weights, lifted very slowly with minimal repetition to maximize muscle metabolism, creating better stress-fighting chemicals in your brain.

10. *Work*. Your work is not your life! If you identify your work as who you are, you are dead already. Our lives are complex; they're supposed to be. We're here to learn, grow, help others, and prosper. Ask yourself this question: who am I without my job, title, possessions, family, or friends? Asking this question often will keep your life and mind in perspective. You are here for a purpose. Finding that purpose is a key to your happiness.

Stress in our lives is actually necessary to be healthy. There is no such thing as a stress-free life. We all have ups and downs. Those who are the happiest are those who put into proper perspective life's turns and twists. Begin your life this minute, this second, to settle for nothing less than your very best in all you do. Follow your heart, your passion, and above all, don't stress about it. And finally, remember that while death is certain, time is not! What is important to you?

About the Author

Randall J. Hammett, DC, is a practicing chiropractor in Kenosha, Wisconsin, with over twenty-six years' experience. He has lectured widely across the United States to other chiropractors on the topics of risk management, practice management, and stress management. He has written for the prestigious *Journal of Clinical Chiropractic* since 1987. His focus of practice is disease prevention and posture correction. His e-mail is in8dc1@execpc.com.

86

Happy Practices

Philip Johncock, MA, MMs

What's the quickest way to improve your health and well-being? Create "happy practices."

A happy practice is an activity done just for the sheer fun of it. It has no practical value at all, really. In the mighty scheme of life, it probably won't lead to you becoming a millionaire, creating a greater impact on the world, or changing someone's life. Wait a minute. Do you mean that there is no value in being happy and having fun?

You be the judge. Here are nine of my favorite happy practices.

Marvelous Greetings

When a person asks me how I am doing, I reply, "Marvelous." I drop my voice and lengthen the letter *a* sound, as in "maaaaaaaarvelous," like comedian Billy Crystal as one of his characters, who says, "Darling, you look marvelous." When I feel down, just saying the word *marvelous* lifts my spirit and the spirits of those around me.

Make Up Songs on the Spot

I make up songs on the spot for special occasions such as birthdays, anniversaries, weddings, graduations, or whenever I feel the urge. I grab my guitar, tune into a rhythm emerging in my body, find a chord progression, then blurt. If I don't know the people we are celebrating, I ask others to tell me their unique, genius qualities and what they appreciate about them. Since I never know what I'm going to sing next, every moment is fresh, new. Often, people attending play instruments and add lyrics.

Last year, I made up songs for relatives and friends on their birthdays. I did this for one of my nieces, Leiah, age five. She is a foster child who I didn't know well. I asked my brother and sister-in-law to describe her genius qualities. I called back and left a song on their answering machine, weaving in what others appreciated about her. When Leiah heard her song on the machine, she stood up on a chair in front of everyone in attendance, beaming ear-to-ear, proud as she could be.

Jiggle

I jiggle during board meetings, long drives, and serious discussions. My favorite jiggling, though, is done lying on my back in one of two positions: completely flat or with my knees lifted. In both positions, I press my feet down like on a gas pedal until my whole body jiggles up and down.

Wiggle

In sitting positions, I rock, wiggle side to side, circle, and spiral. Like most adults, I suffer from repetitive, linear movements, straight forward and backward. I sit in front of a computer keyboard for long periods of time. The result is a stiff neck and sore back. A friend was a secretary to the president of one of the nation's largest universities. She sat for long hours at her desk. One day, she brought a large gymnastic ball to work. As she typed, answered the phone, and performed her duties, she bounced softly on the ball and rotated her pelvis gently in round movements. When I do this on my gymnastic ball for long periods of sitting in classes, I enjoy as much energy flow, concentration, and focus at the end of the day as I did at the beginning.

Giggle

According to Webster's, *giggling* is defined as "laughing with repeated short catches of the breath." When was the last time you giggled? I surround myself with genius gigglers who enjoy catching me off guard when I take myself too seriously.

Joint Massage

Want to increase energy flowing through your body? Give and receive a joint massage. Focus on every joint in your body, starting with the extremities, like fingers and toes. Rotate the bones on both sides of the joints in circles and different directions, varying speed. Do this at a stop light with your finger and wrist joints or on the sofa watching TV with your toes and ankles. Want to give a friend a special treat? Invite him or her to lie down with eyes closed. You (and a few friends, too, if you wish) play with each joint in the person's body and gently massage and move the joints. This practice relaxes and increases the flow of synovial fluid, which lubricates the joints.

Create Money Games

Being happy around my finances is as important to me as a healthy body, mind, and spirit. Did you know that money is the most frequently discussed problem area in relationships? More fights happen because of money issues than anything else, including sex. How's your relationship with money? Serious? Fun?

One way to loosen the serious grip I have around money is by creating fun money games like this one. Eight years ago, I started noticing coins on the ground. I got this brilliant idea to start collecting them. For a container, I used a special mug. When I found a penny, nickel, or dime on the ground, I picked it up and put it in the mug. Over time, the mug gradually filled up. One day, an amazing thing happened. The mug completely filled and began overflowing. Almost to the exact day when the first penny overflowed, I noticed in my accounting system that I had moved from sixty thousand dollars in debt to one cent in assets.

I shared this game with a friend, who decided to play. A Feng Shui master had recently consulted with her to align the energy flow of her house. According to the Chinese Bagua system, the wealth section of her home was in the bathroom. So that's where she placed a bowl for the coins she found, on the shelf in the bathroom. After a few weeks, she noticed that the amount of money in the bowl had grown substantially. Her guests had been using the bathroom and making their own contributions.

Belly Laughs

Have you ever laughed so hard that you got stitches in your side? A colleague told me he got rock hard abdominal muscles by belly laughing. I recommended he patent it and make an exercise DVD. Belly laughing helps digestion and deepens breathing, too. Just last night, a friend noticed that her voice had deepened after laughing for only a few minutes. I laughed recently at a winter solstice celebration when it was announced that the type of Christmas tree in the middle of the room was called a Fat Albert. "Hey, hey, hey."

Funny Voices

As a child, I used to imitate comedians such as Steve Martin and George Carlin. To this day, I can easily recall routines and imitate funny voices. I like to discover new characters and personas. This summer, when I was coauthoring *Power of Living Genius*, about two thirds of the way through the book, we took a break. In the kitchen, preparing something to eat, my coauthor spoke with a funny Cheech and

Chong voice. I responded with my Indian guru accent. We laughed so hard, we cried.

Conclusion

What are your happy practices?
Ask others about their happy practices, too. Want to increase the energy level in any group? Ask about people's happy practices.
Want to increase your vitality on a regular basis? Create a new happy practice every month!

About the Author

Philip Johncock (http://johncock.com) collaborates with people interested in generating health, wealth, and success. His popular online and teleconference courses include Genius Course Online (http://GeniusCourse.net), Genius Calls (http://GeniusCalls.org), Grant Writing Basics and Locating Funders (http://4Grants.net), and Tantra at Home (http://TantraAtHome.com). He has authored twelve books that inspire greatness and cover such vital topics as sex, money, integrity, and life. Some of these include *The Sexual Ecstasy Workbook*, *Dream-Making to Billions*, *Power of Integrity*, and *Book of Life* (http://FunUnlimitedInc.com). He is a PhD candidate in ethical and creative leadership with two master's and two bachelor's degrees. Want to receive a free newsletter of happy practices and how people are even making money doing their happy practices? Go to http://HappyPractices.com.

87

What Does Feeling Have to Do with Healing?

Dr. Andy Kuecher, DC

Beliefs, Payoffs, and Effects

As a society, we reward illness. Think back to when you were a child. When you were sick, you undoubtedly received special treatment from Mom and Dad. You got to lay in a warm bed while you should have been standing outside waiting for the bus on a cold morning. You were entitled to lie around in your pajamas, watch TV, and eat popsicles for lunch.

As children, we are also taught that if we feel ill, there is a pill to combat every one of those bad feelings. Then, as we grow older and become parents ourselves, we pass these same myths on to our own children. Suddenly, we are baffled as to why some perfectly good kids turn to drugs to remedy the emotional turmoil of adolescent metamorphosis. The answer to the mystery is the programmed solution to counteract any and all bad feelings with a pill. We are taught to seek pleasure or relief and avoid pain. Thus we are in part responsible for producing that behavior in our children. We must realize that if we are ever to win the war on drugs, it starts with us and our belief systems, not the streets or even our own medicine cabinets. Our belief systems dictate our actions and thus results throughout our lives.

From a very early age, we have been conditioned to equate feeling bad with illness. B. J. Palmer, the developer of chiropractic, once stated, "When man violates man's laws, we send him to jail. But, when man violates nature's laws, we send him flowers." His words are simple, yet paradoxically and powerfully true. If your belief system dictates that if you feel bad, then you will receive attention, we are psychosomatically (mind-body) creating a sick society. Sick people comprising a sick society contribute to or make a sick world. In a sick world, sick people make sick decisions. This is evidenced in every major newspaper today. The encouraging part is that your belief systems, and thus your results, are not fixed. They can change through conscious effort.

Recognize that if you have a headache, your body is not suffering from a lack of aspirin. I know that sounds ridiculous, but think about that for a moment. Our beliefs determine our responses. In this example, the typical response to a headache is to take an aspirin. But why? Once again, the purpose is to counteract the sign or symptom. But did you know that that your body naturally produces every drug artificially produced? Furthermore, it does so in the proper quantities, at the right time, and in the right place.

Feeling and Healing

How you feel is often indicative of a healing process. Your body exhibits many different healing cycles to completely heal. One such cycle is known as the cardinal signs of healing. One of the signs in this cycle is inflammation or swelling. The caveat is if one were to continually interrupt this cycle with, for example, an anti-inflammatory, it will reset. The end result is that the body is never fully allowed to heal.

Because our bodies engage in cyclic healing, health, just like life, is a journey, not a destination. Remember, both health and illness are a result. They are an accumulation of all the decisions you've made to this point in your life. Consider an onion. Imagine, if you will, that the core of the onion represents your health potential. As you go through life, using and abusing your body, you build up layers of damage. To get back to your inborn health potential, you must first travel through those outside layers. In other words, on the road back to health, you may reexperience those same things you encountered or felt on your journey away from health. In chiropractic, we call this retracing. This sometimes is a part of the healing process and should not be confused with illness.

A New Paradigm

Therefore the question is not how we stop or counteract the sign or symptom from the outside-in, but why it is present in the first place. Earlier, we discussed how feeling can be related to healing; however, it is not necessarily a reliable gauge of your overall health. For example, what is the number one sign or symptom of a heart attack? Chest pain, jaw pain, shortness of breath? The answer is none of the above. Statistically, the number one sign is death because in just over half of all first-time heart attack cases, the person does not survive. The damage to the heart was already beyond the point of no return. This same concept also explains why many forms of cancer are so lethal. Most people with cancer feel fine for months, even years, before it is detectable. As you can see, if we strictly use how we feel as a gauge of our health, it is not always accurate, and in some cases, it can have devastating consequences. Therefore we should not confine our view of health to how we feel, but moreover to how we are functioning or working from the inside-out because health is actually defined as function.

Facts

It is a scientific fact that every function in your body is under the control and influence of your nerve system. In fact, the central part of your nerve system is so important and delicate that it is completely encased in hard bone. Small bones that comprise your spine or backbone are known as vertebrae. Their job is to protect your nerve system. Shifts in these vertebrae can produce endangering pressure and stress on both the spinal cord housed inside the spine as well as on the nerves that come out both the right and left side of the vertebrae at every spinal level. This is known as subluxation. The result of this pressure is a lowered level of function and thus a lowered state of health.

Your body is not a static machine that is prone to breakdown. Your body is self-healing and self-regulating. In chiropractic, we recognize that health itself is a product of life. We call this your innate intelligence. Innate intelligence's job is to continually adapt, heal, and grow your body. Chiropractors seek to free your nerve system of interference as it is the primary wiring system in your body and communication route for the innate intelligence that coordinates all the functions of your body. This is called the adjustment.

Replacing Feeling with Healing

The first step in any change is recognition. Recall, monitoring your beliefs about health and healing, is imperative because this is the foundation for your actions. Many times, when we feel bad, our bodies are actually exhibiting intelligent healing signs such as sneezing, coughing, and vomiting. Therefore we need to expand our view of health to encompass more than just feeling. Rather than using feeling as the sole indicator of health, we need to focus on function or how our bodies are working from the inside-out. Your nerve system is the master system of your body and is responsible for controlling function. Therefore, to achieve true health, it is essential that you have a clear and healthy nerve system. This ensures that your innate intelligence is fully expressed to coordinate, adapt, and heal your body. This is why chiropractic adjustments are a necessary component to everyone's health regiment. Instead of being reactive or even preventative with our health, we must be proactive and actively seek to maximize our natural inborn health potential.

Of course, no one likes to feel bad, and the great thing is that the healthier your body grows, the less adaptive healing signs it will exhibit and for a lesser duration. In other words, the healthier you are, typically, the better you will feel overall.

Following are four important action steps you can take right now:

1. Reevaluate your belief systems about feeling in relation to healing and health.
2. Continually monitor, recognize, and, if necessary, change the way you look at illness and health.
3. Ensure that your nerve system is clear of interference through chiropractic adjustments. This will allow your innate intelligence to be fully expressed and will improve function and overall health.
4. Consciously make healthier decisions every day.

By engaging in the actions listed above, you can continually create health and allow your body to function fully, as it was intended to—not just for now, but for a better tomorrow as well. I wish you a healthier, more fulfilling future.

About the Author

Dr. Andy Kuecher, DC, is a family chiropractor who practices in Brainerd, Minnesota. He is a fellow of the International Chiropractic Pediatrics Association and a member of many other chiropractic organizations. Dr. Kuecher is an author and speaker in the realm of health, philosophy, and human potentiality. His purpose is to empower others with the principles of life and assist them in achieving their maximum inborn potential. He has a vision that one day, empowerment coupled with conscious action will collectively move humanity toward an elevated and enlightened state of being. To schedule a private appointment with Dr. Kuecher, call (218) 828-4166. If you are interested in his workshop series offered to the public as well as to private groups and organizations, visit http://www.telicfamilychiropractic.com. Be sure to watch for his upcoming books.

88

Change Your Story . . . Change Your Life

Annie Benefield-Lawrence, PhD, CHT, HHP

Dianne first entered my office three years ago, withdrawn and hopeless. Countless doctors, psychiatrists, and other specialists had offered her medications with no lasting relief. Her compulsion was to find a cure for depression, anxiety, and sleepless nights. She was consumed by various complaints and dis-ease and obsessed with finding the perfect man to rescue her from her "drama." Dianne wanted to find inner peace and health without the numbing prescription drugs her doctors prescribed for sleep and to reduce anxiety.

I share Dianne's story and the solutions we followed to restore her health to offer you solutions to reclaim your own health.

Pursuit of Health

Our health program had Dianne monitor her thoughts, feelings, and her body's response on a daily basis. She discovered that the anxiety, constant anger, and despair were the same emotions she experienced daily as a child. We discovered that an addiction to toxic emotion drove her to co-create toxic intimate relationships and chronic dis-ease.

Hidden beliefs and fears recreated situations perpetuating feelings of sadness and depression. Her body now secretly craved the chemicals associated with these emotions. Already through her second divorce and countless toxic relationships, both personal and at work, her emotions kept her yo-yoing in emotional pain, despair, and chronic dis-ease.

Recent research has found emotions created through life situations and relationships on a daily basis to be as strong an addiction as heroin. Infrared brain mapping reveals that the part of the brain addicted to heroin is the part producing chemicals as a response to emotions. *Cravings for emotions and their addictive chemicals become an addictive compulsion.*

Excessive Stress Hormones Rob Your Health

Excessive stress hormones were causing reactions in Dianne's body that created nervous tension, anxiety, tight muscles, and loss of sleep. Imminent or imagined, a threat causes your limbic system to respond via your autonomic nervous system, flooding your system first with adrenaline; after a few minutes of sustained stress, cortisol is released. The hippocampus (brain gland) signals when to shut off production of stress hormones, called cortisol. However, these hormones can damage the hippocampus. A damaged hippocampus causes cortisol levels to get out of control.

A threat immediately causes physical reactions, increasing adrenaline flow and cortisol, tensing muscles, and increasing heart rate and respiration. Stress hormones make it harder to sleep. CRH is a stress hormone that makes you stay awake longer and sleep less deeply. In this way, stress is also linked to depression because people who do not get enough slow-wave sleep may be more prone to depression.

Cells Become a Living Toxic Dump

In 1933, a New York doctor named William Howard Hay published a book titled *A New Health Era*, in which he maintained that all disease is caused by autotoxication (or "self-poisoning") due to acidosis in the body.

Reactions to chronic stress were creating a vicious cycle in Dianne's body. When she was upset in any way, her breath became shallow and constricted, depriving her cells of oxygen. Shallow breathing and stress hormones were creating autotoxication, robbing Dianne of her health. Other symptoms Dianne complained of were fatigue, foggy thinking, and lowered immune resistance. Dr. Hay's research showed that cells deprived of oxygen become a living toxic dump, hosting toxic bacteria, viruses, and chronic dis-ease.

Mechanically Moving through Life Disconnected

By following our awareness program, Dianne realized that she moved through her days on autopilot, reacting to life. She reacted to life by tightening her upper back, neck, and shoulders and shortening her breath. A part of her outdated survival response, tightening her body was wired to her nerve pathways as a feeling of being safe.

Reconnecting to Her Body and Learning to Feel Safe

Buried deep in her cells as a survival response, Dianne had a belief that the world was not safe. It felt normal for Dianne's body to feel tight—her body was always ready to react. As a survivor of emotional and physical abuse, her mom never felt safe and passed on a belief that it was not safe to relax. Perceived threats in her life stimulated an immediate tightening response and toxic flooding of stress hormones.

Our program taught Dianne to change her response. To reconnect to her body and check in, she set her watch to beep each hour. With each beep, she checked her neck, upper back, and shoulders and monitored her breathing and inner feelings. As she checked in, she would send a new message to her body to relax. Mentally, she said, "I am choosing to feel safe and soften my neck, upper back, shoulders, and body."

Conscious Breathing Adds Years to Your Life and Life to Your Years

Breathing became an anchoring tool to focus Dianne's awareness and change her life story. Each time her watch beeped for her hourly check in, she breathed deeply for one minute. At first, she felt challenged to be present and take control of her habits. With practice, however, she found her body responding by relaxing and softening. A new feeling of being safe was expanding as she consciously released her inner response of tightening.

Dianne learned to make breathing deeply and feeling safe to relax automatic habits. Each time her watch beeped for her check in and breath break, she anchored the feeling of being safe by visiting her inner peace sanctuary. She also took a moment to mentally sing her cells a health mantra: "Every little cell in my body is healthy, every little cell in my body is well. I'm so glad every little cell is feeling safe, relaxed, happy, and well." Dianne felt her body relaxing, softening, and glowing with energy.

Be Conscious When You Look in the Mirror

Dianne was shocked to find negative thoughts racing through her head as she consciously looked in the mirror. She found herself focusing on wrinkles, dingy teeth, the shape of her nose, and the extra pounds she carried. Mirrors weren't fun for Dianne, but she had never been present to hear her inner critic. Her inner critic created constant inner turmoil, creating toxic emotional chemicals from the inside.

Fire the Inner Critic

Awareness helped Dianne recognize inner turmoil and the reactions in her body as she criticized herself. She fired her inner critic and practiced sending herself love and acceptance as she looked in the mirror. The mirror became another anchoring tool for her healthy habits. She picked one thing every day to focus on that she loved about herself. Post-it notes on her mirror were a reminder to breathe, relax, and focus on love.

A Healthy, Vibrant Life

Dianne replaced childhood beliefs and hidden fears perpetuating destructive emotions, their toxic chemicals, and chronic dis-ease. Her spiritual retreat and monthly coaching sessions reinforced healthy habits. Happiness, inner peace, and passion grow each day for Dianne, and a wonderful man shares her life. She sleeps soundly and feels calm and peaceful throughout her day—without the aid of medication.

Sixty billion dollars were spent on antidepressants in the 1990s. About 95 percent of our retreat guests are women, and 50 percent are on antidepressant medications. We have found depression to result from stress and its related hormones and from unhealthy reactions to life, including stuffing emotions. Retreats offer a time to reflect and change your story to reclaim vibrant health.

About the Author

Annie Benefield-Lawrence, PhD, CHT, HHP, is co-owner of Retreat and Heal, located in Sedona, Arizona. Annie's new books, *Love's Secret—Stop Fighting and Make Love* and *Change Your Story—Change Your Life*, will be available in early summer 2007. Annie's mission is to empower others through spiritual life coaching, EFT, clinical hypnotherapy, meditation, shamanic ceremonies, and Reiki. Retreat and Heal offers spiritual retreats that contain "Life Solutions for Vibrant Living" and are available year-round. Annie and her husband, Jerry Lawrence, PhD, operate the center and have years of experience. They may be reached through their Web site at http://www.retreatandheal.com.

89

Eleven Tips to Get Through a Stressful Workday

Ronnie Nijmeh

Stressed? Finding it hard to cope? Unfortunately, this is becoming the norm.

In a recent survey conducted by ACQYR, almost four in five people felt inadequately trained to cope with stress. Respondents felt that their organizations weren't providing sufficient training and tools to effectively manage increasing stress levels.

The good news is that you're *not* broken. You're fully competent and capable, but you may be negatively handicapping yourself without realizing it. If you focus on your inability to manage your stress, you're actually ignoring the things you *can* do and the strengths and talents you *do* have. By boosting your confidence, you're actually telling yourself, "Yes! I *can* manage the stress in my life!" But before you set out to change your entire life, let's start with a single workday.

Before the Day Begins: Start Strong

Give your body and mind the fuel they need to get the day started, and that means quality sleep and a healthy breakfast. If you're tired before setting foot in the office, you won't be able to cope with the rest of the day.

It sounds simple enough, yet you may forget that each day is interconnected. The decisions you make tonight will directly affect how you feel tomorrow morning. For example, eating and sleeping well *tomorrow* requires you to plan your meals and bedtime *tonight*. So that extra hour watching late night television may seem like a great idea, but it may affect your attitude, energy, and motivation tomorrow.

9:00 a.m.: Manage the Easy First

The day has just begun, but you're already stressed. It's easy to be overwhelmed in anticipation of a busy day, except nothing positive is accomplished by worrying. Don't focus on the challenges; instead, start moving, and allow momentum to build. Strive to tackle the smallest tasks first. Each action you take, however small, will build momentum and move you one step closer to accomplishing your overall goal.

10:00 a.m.: Find Something to Anticipate

Working constantly without any other mental stimulation is draining. This is where you need to have something to get you—and keep you—motivated. For example, you might want to pack an extra special snack or lunch, or perhaps you can plan a dinner date. By infusing some excitement into your day, you will have a positive reward to work toward.

11:00 a.m.: Recharge Your Batteries

Take a moment to rejuvenate your body and mind. It may seem unproductive to take a break with lots on your plate, but it will help you absorb more information and allow you to work more effectively on your return.

You can take a ten-minute walk for some fresh air or play a brain puzzle like Sudoku. The goal is to allow your mind to see something other than the stacks of papers, e-mails, or phone calls that demand your attention.

12:00 p.m.: Refuel Your Body

Lunch is about relaxing, reflecting, and refueling. While your mind affects your body, the nourishment of your body affects the state of your mind. Eating a healthy lunch will give you the energy you need to think and act.

There are enough distractions and problems that pull you away from enjoying your day, so the least you can do is ensure that your body has the fuel it needs to handle whatever comes your way. If you don't eat well, you can't expect to be well equipped to manage your stress.

1:00 p.m.: Take an Observable First Step

As you begin your afternoon, you may need to rebuild momentum by seeing yourself make positive progress.

When you take an observable and positive step, your progress will inspire you to continue. By using stress as a *motivator*, you'll be driven to solve any problem that comes your way to finish what you started. You will work harder and smarter, not because you have to, but because you are seeing results and you want to continue.

2:00 p.m.: Switch Gears

If you become easily distracted, it's a sign that you need to switch gears.

Your brain needs a variety of things to do, so you might want to shift your attention to another task that requires a different thinking process or skill. This will help prevent boredom and keep your mind sharp and active.

Don't get caught up on a single task or let the frustration of a small problem turn into a big deal. Keep moving instead.

3:00 p.m.: Rechannel Your Energy

It's challenging to remain focused when conflict, stress, or your workload begins to eat away at your patience and confidence. Stop wasting precious energy feeling anxious, angry, scared, or worried, and certainly don't waste your energy fighting fruitless battles with others.

Rechannel your energy into useful and productive thoughts and actions. For example, when you pray, meditate, journal, or reflect, you will refocus your mind and rechannel your negative energy into seeking peace and discovering solutions.

4:00 p.m.: Anticipate the Big Push at the End

With last minute deadlines, meetings, or calls, the day never seems to end. Try to anticipate the additional stress as you approach the end of the day. When you do, you'll be able to lighten your load and mentally prepare yourself.

Don't expect that all will go without a hitch, either. There will be challenges and loose ends to tie, but don't worry, things tend to work out whether you're stressed out or not, so why add unnecessary pressure on yourself?

5:00 p.m.: Focus on What You Did Accomplish

You've made it through a stressful day, so it's time to celebrate!
It may seem like you have nothing to show after a long and grueling day, but that's not true. Focus on what you *did*, not what you have *yet* to do. You will never run out of things to do, so don't wait for the perfect time to bask in your own glory.

By recognizing and celebrating your accomplishments, you're giving yourself that extra spark for the rest of the week.

At the End of the Day: Leave Work (and Thoughts of It) at Work

Your life is stressful enough as it is, and if you never escape from the job—both mentally and physically—you'll burn out fast.
Stress is also contagious. Bringing your work baggage home with you will put your family and friends at risk of carrying your stress burden. Be aware of your tone and body language so your loved ones don't feel like they need to tiptoe around you. Besides, when you enjoy your time away from the office, you'll feel refreshed and more productive on your return.

As the cycle repeats each day, ensure that you're proactively managing your stress. Seeking professional advice may also help to keep you on track through customized stress management plans and dedicated support.

Most of all, remember that you're fully competent and capable of managing your stress.

About the Author

Ronnie Nijmeh is the president and founder of ACQYR (pronounced like *acquire*), a personal skill development firm based in Toronto, Canada. ACQYR collaborates with management consultants, stress management experts, and medical researchers to provide its series of reports on transferable skills. Ronnie is the author of the tool kit at the core of the ACQYR Stress Busters program, a 180-page binder packed with tips for handling stress, solutions to thirty common stress triggers, self-assessments, and case studies. To learn more or to access free resources on stress management, visit ACQYR online at http://www.acqyr.com or call (877) 438-3048.

90

Hypnosis: Taking Performance to the Next Level

Dave Oreshack

"So, Doc, you gonna make me bark like a dog or quack like a duck?"

Kevin handed me the clipboard with his pre-session questionnaire as he sat down in my "client recliner."

"No, I think we'll skip that today," I said smiling. "And please call me Dave. I'm not a doctor."

I could see he was nervous but was trying to put up a brave front by joking. It was his first visit to a performance hypnotist.

Kevin was a tall, muscular seventeen-year-old, his baseball team's ace pitcher. He had suffered a shoulder injury in his throwing arm at the end of last season. Even though it had healed physically over the off season, his performance this season had not come back to where he and his coach thought it should be.

His coach had called me and asked if I could help Kevin. "He seems to be holding back, afraid to throw hard. He hasn't made it past the second inning, maybe thirty pitches, in any game he's started this year."

Kevin and I chatted for a while about school, baseball, his social life. I wanted to establish trust and get him to relax. Finally, he couldn't hold it in any longer.

"Just what is it that you're gonna do to me?"

"Before I answer that, let me ask you a question. Why do you think your pitching skills aren't back to where they were before your injury?"

Kevin explained that even after his shoulder had healed, he didn't feel comfortable or confident on the mound. He didn't have his usual "stuff," and he felt he was letting his team and his coach down by not performing as well as he had in the past.

"That's what I'm going to help you with," I said. "Your performance issues seem to be more mental than physical."

"Doesn't that make me a head case?" he asked with a pained look on his face. Another stereotype. Many athletes think they will be seen as "head cases" if they talk to a performance consultant.

"Not at all. Have you ever been hypnotized?"

"A hypnotist came to our school once, and he had kids doing all kinds of goofy things. I was too embarrassed to go up on stage."

I explained that what he saw was stage hypnosis used for entertainment. But hypnosis is a very powerful tool and can be used to help people in many different ways such as controlling pain or producing anesthesia (helpful for a visit to the dentist); reducing stress and anxiety; improving sleep and inducing relaxation; developing better focus and concentration; increasing motivation, self-confidence, and self-esteem; even helping to regulate blood pressure and bleeding.

"I could use some of that. But the trance thing makes me nervous. It reminds me of one of those zombie movies I saw as a kid."

Yet another stereotype. I told him that hypnosis is not mysterious or supernatural and has been used for thousands of years in various forms. It is a natural state that he had probably entered into perhaps hundreds of times.

"Do you ever daydream?" I asked.

"Sure, doesn't everyone?"

Most people don't realize that daydreaming is the most common form of hypnosis. They get lost in the image or fantasy and tune out external distractions. Another example is driving somewhere regularly and seeming to be on autopilot, eventually arriving at a destination without conscious awareness of the process of getting there.

"Yeah, I've had that happen. So that's hypnosis, huh?"

"That's a light level of hypnosis. You probably go in and out of a light hypnotic trance several times a day."

Hypnosis can be defined as "focused concentration," a relaxed state during which the filters of the conscious mind are bypassed and suggestions are made directly to the subconscious mind. These suggestions can get rid of negative, destructive, or habitual thought patterns that block the mind-body connection. By adjusting and adapting these filters through suggestion, hypnosis can help us feel better, both mentally and physically.

"That all sounds great, but this trance thing still has me spooked."

I walked him through some of the most commonly asked questions about hypnosis:

- *Will I turn over control of myself to the hypnotist?* Actually, you have more awareness and control of yourself during hypnosis, and you may come out of the trance anytime you wish if you feel uncomfortable.
- *Can the hypnotist make me do something I don't want to do?* Again, no. You cannot be made to do anything in a trance that you would not do when you are conscious.
- *Will I remember anything after I come out of the trance?* Normally, you remember everything that happens during a session, unless the hypnotist suggests that you not remember, as in the case of a traumatic memory that surfaces during a session.
- *Can I stay "frozen" in a trance?* If something should happen during a session and the hypnotist is not able to bring you out of the trance, you would either awaken on your own after a few minutes, or you would fall into a natural sleep and awaken after a short nap.

363

Finally, Kevin seemed satisfied. "So how is all this gonna help me?"

I explained that I use "performance hypnosis," which provides the athlete or performer with tools and techniques they can use during practice or competition to control focus, concentration, breathing, and psych, or arousal, level. Your psych level is how excited, or psyched, you are during an activity. A football linebacker needs a higher psych level to reach peak performance during competition than, say, a golfer.

We identified three things that Kevin wanted to accomplish both before and during practice and competition :

- relax his mind and body
- control his psych level
- eliminate distractions and focus on each pitch.

Kevin felt that these things would allow him to regain the self-confidence he had lost.

I worked with Kevin in the office and observed him during practice, giving him reinforcement suggestions when necessary.

I taught Kevin deep breathing exercises, a progressive relaxation technique, and how to use self-hypnosis to aid him in using imagery and visualization. With Kevin in a trance state, I regressed him back to events when he felt successful, confident, and in control. Then I embedded specific suggestions and triggers to bring back these feelings when he needed them. I also embedded specific triggers for relaxation, focus, and controlling his psych level. These triggers could be fired at any time using a combination of specific mental and physical cues. We rehearsed these tools several times in both a trance state and on the practice field with great success.

In his next game as starting pitcher, Kevin pitched the entire game, throwing a total of 128 pitches with no physical problem. He struck out five batters and gave up three runs on four hits. He got his first win of the season.

Kevin continues to use the tools and techniques we worked on not only in baseball, but in other areas of his life. He, his team, and his coach are delighted with his performance.

About the Author

Dave Oreshack is a certified hypnotherapist, energy therapist, and performance consultant. He serves his clients through MindSet Performance Solutions and can be reached via his Web site at http://www.mindsetperformance.com.

91

Simple Solutions to Healthy Habits . . . for Life!

Tammy Parkinson, ACSM, CPT, NASM

It seems for so many of us that life gets reprioritized, and our health is rarely at the forefront of our to-do lists. By the time I meet with clients, they are usually at a point where they have tried four or five diets, hoping for a quick and motivating change. Unfortunately, they were looking for something that was fast and supposedly worked for the masses, without taking into consideration that they are very special individuals with individual needs and personal habits.

In the past, you might have decided, "OK, I'm going to go to the gym *every* day and have *no* sugar and only salads for dinner!" You've just jumped from a very long time of creating bad habits to completely wiping the slate clean and going to an extreme level, expecting to create several new habits overnight. This is a disaster waiting to happen because coupled with this extreme remodeling, you expect to lose weight immediately and get back what you had five years ago in thirty days.

To achieve your goals *for life*, we first need to understand what got us to where we are, dissolve those unhealthy habits, and create new, healthy ones. I mentioned above that I believe in taking small baby steps toward this thought process. If we try to leap, usually, we jump too far and fail, so be patient, and take only a couple of challenges at a time. I continually see that those who are dissatisfied with their health don't exercise consistently, nor do they have healthy snacks available to them. During the next couple pages, I will be suggesting ways to create new habits one week at a time.

It takes twenty-one days to create a habit and three days to break it.

Let's create a new habit by committing to exercise two times per week for thirty minutes during the first week you enter a program. Now you might be thinking that two times is not enough to meet your goals, but what it does do is create an easy, attainable habit that doesn't feel overwhelming, and once two times a week is easy, then consider three times a week—but no rush!

Now that you're on your way to feeling stronger, consider adding more antiaging foods into your diet. If you have a habit of having chips or a cookie with your lunch, change your habit and grab an apple or pear.

Last, drink three cups of water a day—again, not a huge amount, but if you are like many of the people I meet, water's an afterthought, so commit to three a day!

Overview suggestion for your first week:

1. Exercise two times for thirty minutes.
2. Replace your mid-day potato chips, French fries, or cookie with fruit.
3. Drink three glasses of water each day.

Another must for each week is to keep a food journal of what you are eating and what time you are eating it. You can write in a nice, tidy journal or on a bunch of sticky notes—whatever works in your world! You don't need to show this to anyone, but it will help you with your own accountability. This is so important; it's a defining success with those who achieve their goals!

When you feel solid with your new habits, consider week 2.

Rolling Your New Habits into Week 2
It takes twenty-one days to create a habit and three days to break it.

In hopes that your first week's challenge has been doable for you, remember that it's all about your commitment! If you slipped, it's OK, but don't let the slippery slope go too far, or the habit's nonexistent. Get right back on it until it becomes natural! Setting short-term and long-term goals is vital in any goal-worthy situation. I recommend you have an accountability partner or coach to help you determine and reach your goals. It's also important to reward yourself (not necessarily with food in this case!) once you've achieved your goals. Some suggestions might be to get a special manicure if you can comfortably fit into an old pair of jeans, or take a half day off and spend time with friends if you've been able to consistently work out three times a week for forty-five days. Pat yourself on the back, and embrace this new lifestyle you are creating!

We want to roll week 1's habits into week 2, so here's your challenge for the next week:

1. Go shopping for healthy food to keep in your car, office, or home, and do this once a week.
2. Eliminate all foods (or most) that contain white flour and/or white sugar (very important with a weight loss program).

3. Do ten push-ups and twenty lunges every day, as long as they can be done safely.
4. Eat a high-fiber breakfast with a little protein.

Having healthy snacks available to you is one of the most important musts in any healthy eating plan! This will set you up for success in any situation and will keep you from ordering the not-so-healthy foods because you are famished by the time you finally eat!

Gaining Momentum Instead of Weight with Week 3
It takes twenty-one days to create a habit and three days to break it.

If you've been integrating weeks 1 and 2 toward creating new habits, you are on a roll now! You're feeling great, building momentum, and probably expecting fast results! Here's a reality check: it takes time and patience. Keep focused, however, because you *will* achieve your goals if you allow your body to adjust to a new healthy way of living. We still want to continue with the past two weeks' goals, but now we have a few more to add or modify:

- Work out three times a week for thirty minutes (adding on a day now!).
- Have a vegetable two times a day.
- Have a fruit two times a day.
- Only choose nonfat versions of milk/soy in your coffee drinks if you have these (lots of hidden calories here!).

With this week, you are starting to add in nutrient-rich choices. These choices will also add fiber to your diet, helping you stay fuller longer, among many other health benefits.

You should be reaching one of your short-term goals by now. Keep the momentum moving, and have fun with these new foods!

Putting It All Together with Your Fourth Week
It takes twenty-one days to create a habit and three days to break it.

Congratulations! If you've been following the four-week plan, you are now well into your twenty-first day of new habits. Drinking more water is easier, working out is part of the day, and having a piece of fruit should be natural for you. I'm also hoping you've taken time to shop for your healthy foods once a week so you're never running to McDonald's because you are famished!

On this home stretch of creating new habits one week at a time, thank yourself for being not only motivated, but disciplined enough to create new choices for your health. This is a big deal and one you should be proud of!

I know you are still doing your food logs (if not, get back on it!), and now I suggest you write down one healthy choice you make every day in your journal as a reminder toward your goals. Be proud of your accomplishments!

- Increase your water to four glasses a day.
- Have fish two times a week in place of a fattier protein (i.e., red meat, pork, dark meat chicken).
- Eat every three to four hours, never being too hungry or too full.

This last week's challenge is the beginning to creating health and wellness *for life*. Every one is different with his habits and goals, and all of the weeks are suggestions to the average, health-conscious person. I invite you to contact me if you are committed to a more individualized plan, but either way, *stay* committed, talk about your successes with your peers, inspire others by your determination, and always remember your bigger goal: living the ultimate quality of life with a healthy body! Congratulations on creating a habit (or several) to make this diet the one that makes a difference!

About the Author

Tammy Parkinson, ACSM, CPT, NASM, is a fitness and nutrition expert and CEO of Body Firm Personal Training and Nutrition Consulting, Los Gatos, CA. For more information about fitness, wellness, and nutritional programs, please visit Tammy and the Body Firm team at http://www.mybodyfirm.com.

PART NINE

*Vitamins, Minerals, and
Nutritional Supplements*

It is easy to get a thousand prescriptions but hard to get
one single remedy.

-- Chinese Proverb

92

Dietary Indoles

G. Merrill Andrus, PhD

Breast cancer rates in Europe dropped dramatically for five to six years, only to rebound at the end of that period. For a while it seemed that breast cancer might be going or gone, but then it came back. What was going on? World War II! The war diminished breast cancer? Could it possibly have been the change in diet?

It took scientists about twenty years to conclude that the decreased incidence of breast cancer in Europe during World War II was probably associated with a change in diet and that one chemical entity in one type of food was responsible. It took time to come to the correct conclusion. No one jumped up in 1950 and said, "It's because we ate so much cabbage." However, during the war, the women and girls in Europe did eat a lot of cabbage. Cabbage was easier to get than sugar, meat, and fat.

From the end of World War II until today, people have wondered if ingredients in cabbage and other vegetables are truly important in the fight against cancer. A lot of work with mice and rats doped with cancer-causing substances has shown that cabbage juice could inhibit the formation and growth of cancers. Furthermore, a lot more work was done to identify a specific component in cabbage juice that could be responsible for a reduction in the occurrence of breast cancer and other cancers.

In cabbage, Brussels sprouts, broccoli, and many other vegetables called cruciferous vegetables, there grows a set of chemical compounds called glucosinolates. One of these glucosinolates is called glucobrassicin. When plant cells of cruciferous vegetables are broken up by chewing, cutting, or grinding, an enzyme called myrosinase is released. Myrosinase will break down the glucobrassicin to produce, among other components, a dietary indole named indole-3-carbinol (I3C).

Literally hundreds of scientists have worked on the physiological effects of I3C and other dietary indoles in the human body and in the bodies of mice and rats. This extensive work has shown unequivocally that what your mother said about broccoli being good for you is absolutely true and scientifically proven.

What Happens to I3C in the Human Body?

The exact mechanism by which I3C does some good for human beings is not completely understood. However, important connections were discovered about 15 years ago.[1] In this chapter we will only describe a small part of what is known. First, we know the chemical structure of I3C.

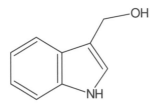

We know that in the presence of acids, such as those in every person's stomach, I3C is quite reactive and is readily transformed into a number of larger molecules that are biologically active. These indoles may undergo changes before interacting with the estrogenic hormones in the body.

What Do Dietary Indoles Have to Do with Estrogens?

Estradiol, a major female sex hormone produced in the ovaries, is carried by blood circulation to various cells in the body, where it is oxidized to produce other hormones that attach to estrogen receptors. Under one set of conditions in a human body, estradiol is normally oxidized to give the product 16-α-hydroxyestrone. This compound is said to be highly estrogenic; that is, it will enhance cell division. We want cell division when a baby is developing. We do not want rapid cell division in a cancer or a growing wart or a growing viral infection.

Another mode of oxidation of estradiol will give 2-hydroxyestrone. This compound will be attached to estrogen receptors, and by doing so, it will block the action of 16-α-hydroxyestrone. Hence 2-hydroxyestrone will suppress the cell division in a cancer or wart. In the normal human body, both these oxidation mechanisms occur, and only the balance between 16-α-hydroxyestrone and 2-hydroxyestrone will vary.

---

[1] J. J. Michnovicz and H. L. Bradlow, "Dietary cytochrome P-450 modifiers in the control of estrogen metabolism," in *Food Phytochemcials for Cancer Prevention I: Fruits and Vegetables*, ACS Symposium Series 546, ed. M.-T. Huang et al. (Washington, DC: American Chemical Society, 1994), chap. 23.

An abundance of I3C or the other dietary indoles appears to favor the formation of 2-hydroxyestrone. The proof of this effect has been thoroughly worked out by large-scale studies in which women were given I3C or a placebo. About sixty-five percent of those taking the I3C were shown to favor 2-hydroxyestrone production significantly.

Why Did Eating Cabbage Prevent Breast Cancer?

Breast cancer is a manifestation of unwanted cell division on a massive scale. If a cancer remains so small that it is not detected, who cares, until it starts to grow and is detected? The women in Europe during World War II might have had some cancers on a submicroscopic scale. These tiny growths did not show themselves because the cells were slow to divide, if they divided at all. The indoles from the cabbage that these women ate suppressed the more estrogenic oxidation of the estradiol, and the receptors that cause rapid cell division just did not get the signal to promote wild growth.

What Other Afflictions Are Responsive to Dietary Indoles?

A number of other cell division processes are inhibited by dietary indoles. For example, a host of diseases can be traced to various strains of papilloma viruses. These viruses are often transmitted from one person to another by sexual contact. This transmission is very widespread, but since most of the papilloma viruses give few or mild aggravating symptoms, less attention is paid to curing this infection. However, genital warts result from some strains of the papilloma virus, and this is a prevalent affliction. Mothers can transmit such viruses to their children during childbirth. Such an infection might show up as warts on the infant's vocal chords, which become a clinical condition in young children.

Warts on the soft tissue of the vocal chords is called laryngeal papillomatosis or recurring respiratory papillomatosis (RRP). This condition responds to dietary indoles taken orally.

Effective in about sixty percent of the children with RRP, dietary indoles are among the most effective and least expensive methods of dealing with this infection.

Prior to the early 1990s, doctors were prescribing cabbage juice as a remedy for RRP, building on the earlier studies growing out of the observations concerning women in Europe during World War II. You can imagine the fuss of getting a five-year-old to drink cabbage juice, maybe pints per day.

Cancer of the cervix in women is known to result from a papilloma infection of the cervix that first manifests as cervical dysplasia. While there is presently a vaccine for cervical cancer, women often find relief from cervical dysplasia by taking dietary indoles.

Since fibromyalgia, symptoms of which include chronic fatigue, is more prevalent in women than in men, it is reasonable to conclude that fibromyalgia is at least partly hormone related. A number of people with fibromyalgia have found that they can sleep much better when they are taking dietary indole supplementation.

About the Author

G. Merrill Andrus, PhD (chemistry), has a major interest in alternative and natural healing that will prolong his active life. At age eighty-one, he still works full-time and intends to do so for years to come. His recent activities in the dietary supplement field include advancing the use of dietary indoles for protection against RRP, cervical dysplasia, fibromyalgia, and other hormone-related conditions. He has also helped show that the use of L-glutathione will enhance the antioxidant requirements of the body. As president of Theranaturals, Inc. of Orem, Utah, he has the opportunity to promote these and other supplement applications.

93

Probiotic Power

Caroline Barringer, NTP, CHFS

Consider yourself a human superorganism, for inside you lives an intimate, highly organized community of microbes. These intelligent beings, including bacteria, yeasts, fungi, and so on, inhabit our digestive, respiratory, and urinary tracts as well as the surface of our skin—in the trillions! They are essential for performing countless metabolic duties, digestive processes, immune-supporting functions, detoxification protocols, and more.

Science tells us that there are over five hundred known species of beneficial, neutral, and pathogenic microbes, and they've been with us since we began inhabiting the earth. The *beneficial* microbes are more commonly referred to as "probiotics," meaning "for life." These microbes share a symbiotic relationship and are abundantly present in our bodies at all times. In fact, they out number our human cells by a ten-to-one ratio, with new species being discovered every day. In the words of Dr. Jeffrey Gordon, gastroenterologist turned full-time microbiologist at Washington State University's School of Medicine in St. Louis, "We are discovering parts of ourselves that we weren't even aware of. It's a whole other planet down there."

The most recognized probiotic strains are from the lacto and bifido species. They are widely used to formulate probiotic supplements and to culture foods like sauerkraut and yogurt (lactofermentation). Transient in nature, they enter our bodies, do their work (if they survive stomach acids), and leave in the stool without colonizing in the intestinal mucosa in large numbers. Mainly acquired through dietary sources, the lacto and bifido species are necessary components of our microbial communities, but they play a much smaller role than previously thought. Largely overlooked until late 2005, the broad spectrum of microbes *actively* colonizing in the intestinal mucosa began to gain some attention. These permanent dwellers are environmental in nature, meaning they enter our bodies via the air, soil, and water supply. Unlike their lacto and bifido cousins, environmental microbes colonize within us in larger numbers and are highly resistant to stomach pH, resilient in the destructive path of antibiotics, and pooocoo powerful antiviral, antifungal, and antiparasitic properties.

Much of the microbiota we carry throughout our lives are acquired at birth as we make our journey through the birth canal from a mostly sterile womb to a microbe-filled outer world. Micro-organisms present in a woman's birth canal mirror the same composition of microbes found in her environment. Those born by cesarean section sadly miss out on this crucial "microbial vaccination" that only a natural birth can provide. A new mother's colostrum and breast milk should also contain a healthy microbial profile, which she will then pass on as a second inoculation during breast-feeding. Essential nutrients in a woman's breast milk, mainly the organic sugars, serve as a food source for the microbes, allowing them to proliferate and colonize in the mucosal lining of a baby's digestive tract. This is the beginning of the immune system.

Beneficial superorganisms transferred during birth should comprise 80 to 85 percent of the total human microbiota. Any other ratio can lead to poor health. Chronic ear, urinary tract or yeast infections, constipation, diarrhea, excess bloating, flatulence or belching, sleepiness after meals, acne, eczema, hormonal imbalances, chronic halitosis, toenail/fingernail fungus, and a white coating on the tongue are just some of the classic symptoms of an imbalanced microbiota. Even a person's weight may be influenced by the microbes he or she carries. Life-giving probiotic organisms help us manufacture vitamins (especially B and K); digest food and absorb nutrients; create end-stage digestive enzymes; balance intestinal pH; fight off parasitic invasions; attack, quarantine, and neutralize toxins; trigger hormones; increase and improve bowel transit time and movement; and protect intestinal walls. They are truly essential to our well-being!

After birth, it is our responsibility to maintain and nourish our inner microbial environment. Unfortunately, a stressful lifestyle, a diet high in refined sugars and carbohydrates, and the overuse of antibiotics, contraceptives, vaccinations, and pharma drugs will permanently alter the delicate composition of the human microbiota. In general, microbes eventually bounce back on their own, but never to their original, healthful composition. Antibiotics, meaning "against life," pose the most serious threat to our microbial partners. Just one or two courses can negatively impact a person's inner ecology. Antibiotics destroy all forms of bacteria, allowing other microscopic organisms, such as yeasts and fungi, to dominate the inner environment. This sort of pathogenic overgrowth weakens the immune system, compromises intestinal function, and stresses the body's natural pathways of detoxification—greatly increasing the risk of disease.

Tips to Restore, Protect, and Maintain
Your Inner Microbial Environment

1. *Take a high-quality probiotic/prebiotic supplement.* When searching for a high-quality probiotic/prebiotic, look for a brand with a broad spectrum of colonizing, environmental microbes blended with or without the more transient lacto and bifido strains. Prescript-Assist™ (P-A) contains over thirty beneficial microflora

and is my probiotic supplement of choice. Often referred to as "Mother Nature's micro-organisms and minerals in a capsule," P-A is a breakthrough in probiotic/prebiotic technology. Four years of clinical trials have shown that just two P-A capsules per day (550 milligrams each) can drastically reduce or even eliminate gastric upset by rapidly restoring balance to the mucosal flora.

2. *Eat cultured foods on a daily basis.* Probiotic-rich superfoods, such as organic kefir, organic cultured vegetables, unpasteurized miso, natto, cultured raw butter, organic yogurt, and other cultured foods, will do wonders for your mind, mood, body, and spirit, and they're incredibly delicious, too! Just three or four half-cup servings per day will provide lasting and profound benefits. Cultured foods—traditionally prepared for thousands of years to preserve food before refrigeration—improve digestion and support the immune system, bringing forth robust health and vitality. Homemade cultured foods are far more economical and therapeutic compared to commercial brands. Cultured foods are rich in lacto and bifido probiotics.

3. *Eliminate refined foods from your diet and reduce your consumption of starchy carbohydrates.* Refined, highly processed foods and starchy carbohydrates quickly break down into sugar—the preferred food source of pathogenic micro-organisms. Depriving these opportunistic microbes of sugar will cause them to starve, killing them or forcing them to leave your body. This allows the beneficial microbes to flourish once again, returning balance and harmony to your inner environment.

4. *Go organic.* Conventional food crops are heavily sprayed with pesticides, insecticides, and fungicides. These hazardous substances have a sterilizing effect on soil, depleting its minerals and killing off the naturally occurring soil-borne organisms. Foods grown in depleted crops carry no beneficial microbes and are deficient in essential vitamins, minerals, and phytochemicals. Going organic protects your health and supports the organic farmers who are dedicated to saving our soil and protecting our precious food supply.

5. *Reduce your exposure to chlorinated water.* Chlorine is a powerful antimicrobial, and it has a grave effect on the human microbiota. Installing a shower filter can reduce your chlorine exposure by up to 99 percent. Quality water filters have become extremely affordable. Cooking with and drinking purified water can protect your digestive tract from the damaging effects of chlorine.

6. *Eat your meals in a relaxed environment.* When we eat on the run, gobbling down our food without chewing it properly, we set ourselves up for gastric disaster. Stress stimulates the human nervous system to shift into a mode of fight or flight, halting digestion until the perceived danger has passed. The foods trapped in the gastrointestinal tract begin to ferment, putrefy, and rancidify. Pathogens multiply, and gases begin to build up, eventually leading to the release of digestive acids into the esophagus. This common condition is known as GERD. When digestion

resumes, flourishing pathogens flood the intestines, causing the gut to become inflamed and hyperpermeable (leaky gut). Conversely, if we sit down to enjoy a meal in a relaxed state, digestion is optimized. The simple act of setting time aside to eat and digest properly can make a world of difference to our intestinal health.

Consuming cultured foods and probiotic/prebiotic supplements, combined with eating a wholesome, organic diet and living a healthy lifestyle, are powerful healing tools in any health improvement protocol. Everyone can benefit from the power of probiotics. Health begins and ends in the gut. What's in yours?

About the Author

Caroline Barringer, cofounder of Immunitrition™ (http://www.immunitrition.com), is a nutritional therapy practitioner (NTP), certified healing foods specialist (CHFS), EFT therapist, body ecologist, and international lecturer. She is best known for creating the Birth Renaissance Foundation™ and the Certified Healing Foods Specialist Program™ in New York. Caroline's mission is to change the way the world eats—one person at a time! She advocates self-care, education, and growth, where an individual has the right to make health decisions based on his or her own intuition and research. Immunitrition's wellness CD series and *Cultured Cuisine*™ DVD will be released in late 2007. To order culture starters, culturing kits, organic cultured vegetables, and Prescript-Assist™, and more, please visit http://www.culturednutrition.com. To register for an Immunitrition event or to sign up for the Certified Healing Foods Specialist Program, please call Immunitrition at (877) 773-9229.

94

Minerals:
Our Connection to Mother Earth

Dr. Brad Case

Our bodies are literally made from earth. Have you ever really thought about that? Every speck that is currently your physical body was once either water from the earth or the very ground that we walk on. What's more, the stuff that you are made of today will one day be part of the earth again. I find this both fascinating and humbling.

Our bodies are not separate from the ecosystem; they are an integral part of it. Because we are made from earth, how we treat the earth is reflected directly in our health as a species. Soil, which we use to grow our food, requires a good balance of minerals, water, and millions of micro-organisms for it to be healthy. Healthy soil is required to grow healthy plants, and we require healthy plants to be healthy humans. Because our bodies cannot manufacture minerals, it only makes sense that our soil must contain all the minerals we need if we're going to be healthy. Thus, when we strip all the naturally occurring minerals from the soil and only replace a few of them (typically, nitrogen, phosphorus, and potassium) using artificial fertilizers, we are creating a gross imbalance in the soil, in our plants, and in us.

Like anything else, our bodies are only as good as the materials we use to make them with. If your body needs iodine to make thyroid hormone, for example, but there's no iodine around, it can't just wave a magic wand and produce some iodine. What your body does in this case is use the next best thing, which will be a mineral that's fairly close in chemical composition to iodine such as chlorine, fluorine, or bromine (all of which are toxic to the thyroid). In other words, your body doesn't just throw its hands up in the air and say, "Well, forget it then." It always does the best it can with the materials you've given it. But the finished product will be substandard, and eventually, this will lead to a breakdown in the body, which we describe as sickness. In the example above, the eventual result will be hypothyroidism because thyroid hormone made with chlorine, fluorine, or bromine doesn't work the same as thyroid hormone made with iodine. People who are hypothyroid end up with a myriad of symptoms including weight gain, low energy, depression, thinning hair, and so on.

And making thyroid hormone is just one single function of one little mineral. Every one of the millions of functions in your body requires a very specific balance of minerals.

Not only do these minerals need to be present in the soil and in our plants, but they need to be absorbed into our bodies as well. Calcium, for example, is one of the most abundant minerals on earth (and in our bodies), but for it to be absorbed, you need to have sufficient hydrochloric acid in your stomach. Without an acidic stomach, you will not be able to break the calcium down and get it into your bloodstream. This means that antacids (including those that contain calcium) actually *prevent* the absorption of calcium. They also prevent the absorption of protein and other minerals.

Besides building bones and teeth and helping in the contraction and relaxation of muscles, calcium has many other roles to play in the body. One of the most important roles it plays is to help buffer the body's pH. While you want your stomach to be acidic, the rest of your body (with few exceptions) prefers to be slightly alkaline. Calcium as well as other minerals help to keep the body in this alkaline range. This is an important step in preventing cancer and a multitude of other illnesses.

Besides an acidic stomach, we also need vitamin D to absorb calcium from the gut. Unlike minerals, though, your body can produce vitamin D, provided you get enough sunlight (without sunscreen) and have enough cholesterol in your skin. To prevent the negative effects of the sun, for example, wrinkles, skin cancer, sunstroke, herpes outbreaks, and so on, it's important that you have plenty of essential fatty acids in your diet. I recommend one to two tablespoons of raw flax seed oil per day for this.

Minerals do not work independently in the body. They all play off each other in an incredibly synchronized dance. Zinc and copper, for example, play off each other on a teeter-totter principle. When copper levels become too high in the body, zinc compensates by becoming too low, and vice versa. Zinc is needed for many functions in the body, including the production of hydrochloric acid, which, as we've just learned, is needed for the absorption of calcium. So having too much copper could lead to having low zinc and calcium levels. Zinc is also needed for immune function, for healthy prostate function, and for melatonin and DHEA production. Thus minerals need to be *in balance* with one another; more is not necessarily better.

Minerals also need to be in an absorbable form. When we get our minerals from plants and animals, this happens automatically. When we rely on manufactured and man-made supplements to make up the difference, the minerals that are used are often forms that are difficult or impossible for the body to break down, absorb, and convert into a usable form. Calcium carbonate, for example (one of the more common forms of calcium), is very hard for the body to break down. This form of calcium is actually limestone. If any calcium carbonate *is* absorbed, it takes the body about a dozen steps to convert it into the form of calcium we can actually use. This requires energy and additional raw materials.

So how do you find out what minerals you need as well as which ones you may have too much of? The best way to do this is with a hair analysis. Why hair and not blood? Because our bodies are designed to maintain certain levels of minerals in the blood at all costs, oftentimes robbing Peter to pay Paul. In other words, if your body detects your blood calcium levels dropping, it will pull calcium from your muscles or bones to bring the blood calcium back up. This is part of your body's self-regulating mechanism that we call homeostasis. Thus you could have a raging calcium deficiency in your bones and tissues and never detect it using a blood test. Also, blood tests only tell you what's happening the second the blood is drawn. With hair analysis, we can see what's been happening, on average, over the past several weeks or months and get a more accurate depiction of your overall mineral status.[1]

Finally, what's the best way to balance your mineral levels once you know what they are? As I mentioned, our bodies like to get their minerals from plants (either directly, or indirectly, through animals), which are grown on soil that contains all the minerals and trace minerals and no pesticides or herbicides. Nature has figured out exactly how to balance minerals in proper ratios for our bodies. So, I recommend eating a diet as high as possible in raw (or lightly steamed) organic fruits and vegetables as well as organic, free-range meats, poultry, and eggs. I also recommend supplementing your diet with whole food concentrates that are grown in similar conditions.

In conclusion, your body needs very specific amounts of all the minerals, and it must get those minerals from the plants, animals, and animal products you ingest. To find your current mineral balance, I recommend finding a doctor or practitioner who uses hair analysis. Balancing your minerals can be a complex process. It's really not as simple as "your iron levels are low; take some more iron." This work requires an in-depth understanding of the many interactions and relationships between the minerals. Once you know what your mineral levels are, I recommend using whole food concentrates (plants and animal parts ground up and concentrated into pills) to get the rebalancing process under way and frequent rechecks to test your hair mineral levels as they improve and change. It can take years to fully rebalance, but the results are often profound, sometimes even resulting in positive changes to your personality. One final bit of advice: be patient, be persistent, and in time, you'll be healthy. Good luck!

---

[1] E. Hamilton, E. Sabbioni, and M. Van der Venne, "Element reference values in tissues from inhabitants of the European community VI: Review of elements in blood, plasma and urine and a critical evaluation of reference values for the United Kingdom population," *Science of the Total Environment* 158 (1994): 165–90; Paul Eck, "Why I prefer hair tests to blood tests," *Healthview Newsletter* 27–29 (1981): 33–34.

About the Author

Dr. Brad Case is the author of the soon-to-be-released series *The Natural Health Care Revolution*. The first book in the series, *Controversies, Conspiracies & Myths of Modern Medicine: How Your Doctor Is Making You Sick and What to Do about It*, is a scathing exposé on the American health care system. Dr. Case also runs a holistic health care clinic on the central coast of California, specializing in nutrition, immune enhancement, applied kinesiology, and allergy elimination. He is a doctor of chiropractic. For more information about either his books or his clinic, or to order a hair analysis kit, please visit his Web site: http://www.drbradcase.com.

95

Hormones for Health: Bioidentical Hormone Replacement Therapy

Frank Comstock, MD, FACEP, FAAAM

As we age, certain hormone levels decline, creating hormone imbalances that increase our risk for many degenerative diseases. These hormone imbalances and deficiencies will accelerate the aging process. Supplementing with bioidentical hormones can restore hormones to youthful levels and restore energy and vitality, greatly enhancing your quality of life.

To appreciate the potential of bioidentical hormone replacement, it is necessary to review what hormones do in the body and understand the diverse role they play in your health and well-being. Hormones are chemical messengers that control all the body's functions. They control our metabolism, our energy production, and our mood and memory and contribute greatly to our libido and sexual performance. Hormones direct cells throughout the human body by giving cells chemical messages, or instructions, to carry out cellular function. Every cell in the body requires interactions with hormones for optimal cell function and health. If hormone levels are deficient, cell function and, subsequently, organ function will suffer. To maintain our health, we must maintain youthful hormone levels with bioidentical hormone replacement.

Understanding the wellness benefits of bioidentical hormones requires differentiating bioidentical hormones from traditional synthetic hormone replacement. *Bioidentical* means that the hormones used are exact replicas of hormones produced naturally in our bodies: same shape, same structure, same effects. Traditional synthetic hormones are not the same as our own hormones; rather, they are chemical substitutes for our hormones: different shape, different structure, different effects. Hormones interact with cells throughout the body by binding onto cell receptors. Cell receptors recognize different hormones based on their shapes and structures. If we want a specific hormone effect in the body, we must use a hormone that is biologically identical to that hormone, not a synthetic mismatch. By supplementing deficient hormones with the exact hormone, we allow the body to utilize the hormone naturally and without side effects.

Let us move on to the specifics of bioidentical hormone replacement. As women age, they produce less estrogen, progesterone, and testosterone hormones. *Estrogen* is a broad term for three main hormones called estriol, estradiol, and estrone. As men age, they produce less testosterone and gradually produce more estrogen. In addition, both men and women release less human growth hormone and dehydroepiandrosterone (DHEA). It is crucial to acknowledge that insufficient levels of some or all of these hormones result in hormone deficiency states that will adversely influence health and aging. Low hormone levels will mean suboptimal metabolism, leading to higher body fat, less muscle, and less bone density. Remember that these hormones interact with every cell in the body. Suboptimal cell function leads to accelerated skin aging, increased risk of heart disease, dementia, stroke, and osteoporosis. Our immune system is adversely affected, so we are less resistant to bacterial and viral illness and cancer. To add insult to injury, mood and libido will suffer from low hormone levels. As hormone levels drop, night sweats, hot flashes, fatigue, depression, dry skin, and insomnia can develop. The end result of a hormone deficiency is decreased quality of life.

A key word in bioidentical hormone replacement is *balance*. Balance means that we correct all deficient hormone levels, instead of focusing only on estrogen supplementation in women or testosterone replacement in men. Unfortunately, isolated hormone replacement with synthetic hormones has been the norm with traditional hormone replacement. All the hormones work together for optimal effect and safety in the body. If we only focus on a few deficient hormones, then we will never restore hormonal balance, and we will never reach optimal health.

Heart disease is a leading cause of death. Bioidentical hormone replacement plays a tremendous role in decreasing many cardiac risk factors. For example, both estrogen and testosterone improve cholesterol panels, improve blood flow to the heart, improve blood pressure, improve blood sugar and insulin levels, and decrease the risk of blood clotting. Most of the benefits of bioidentical hormones on heart function also apply to brain function, with improved memory, mood, and decreased risk of dementia and stroke. With traditional hormone replacement we tend to focus only on symptom reduction, that is, night sweats, hot flashes, and so on, while ignoring the huge impact of hormones on heart and brain health. Bioidentical hormones are also natural anti-inflammatories and antioxidants, and these attributes decrease the risk of every degenerative disease. Because of the crucial role bioidentical hormones play throughout the body, it is essential to understand that there is no physiologic benefit to maintaining deficient or low hormone levels. For optimal health we must measure our hormone levels and correct deficiencies as they develop.

We identify hormone deficiencies by a combination of reviewing symptoms and hormone blood levels. We correct hormone deficiencies by working with compounding pharmacies. Compounding pharmacies allow us tremendous flexibility in dosing as well as routes of hormone administration. Depending on the hormones that are deficient, we can offer hormone replacement as topical creams, oral capsules, troches (wafers that dissolve under the tongue), or injections. Flexible dosing options allow us to meet individual patient requirements. The multiple dosing and route options make bioidentical hormone replacement a unique, individualized program for each patient. This allows improved patient compliance and results. We monitor each patient with serial reviews of hormone deficiency symptoms as well as with serial measurements of blood hormone levels to ensure patient safety and success.

Keys to bioidentical hormone replacement include the following.

1. Obtain blood tests for specific hormone levels both at onset of therapy and with serial follow-up. A hormone panel for men includes total and free testosterone, DHEA, IGF-1 (measure of growth hormone), and estradiol (main estrogen). A hormone panel for women includes testosterone, estradiol, progesterone, IGF-1, and DHEA. Both men and women should check a thyroid panel (TSH, free T4, and free T3).
2. Work with a physician trained in bioidentical hormone replacement therapy.
3. Supplement deficient hormones with bioidentical hormones (no synthetic substitutes). Remember balance.
4. Optimize results by combining symptom reduction with hormone blood levels to gauge dose adjustments.
5. Custom dosing and routes with compounding pharmacies.
6. Eat a whole-food diet rich in healthy protein (lean meats, fish, eggs), healthy fats (olive oil, avocado, raw nuts, seeds, fish oil), and healthy carbohydrates (fruits and vegetables).
7. Avoid or minimize processed foods, chemical food additives, and artificial sweeteners.
8. Participate in a moderate, consistent exercise program.[1]

Bioidentical hormone replacement offers a modality that slows the aging process, improves health, and decreases the risk of many degenerative diseases. It will add quality years to your life.

About the Author

Frank Comstock, MD, FACEP, FAAAM, is board certified in antiaging medicine and emergency medicine. He is now into his twentieth year of emergency medicine and his seventh year of antiaging medicine. At Lifestyle Spectrum in Tucson, Arizona, he offers private consultations for programs including healthy diet, exercise, bioidentical hormones, and supplementation. Contact www.skinspectrum.com or LifeStyle Spectrum, 6127 North La Cholla, Tucson, AZ 85741.

---

[1] Healthy diet and exercise programs maximize results with hormone replacement programs.

96

Hudor:
The Miracle Substance

P. J. Glassey, CSCS

Have you heard of *hudor?* Its effects overshadow even the most potent ancient Chinese herbs. Its healing capabilities outperform wonder drugs from deep in the Amazonian rain forest. It holds the key to countless health benefits and wellness miracles.

Hudor can make your nails stronger, hair healthier, and teeth whiter. It greatly reduces skin problems and acne. It can even take away wrinkles and make your lips fuller. It promotes better skin circulation and tone, while often adding color as well. *Hudor* can heal chapped lips and dry mouth. Even chronic bad breath is often neutralized with proper doses.

Hudor acts as a catalyst for transporting essential nutrients throughout the body and performs as a solvent for all products of digestion, aiding absorption through the intestinal walls into the bloodstream.

Hudor promotes protein metabolism better than anabolic steroids. It also metabolizes energy-producing carbohydrates. It prevents muscle cramping; increases physical performance, strength, and endurance; and can lower your pulse rate and blood pressure. It is the best substance for maintaining electrolyte balance. It is the only proven ergogenic aid with no side effects or restrictions from the Food and Drug Administration.

The minerals potassium, sodium, magnesium, and calcium are essential for conducting electrical currents from the brain to the nervous system and then to the muscles signaling contractions. *Hudor* promotes this more effectively than any other element, even to the extent of preventing heart attacks.

Hudor also removes waste products from the body while simultaneously regulating its temperature. It is the key ingredient in chemical reactions that metabolize stored fat—especially when taken just before a meal and again right after. It can also act as a potent appetite suppressant, filling you up without any chemical side effects.

It promotes healing of injuries as well as illness. It boosts the immune system's defenses better than any drug on the market. It holds the key to transporting antioxidants and aids in their effectiveness to fight cancer. It improves general comfort, mood, and well-being, while decreasing irritability and nervousness. It helps prevent fatigue and improves concentration, memory, and alertness.

Cuts, bruises, and even tendonitis are healed up to twice as fast with proper amounts of *hudor*, and chronic daily headaches are often permanently cured. Muscle soreness from injury, overuse, or exercise is cut in half or less with *hudor*. It also lengthens the life of all vital organs—especially the liver and kidneys—and is still available over the counter!

The significance of liver and kidney health is especially important to fat loss. If the kidneys are functioning properly, the liver doesn't have to help them out and can concentrate on its job of taking fat out of your tissues to be burned off. *Hudor* directly affects both kidney and liver health in a very specific way, which in turn accelerates fat loss.

Where do you get *hudor*? It has been around since before man existed. Your body is made up of 65 percent *hudor*. It takes up more than 70 percent of the earth's surface, and the nearest source is your tap. *Hudor* is the Greek word for water, and you're probably not getting enough.

The average person loses two cups of water through normal perspiration. Another two cups is exhaled as water vapor during the process of breathing. Together, the intestines and kidneys use about four cups a day. That's eight cups used just for living, not counting anything extra we might do during the day.

If you drink at least three quarts or more a day, you're already experiencing its wonderful effects. If you are like most Americans, who drink dehydrating beverages like coffee, soda, and alcohol with very little water, the effects of three quarts or more daily will truly be miraculous. You may find yourself in the restroom more frequently, but just ask yourself, which is more inconvenient: finding a bathroom more often, or carrying around extra weight and being less healthy *all* the time?

Make sure you're drinking it plain, too. Mineral and sparkling water often contain too much sodium. Soft drinks are even worse. Although their main ingredient is water, less than 10 percent of it will be absorbed because of all the preservatives, dyes, flavoring agents, sugar, sodium, and additives.

Pure, clean water is absorbed through the lining of the intestines. Juice, coffee, or soda is held within the intestines for further digestion. The process of digesting these other drinks can require even more water than originally found in the beverage! These drinks may further encourage dehydration, rather than relieving it. Try to get filtered water whenever possible. Reverse osmosis systems are the best and most effective at taking out the chemicals and sediment often found in municipal sources.

If additional water is not consumed to make up for a deficit, the body may be forced to draw on itself from the areas of richest supply, namely the muscles. When muscle tissue dehydrates by even as little as 3 percent, it will lose 10 percent of its contractile strength and 8 percent of its speed. Dehydration also adversely affects the structure and function of the nervous system, producing a miniscule but crucial shrinkage of the brain resulting in decreased concentration, coordination, performance, and sometimes a headache.

To obtain the benefits of the wonder fluid, go straight to the source and get the real thing in its cleanest form. The next time you find it hard to move off the couch, can't concentrate, or are having a bad day, pour yourself a big glass of filtered water. It may also be the key to losing those last few stubborn pounds or the cure to a frustrating fitness plateau. It's worth a try. It may be just that simple.

About the Author

P. J. Glassey, CSCS, started personal training in 1987 and phased into it full-time as an in-home trainer after receiving his B.S. degree in Exercise Science in 1989. P. J. and his wife Sharmon opened their own personal training studio in 1998 called the X Gym. The business has since grown to 3 studios in the Seattle area. Their program is so effective, 90 percent of their new clients come via word-of-mouth referrals from present and past satisfied customers. Visit their Web site at http://www.xgym.com.

97

The Magic of Fulvic Acid

Susan Lark, MD

Dear Friend,

I am always on the lookout for new and exciting products that help enhance health and wellness. So, I am thrilled to let you in on a little-known but very exciting substance called *fulvic acid*. Don't be surprised if you've never heard of fulvic acid. I have only been researching it for a year or so, and most people in the complementary medicine field don't even know what it is. What makes this substance all the more intriguing is that it has been around for centuries, but only in the last few years have research studies supported what traditional use had already shown—fulvic acid is a miracle healer.

The history of fulvic acid is quite interesting. Originally discovered in New Mexico, fulvic acid was comprised of ancient organic, compacted vegetation rich in trace minerals. Hundreds of millions of years ago, New Mexico was more like a tropical rain forest than the desert it is today. Like a rain forest, this area was vibrant with tree and plant matter as well as swampland. As the trees and plants died, they often fell into the water, amassing at the bottom of the swamp floor.

Because the swamps were most often stagnant, they were not well oxygenated, which meant that decay was less likely to take place. As a result, the trees and plants didn't decompose as they would under normal conditions. Instead, the leaves and softer shoots broke down into a jelly-like substance, while the harder, woody parts, like branches and trunks, turned into peat. This combination created the initial components of fulvic acid.

Over the course of many, many centuries, the waters of these swamps receded, and this mineral-rich jelly and peat became visible. By the early 1600s, the Native Americans living in the New Mexico area as well as the Spaniards that also resided in the Southwest discovered this biomass mineral material, wrongly assuming that it was coal. However, they quickly learned their mistake when the "coal" wouldn't burn.

One Spaniard in particular, a Catholic priest by the name of Fray Benavides, was not content simply to overlook the possible benefits of this thick, lush material. He studied it, pulverized it, and even sprinkled some of it on his food. Surprised by the lack of taste, he almost determined that it was nothing more than dirt. Almost.

During a walk, Father Benavides bumped up against a cactus, impaling several of the spikes into his foot. While he was able to remove most of the thorns, several were too deep and began to fester. He decided to sprinkle some of the pulverized material onto his injured foot. He continued to use it for several days, and much to his amazement, the infection cleared up, and his foot healed completely.

Modern research has begun to examine both fulvic acid's nutrient content and its physiological benefits in cells and tissues. While clinical research has yet to be done, some practitioners are beginning to recommend fulvic acid–based nutritional products and are amassing anecdotal information about its benefits. For instance, fulvic acid shows promise in promoting healing in patients with a variety of serious health conditions for which mineral deficiency plays a much underreported role. People using fulvic acid report healing benefits for chronic fatigue, acute muscle aches and pains, fibromyalgia, arthritis, wound healing, and Bell's palsy. There also have been some amazing testimonials from people who have used fulvic acid to help recover from other, more serious conditions such as cancer, autism, and chronic pain. Fulvic acid also appears to promote healthier, more efficient detoxification within the body—a crucial function that's needed if we want to enjoy optimal health. In this article, I'd like to talk more about fulvic acid and tell you how it can promote, protect, and restore vigorous health for us all.

The Magic of Fulvic Acid

Fulvic acid, a natural component of rich, organic humus, can be found in any nutrient-rich, organic soil. It is created by micro-organisms that live in decaying organic matter, such as centuries-old deposits of composted vegetation and manure. Fulvic acid is not actually an acid—nor is it a mineral. It is, rather, a complex compound that can attract and hold both negatively and positively charged ions. As such, it can bond and hold ionized minerals—such as calcium, magnesium, and zinc—incorporating them into its own molecular structure. This creates a new fulvic acid–multimineral compound that plants, animals, and humans can easily digest, absorb, and utilize to support vibrant health.

This is the real magic of fulvic acid—its ability to dissolve elemental minerals present in the soil and convert them into a form that is highly absorbable by the roots of plants. Once absorbed, those minerals are in the perfect form for feeding, strengthening, and growing the botanical, whether it's an herb, cherry tree, or tomato plant. When ingested, these nutrient-rich minerals that are now present in the fruits, vegetables, and herbs pack a powerful nutritional punch. Obviously, this is how our bodies are designed to meet our daily mineral needs—by eating well-nourished foods. But there's a problem.

For soil to contain significant levels of fulvic acid, it must provide a friendly, nutrient-rich environment for the micro-organisms that produce it. However, those who practice conventional farming methods have neither the inclination nor the patience to maintain their fields organically, therefore creating an environment unsuitable for the formation of fulvic acid.

Unfortunately, conventional farmers don't even look at soil as the living, bustling community of important micro-organisms that it is. To them, soil is simply a medium in which to plant seeds, add chemical fertilizers, and grow mass-marketable, nutrient-deficient produce. On top of that, the harsh chemical environment that grows most mass-produced fruits and vegetables not only fails to nurture the micro-organisms that produce fulvic acid, but it actually kills them.

As I've discussed many times in the past, the makeup of fruits and vegetables depends on the soil they are grown in. A plant growing in a garden that is enriched by organically produced compost, rather than chemical fertilizer, and cultivated organically, rather than with chemical herbicides and pesticides, has its roots in luxurious soil teeming with fulvic acid–producing microbes. These beneficial soil "bugs" thrive in this nutrient-rich environment, and in turn, they lavish the soil around the plant's roots with fulvic acid.

Why Minerals Matter

As you know, there are many key minerals that are essential for good health. Unfortunately, the typical foods and supplements in most supermarkets simply can't provide the quantity and quality of minerals our bodies need to be strong and healthy. The epidemic of osteoporosis and osteopenia in America—even among women who religiously take bone-building supplements—is a perfect example.

However, this issue goes way beyond bone health. Minerals are vital for literally every biochemical function in every organ system in the human body—from transmitting a nerve impulse to making a muscle fiber twitch, neutralizing a toxic free radical, regulating thyroid hormones, and recharging a red blood cell with oxygen. And there is a growing body of evidence to suggest that deficiencies of minerals are at the root of many major health problems, including thyroid disease, cancers, neuropathies, immune deficiencies, and fatigue disorders. For example, according to a report from the A-D Research Foundation published in the November 2003 issue of the *Journal of Carcinogenesis*, there is a significant link between cancer and mineral deficiencies. The report suggests that providing cancer patients with specific, critical nutrients could lead to a reversal of the disease.

Enrich Your Body with the Minerals It Needs

Fulvic acid is one of the many reasons I recommend eating and feeding your family organic food. In addition to the well-recognized perks—freedom from herbicides, pesticides, and chemical fertilizers—organically grown food is richer in chelated fulvic acid and mineral compounds that provide the nourishing, alkalinizing minerals your body needs to thrive.

Fortunately, there are a growing number of small-scale organic farms that provide produce rich in fulvic acid and countless other nutrients. Visit http://www.ams.usda.gov/farmersmarkets and click on "Find a Farmers Market in Your State" to find such farms near you. There are also a growing number of online outfits, such as http://www.diamondorganics.com, where you can buy organic food. It may cost more than supermarket produce, but the health benefits of eating organically are immeasurable.

However, because it took eons for many of this country's soils to become mineral-rich, and only a few generations to deplete them, you can't rely strictly on good-quality food to provide the minerals you need. I recommend enhancing your mineral intake with top-quality fulvic acid supplements. What do I mean by top quality? Let's revisit calcium as an example. Typical supplements are chock full of calcium, but much of it goes right out of the body because it's so difficult to absorb (the same goes for other minerals). Even when some of the calcium does manage to gain access to your bloodstream, it must then pass into and through complicated, maze-like membranes and cell walls to get into your cells and actually work.

Minerals chelated to fulvic acid are very good at getting all the way into cells. But it's important that the quality of the fulvic acid compound be beyond reproach. While fulvic acid increases the availability of essential minerals, it also can increase the intake of some minerals that may be toxic. Therefore it's crucial to find fulvic acid mineral complexes that are extracted from pure, unpolluted sources and tested for toxic heavy metals. I've carefully researched the fulvic acid products currently available and recommend the following:

- Fulvic Mineral Complex from Vital-Earth Minerals, LLC (866-291-4400 or http://www.vitalearth.org) is a potent liquid complex containing a multitude of plant-derived minerals in a fulvic-chelated formulation. Another plus is this product's alkaline pH of 7.0–7.8.
- Energy Boost 70 from Morningstar Minerals contains organic mineral complexes and amino acids in an organic fulvic acid base. Also available are Fruitland Agriculture Products, designed to replenish the soil of your organic garden with essential humic and fulvic acids. To order, call (866) 898-4467 or visit http://www.msminerals.com.

About the Author

Susan Lark, MD, is one of the foremost authorities in the fields of clinical nutrition and preventive medicine. A graduate of Northwestern University Medical School, she served on the clinical faculty of Stanford University Medical School from 1981 to 1983 and taught in Stanford's Primary Care Associate Program in the Division of Family and Community Medicine from 1991 to 2002. Dr. Lark is a distinguished clinician, author, lecturer, and innovative product developer. Throughout her thirty-two years of clinical experience, she has pioneered the use of self-care treatments, such as diet, nutrition, exercise, and stress management techniques, in the field of women's health and has lectured extensively throughout the United States on topics in preventive medicine. She has also authored and published several books, her most recent being *Eat Papayas Naked: The pH-Balanced Diet for Super Health and Glowing Beauty*. For more information, visit http://www.DrLark.com.

98

Healing the Addicted Brain with Amino Acids

Merlene Miller, MA

We are all affected in some way by addiction, whether our own or that of someone we care about. Yet no physical disorder that affects so many of us in so many ways is so little recognized and so little understood. Other efforts to be healthy will fail as long as addiction—whether to alcohol, illegal drugs, sugar, nicotine, or prescription medications—is actively affecting our lives.

What is not recognized about addiction is that it is a *physical* disorder originating in the brain.[1] Another little understood aspect of the nature of addiction is that there are painful symptoms that occur during abstinence that interfere with the ability to stay sober: craving, obsession, compulsion, stress sensitivity, anxiety, depression, mental confusion, and hypersensitivity to the environment.[2] Most people are unaware that the pain of staying sober can be, and frequently is, so severe that it interferes with the ability to function, even when the desire for and commitment to recovery is strong.

Neurotransmitters and Addiction

We all seek physical and emotional comfort. We want to feel good. Chemicals in the brain called neurotransmitters play a significant role in feelings of pleasure and well-being. A deficiency or excess of any neurotransmitter will give rise to uncomfortable feelings. Most of the actions we take are chosen to produce good feelings or relieve bad feelings. We eat because it produces a reward of good feelings. We eat *certain* foods because they produce a better reward than others (chocolate produces more reward for most people than parsley). We have sex because it produces a powerful release of pleasurable chemicals. We work because the work itself is rewarding for us or because the end result produces a reward. We refrain from certain actions because they do not produce the feeling of reward we

---

[1] Kenneth Blum and James Payne, *Alcohol and the Addictive Brain* (New York: Free Press, 1991).
[2] Terrence Gorski and Merlene Miller, *Staying Sober: A Guide for Relapse Prevention* (Independence, MO: Herald House, 1986).

are seeking. We all differ in what gives us satisfaction and in the depth of satisfaction we experience, but we are all motivated by chemical actions in the brain that nature uses to keep us alive, motivated, functioning, and reproducing.

An imbalance in the interaction of neurotransmitters can result in a reward deficiency[3] that can manifest as restlessness, anxiety, emptiness, lack of satisfaction, and vague or specific cravings. This is the brain's message to us to take action to right the imbalance. This need can lead to use of a mood-altering substance or behavior to self-medicate the discomfort.

There are substances and activities that change our biochemistry so much that we want to do them over and over. And if the person has a reward deficit that predisposes to addiction, the activity that *works* will be repeated as often as necessary to get the desired reward. For the person predisposed to addiction, the chosen activity will rapidly go from self-medication to addiction.

But because a substance does not lead to out-of-control behavior does not mean that it is not dangerous. Many socially acceptable addictions can lead to serious health problems and even death. Nicotine usually does not lead to intoxication but does lead to serious health problems. It is far more addicting than alcohol or illegal drugs and is usually accompanied by severe withdrawal symptoms when smoking ceases and can be as painful as withdrawing from alcohol or cocaine. Prescription painkillers and antidepressants can be highly addictive. Withdrawal, especially from benzodiazepines, can be very serious and can even lead to death. For some people, food is the most powerful mood-altering substance available. Most people believe that overeating is a lack of willpower or self-discipline. But the people most susceptible to it often have a physical condition that keeps them from feeling satisfied from normal eating. Some addictions are not to substances but to behaviors such gambling, compulsive working, or excessive spending. The problem does not lie in the behavior itself, but in how it is done. If any behavior is accompanied by compulsion, obsession, and negative consequences, it is a problem and requires some action to learn to manage the behavior in a healthy way.

Healing the Addicted Brain

While research has opened doors to new understandings of the nature of addiction and its effect on the brain, little of this information has been applied to actually helping people get well from this devastating disease. There are scientifically

---

[3] Kenneth Blum, Eric R. Braverman, Jay M. Holder, Joel F. Lubar, Vincent J. Monastra, David Miller, Judith O. Lubar, Thomas Chen, and David E. Comings, "Reward Deficiency Syndrome: A Biogenic Model for the Diagnosis and Treatment of Impulsive, Compulsive, and Addictive Behaviors," *Journal of Psychoactive Drugs* 32 (2000): 1–11.

based strategies that change the brain chemistry of the addicted person, removing the discomfort of withdrawal, eliminating cravings, and relieving the abstinence-based symptoms of addiction. These include nutritional therapy, acupuncture, auriculotherapy, and brain wave biofeedback. The most important is the nutritional approach, especially with the use of amino acids, which is the focus of this discussion.

Amino Acid Therapy

Neurotransmitters are made from amino acids, the building blocks of protein. The nervous system is regulated almost entirely by amino acids and their biochemical companions, vitamins and minerals. There are key neurotransmitters that are affected by addiction and need to be restored to their normal state for the recovering person to be free of cravings and anxiety. The amino acids, precursors to neurotransmitters, can be taken separately, as a formulated compound, or intravenously. Intravenous delivery has the advantage of bypassing the digestive system. This offers hope for the thousands of people whose digestive systems have been damaged by addiction to alcohol or drugs, caffeine, or junk food. Certain vitamins—especially B vitamins—activate and potentiate the effects of amino acids. There are treatment centers that offer nutritional therapy intravenously. This form of treatment is extremely effective in relieving withdrawal symptoms and in helping people maintain long-term sobriety.

Nutrition

Amino acids and vitamin supplements are essential for nourishing the brain recovering from addiction. But supplements are not more important than the foods you eat daily. Long-term recovery from addiction requires healthful eating and an adequate supply of amino acids, vitamins, and minerals—not for a short period of time, not just until you are feeling better, and not just until the initial withdrawal and craving are gone. A person seeking freedom from the discomfort of addiction must make the same kind of commitment to healthful eating that a diabetic must make. At this point in time, we have no magic bullet to fix either the pancreas or the brain once and for all. Dysfunction of both takes special care on a regular basis.

Depending on what amino acids they contain, some foods increase mental alertness, concentration, and energy, while others are natural tranquilizers that calm feelings of anxiety and stress. The neurotransmitter tyrosine synthesizes to dopamine and norepinephrine, increasing energy and alertness. Foods highest in tyrosine are foods derived from animal protein: chicken, turkey, pork, beef, dairy, and eggs. Moderate amounts of tyrosine are found in plant foods such as beans, corn, spinach, oatmeal, nuts, and seeds.

The neurotransmitter tryptophan synthesizes to serotonin, producing relaxation and sleep. Foods high in tryptophan are turkey, green leafy vegetables, dairy products, bananas, pineapple, avocado, soy, lentils, sesame seeds, and pumpkin. There is not an abundance of foods that contain tryptophan, and those that do may not contain amounts sufficient to make it into the brain if they are competing with other amino acids, especially tyrosine. However, carbohydrates help carry the tryptophan to the brain. But if you eat a carbohydrate-rich meal early in the day, it can cause drowsiness. It is better to eat tryptophan-rich foods and carbohydrates in the evening when you want to relax and prepare for sleep, rather than for breakfast, when you want to become alert and energized.

A very important thing to know about a diet for recovery is that protein contains all the essential amino acids. Therefore a high-protein diet will give your brain more of what it needs. Complete protein foods include meat, poultry, fish, eggs, and dairy products. The body stores very little protein, so you should eat it at least three times a day. And for the sake of both energy and your brain, we recommend three meals and three snacks daily.

Supporting Recovery

To support healing of the brain, other healthy lifestyle choices are important. A support group such as Alcoholics Anonymous or Overeaters Anonymous, regular exercise, yoga, rest, relaxation, fun, and creative living are important to reduce stress and increase a sense of serenity and well-being.

Healthy living with good nutrition at its center is the key to recovery from addiction. For people who have given up hope that they can ever overcome the compulsion and obsession related to an addictive substance or the agony of abstinence, there is a way they might not have tried. If you or someone you know is looking for an addiction treatment center, find one that offers nutritional therapy (preferably in the form of intravenous nutritional therapy). The miracle of amino acid therapy combined with other healthy ways of living has given hope to many for regaining freedom from addiction and for enriching their lives.

Bibliography

Gant, Charles, and Greg Lewis. *End Your Addiction Now.* New York: Warner Books, 2002.
Miller, David, and Kenneth Blum. *Overload: Attention Deficit Disorder and the Addictive Brain.* St. Louis: Miller, 2000.
Miller, Merlene, and David Miller. *Staying Clean and Sober: Complementary and Natural Strategies for Healing the Addicted Brain.* Orem, UT: Woodland, 2005.
Ross, Julia. *The Mood Cure.* New York: Penguin Books, 2002.

About the Author

Merlene Miller, MA, is an educator and author with 25 years in the addiction field, specializing in relapse prevention. She works with LIfeStream Solutions (http://www.lifestream-solutions.com) to promote the use of intravenous nutritional therapy. She is director of educational development for Bridging the Gaps, an addiction treatment center in Winchester, Virginia that utilizes complementary treatment methods, including intravenous nutritional therapy (http//www.bridgingthegaps.com). She has authored or co-authored numerous books including *Staying Clean and Sober: Complementary and Natural Strategies for Healing the Addicted Brain,* (with David Miller), *Reversing the Regression Spiral* (with David Miller) , and *Learning to Live Again: A Guide to Recovery from Chemical Dependency* (with Terence Gorski and David Miller). Visit http://www.miller-associates.org.

99

Caring for the Whole Body with South American Herbs

Dr. Viana Muller

Despite the environmental stresses we face daily, our less than ideal lifestyle choices, and our genetic challenges, we can reap impressive health results through consistent use of therapeutic herbs, which can strengthen the structures and functions of our bodies. Many Americans are familiar with some North American herbs like Echinacea, used to help prevent colds and flu, St. John's wort, used for mood support, and the Chinese herb ginseng, taken for energy support. But for most of us, knowledge stops with fewer than five herbs. In this article, I will introduce you to a handful of very impressive Peruvian herbs, now just becoming available in the larger health food stores, in specialty herb shops, and on health-related Web sites. Unlike Chinese and Ayurvedic herbs, they are easy to understand. Clinical experience and scientific studies have shown them to be highly effective in greatly improving many health issues when used on a frequent or regular basis. Following are some examples of how to use a few of these herbs to support your body.

Hormonal Imbalances

Difficult menstrual periods, PMS, ovarian cysts, difficult menopause, or, in the case of men, issues with early andropause and erectile dysfunction as well as those suffering from chronic adrenal, thyroid, or pancreatic problems may find a stunning herbal helper in a Peruvian root vegetable from the Andes called maca or maca root.[1] Not only has maca clinically proved to be a superb hormone balancer, it appears to strengthen the immune system and to help with the healthy production of neurotransmitter hormones such as serotonin (regulating mood) and melatonin (regulating sleep).[2]

---

[1] Morton Walker, "Effects of Peruvian Maca on Hormonal Functions," *Townsend Letter for Doctors and Patients* (November 1998).

[2] Artemio Chang and Viana Muller, "Effects of Cooked Maca on Serologic Serotonin Levels in Mice" (unpublished study, San Luis Gonzaga University, Ica, Peru, 2004). There have also been many reports from clinicians on the improvement in sleep by their patients after beginning maca therapy.

Mood Balance

People who are prone to depression or anxiety can often find nutritional/herbal support surprisingly effective. Maca root, by improving hormone balance, also improves serotonin levels.[3] The Amazonian wild fruit camu-camu, with more natural vitamin C than any other botanical, also contains phytochemicals that improve mood and has been shown in clinical practice to often work the same day.[4]

Digestion and Elimination

Cat's claw (*Uncaria tomentosa*) ingested as a tea or a water-alcohol extract is considered by many master herbalists to be the herb par excellence for flatulence, headaches (digestion-related), constipation, diarrhea, leaky gut syndrome, Crohn's disease, and ulcers—conditions reflecting chronic inflammatory processes in the stomach and intestines.[5] Dietary changes are also essential as a high-sugar, low-fiber diet contributes to the loss of a healthy bowel ecology.

Liver and Gall Bladder

The Peruvian herb *chanca piedra* or break-stone (*Phyllanthus niruri* and related species) is the most important herb for people with common liver and gall bladder issues, including gall stones and hepatitis. Both clinical practice and research demonstrate break-stone's antiviral (hepatitis) properties[6] and its ability to improve the digestion of fats.[7]

People with particular risk factors for liver problems but no demonstrated liver disease would also do well to use break-stone regularly. These factors include a history of hepatitis, obesity, or alcohol use; the regular use of drugs, pharmaceuticals, or hormone therapy; and anyone with regular exposure to environmental toxins, including car exhaust, chemical cleaning, or printing

---

[3] Ibid.

[4] James Duke, "Ethnobotanical Database," http://sun.ars-grin.gov:8080/npgspub/xsql/duke/pl_act.xsql?taxon=1241. See also Gary Null, *A Woman's Encyclopedia of Natural Healing* (New York: Seven Stories Press, 1997) and Null, *The Clinician's Handbook of Natural Healing* (New York: Kensington Press, 1998).

[5] J. L. Aguilar et al., "Anti-inflammatory Activity of Two Different Extracts of *Uncaria tomentosa* (Rubiaceae)," *Journal of Ethnopharmacology* 81 (2002); R. Aquino et al., "Plant Metabolites: New Compounds and Anti-inflammatory Activity of *Uncaria tomentosa*," *Journal of Natural Products* 54 (1991).

[6] M. X. Wang et al., "Efficacy of *Phyllanthus* spp. in Treating Patients with Chronic Hepatitis B," *Zhongguo Zhong Yao Za Zhi* 19 (1994).

[7] A. K. Khanna et al., "Lipid Lowering Activity of *Phyllanthus niruri* in Hyperlipemic Rats" (unpublished study, Division of Biochemistry, Central Drug Research Institute, Lucknow, India, n.d.).

products.[8] Liver weakness may show up as a feeling of heaviness in the liver, a loss of energy, liver or gall bladder pain, elevated liver enzyme levels, or cirrhosis (scarring) of the liver.

Kidney and Bladder

Break-stone is also the herb of choice for urinary organ issues, including kidney stones,[9] recurrent kidney or bladder infections,[10] diabetes,[1111] and high uric acid levels (gout).[12] The kidney and bladder are also highly sensitive to toxic chemicals, and people with high exposure to toxins may benefit from regular use of *chanca piedra*. Scientific research demonstrates break-stone's reduction of elevated aldose reductase levels, the chemical compound that causes peripheral nerve and kidney damage in diabetics.[13]

Immune System and Autoimmune Conditions

There are a number of Peruvian herbs that *support* the immune system without *stimulating* it. These include the Peruvian rainforest botanicals cat's claw,[14] maca,[15] and camu-camu.[16] Research on *Uncaria tomentosa* (the most effective species of cat's claw) shows that its use is linked to an increase in the number of killer T-cells and

---

[8] K. V. Syamasundar et al., "Anti-hepatotoxic Principles of *Phyllanthus niruri* Herbs," *Journal of Ethnopharmacology* 14 (1985).

[9] A. M. Freitas, N. Schor, and M. A. Boim, "The Effect of *Phylanthus niruri* on Urinary Inhibitors of Calcium Oxalate Crystallization and Other Factors Associated with Renal Stone Formation," *British Journal of Urology International* 89 (2002); J. Nishiura et al., "*Phyllanthus niruri* Normalizes Elevated Urinary Calcium Levels in Calcium Stone Forming (CSF) Patients," *Urology Research* 32 (2004).

[10] A. Mazumder et al., "Antimicrobial Potentiality of *Phyllanthus amarus* against Drug Resistant Pathogens," *Natural Products Research* 20 (2006).

[11] N. Srividya and S. Periwal, "Diuretic, Hypotensive and Hypoglycemic Effect of *Phyllanthus amarus*," *Indian Journal of Experimental Biology* 33 (1995).

[12] V. Murugaiyah and K. L. Chan, "Antihyperuricemic Lignans from the Leaves of *Phyllanthus niruri*," *Planta Medica* 72 (2006).

[13] M. Shimizu et al., "Studies on Aldose Reductase Inhibitors from Natural Products. II. Active Components of a Paraguayan Crude Drug 'Para-parai mi,' *Phyllanthus niruri*," *Chemical Pharmacology Bulletin* 37 (1989).

[14] I. Lemaire et al., "Stimulation of Interleukin-1 and -6 Production in Alveolar Macrophages by the Neotropical Liana, *Uncaria tomentosa* (Uña de Gato)," *Journal of Ethnopharmacology* 64 (1999).

[15] Walker, "Effects of Peruvian Maca."

[16] Duke, "Ethnobotanical Database."

macrophage cells produced by the body.[17] Clinical experience also suggests that *Uncaria tomentosa* helps create a healthier blood ecology by reducing the C-reactive protein level in the blood (a primary marker for inflammation)[18] and can reduce tumors,[19] arthritis, allergies, and the symptoms of lupus. Maca, through improved hormone balance, has also been found in clinical practice to improve autoimmune conditions like arthritis and psoraisis.[20]

Heart and Circulatory System

A high C-reactive protein level—the greatest predictor of heart attack or stroke—can be substantially reduced by regular use of cat's claw.[21] Cat's claw and break-stone can also help reduce blood pressure.[22] Camu-camu, a wild Amazonian fruit supplement, is an extremely rich source of natural vitamin C, the most important vitamin for heart health.

Brain

Research suggests that cat's claw, which has been shown to inhibit inflammation up to 89 percent, may be useful in preventing the formation of the amyloid plaque

---

[17] Y. Sheng et al., "Enhanced DNA Repair, Immune Function and Reduced Toxicity of C-Med-100, a Novel Aqueous Extract from *Uncaria tomentosa*," *Journal of Ethnopharmacology* 69 (2000); Y. Sheng et al., "DNA Repair Enhancement of Aqueous Extracts of *Uncaria tomentosa* in a Human Volunteer Study," *Phytomedicine* 8 (2001).

[18] Karen Paris, Atkins Clinic, New York, personal communication, 2003. Paris attested to the dramatic reduction in C-reactive protein level of her coronary patients with the use of a water-alcohol extract of *Uncaria tomentosa*. Also see A. M. Yepez et al., "Quinovic Acid Glycosides from *Uncaria guianensis*," *Phytochemistry* 30 (1991).

[19] E. L. Salazar et al., "Depletion of Specific Binding Sites for Estrogen Receptor by *Uncaria tomentosa*," *Procedures of the Western Pharmacology Society* 41 (1998); Y. Sheng et al., "Induction of Aptosis and Inhibition of Proliferation in Human Tumor Cells Treated with Extracts of *Uncaria tomentosa*," *Anticancer Research* 18 (1998).

[20] Antiarthritic effects of maca are widely reported in the native population in the Sierra Central of Peru. Perhaps four or five women whom I have interviewed have reported a dramatic improvement in their psoriasis after several weeks of using an organic, sun-dried, precooked maca root powder or capsules.

[21] C. Chan-Xun et al., "Inhibitory Effect of Rhynchophylline on Platelet Aggregation and Thrombosis," *Acta Pharmacologica Sinica* 13 (1992). Substantial research documents that the most accurate predictor of future heart attack or stroke is an elevated C-reactive protein level in the blood. Dr. Karen Paris (pers. comm., 2003) told me that the daily use of a water-alcohol-based extract of *Uncaria tomentosa* resulted in a great reduction of the C-reactive protein level of their coronary patients.

[22] S. Yano et al., "Ca_2, Channel-Blocking Effects of Hirsutine, an Indole Alkaloid from *Uncaria* Genus, in the Isolated Rat Aorta," *Planta Medica* 57 (1991); Srividya and Periwal, "Diuretic, Hypotensive."

in the brain associated with Alzheimer's disease.[23] The elevation of a particular liver enzyme level has also recently been implicated in the formation of this plaque. Since break-stone helps normalize elevated liver enzyme levels, it is possible that its regular use may be useful in preventing amyloid plaque formation.[24] Camu-camu's high natural vitamin C content helps chelate out heavy metals, believed to play a role in the development of Alzheimer's.

Vitamin/supplement departments in the health food stores have been around for more than thirty years, but their full potential as herbal apothecaries are just beginning to be explored. As Peruvian herbs become more accessible through these stores and herbal Web sites, and as consumers start to use them based on their friends' recommendations and the research findings, their remarkable effects on health will soon be recognized.

About the Author

Dr. Viana Muller is a cultural anthropologist who set up bilingual, bicultural training programs in Mexico, taught African and Latin American cultural studies in several universities, and was a college administrator before she discovered her life's mission in Peru while studying the plant medicines used by native peoples in the Andes and rainforests. Going through a difficult menopause, she stumbled across the maca root, which was virtually unknown in the U.S. at the time. It changed her life in just a few days. Returning to the United States, she cofounded Whole World Botanicals (http://www.wholeworldbotanicals.com) to make maca available along with cat's claw and other amazing botanicals that she encountered both through her native guides and Peruvian plant pharmacologists.

---

[23] M. Sandoval-Chacon et al., "Anti-inflammatory Actions of Cat's Claw: The Role of NF-ϰB," *Alimentary Pharmacology and Therapeutics* 12 (1998). There is a large body of research documenting cat's claw's anti-inflammatory properties. Two have previously been cited here (Aguilar et al., "Anti-inflammatory Activity"; Aquino et al., "Plant Metabolites"), P. J. Van Ess et al., "Elevated Hepatic and Depressed Renal Cytochrome P450 Activity in the Tg2576 Transgenic Mouse Model of Alzheimer's Disease," *Journal of Neurochemistry* 80 (2002).

[24] Duke, "Ethnobotanical Database."

100

Newly Discovered Nutrients Significantly Impact Overall Health of 98 Percent[1]

Victoria Smith, BSHT

Today, we are living in a society riddled with disease, illness, and disorders, and many of these are a result of a malfunctioning immune system. In fact, just about everybody seems to have a condition or disease that they are being treated for, even children. This was not the case just a decade ago. On reflection, it is apparent that something vital to good health is missing.

A Breakthrough in Medicine

The missing link was discovered in the 1980s. While doing research for a pharmaceutical company, a scientist discovered a nutrient that was not previously identified while looking for the active ingredient in aloe vera. Mannose, a previously unknown sugar molecule, was identified as the constituent in aloe responsible for the natural healing properties. (Yes, a sugar with healing properties!)

The discovery may have eluded scientists because once the aloe is processed, an enzyme in the plant quickly metabolizes the mannose, rendering it nonexistent. A (patented) process was developed to extract the mannose from the aloe, thereby making some of the aloe supplements available mannose-rich.

In the years following this groundbreaking discovery, over two hundred nutrients were identified in this newly discovered class of carbohydrates. The science and study of glycobiology emerged, and today, the function of glyconutrients is understood as impacting the natural workings of the human body.

Simply stated, a glyconutrient is a biochemical that contains a sugar, and some glyconutrients are vital for cell-to-cell communication. This is new knowledge, as sugar

---

[1] The products, science, and technology behind glycobiology are nutritional supplements designed to support the body. They are not meant to be used in place of standard therapy or proven medical care. However, science has recognized a connection between better nutritional intake and improved health.

was always thought of as only being beneficial for energy production. Glyconutrients are a class of carbohydrates that provide raw material for cellular health and do not increase blood glucose levels. Glyconutrients are not minerals, vitamins, fats, proteins, or enzymes, and not all glyconutrients are vital for cellular health.

Eight of these over two hundred glyconutrients have been validated as essential for cellular health. Pesticides, green picking practices, soil depletion, genetic modification, food processing and farming practices have all played a role in the depletion of the nutritional loss of our foods. This includes glyconutritionals. Our diets are deficient in six of the eight essential glyconutrients that are vital for good health.

The eight sugars essential for health follow:

- *Glucose* is overabundant in our diets. Our bodies convert white sugar, frutcose, and starchy foods into glucose.
- *Galactose* is also available in our diets, obtained through the conversion of lactose (milk sugar). It is easily obtained from dairy products, unless you happen to be lactose-intolerant.
- *Fucose* is found in breast milk and several medicinal mushrooms. It has numerous well-documented benefits for the immune system. It is not readily available in our diets.
- *Mannose* is also not found in our diets. Mannose has a profound impact in cellular interactions. This sugar is absolutely vital for proper immune defenses.
- *Xylose* is not found in our diets, but it is said to have antifungal and antibacterial properties.
- *N-acetyl-neuraminic acid* is not found in our diets, but it is one that is also abundant in breast milk. This sugar dramatically impacts brain function and growth. In certain disease states, the ability to digest this sugar is impaired.
- *N-acetyl-glucosamine* is not in our diets. This is a precursor for glucosamine, which is well known for cartilage regeneration and joint inflammation. Malfunction of this sugar has also been linked to diseases of the bowel.
- *N-acetyl-galactosamine* is the least known of the eight sugars that are essential for cellular health, although it appears to inhibit the growth of some tumors, and like other sugars, it plays its individual role in keeping all cellular communication clear and promptly delivered.

These last six sugars listed are not present in our diets at all or in adequate amounts to support our bodies' needs. Since our food supply is no longer supporting our needs for these nutrients, it is beneficial to supplement the diet.

When these eight glyconutrients are present in our diets, glycosynthesis may occur; that is, these nutrients bind with fat (lipids) and protein molecules to form glycoforms on the surface of our trillions of cells.

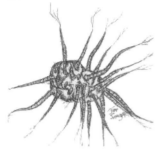

There are two types of glycoforms. When one or more of these eight essential sugar nutrients bind with fat, they are called glycolipids. When they bind with protein, they are called glycoproteins. These glycoforms attach to receptor sites on the cellular surface. When all of the receptor sites on the cellular surface have been filled with a glycoform, they are said to be glycosolated—saturated—and our immune systems may become fully functional.

Figure 1: A glycosoluated cell has many glycoforms, which enhances cellular communications and regulates the immune system. Without the proper raw materials in the diet, cells are without glycoforms, and glycodeficient cells are unable to efficiently communicate.

These hair-like glycoform structures create a protective barrier against viruses, bacteria, cancer, and other invasive pathogens and also act as a communication system. The glycoforms operate as a telephone wire might, sending messages throughout the body. Simply put, these sugars are absolutely vital to cellular survival and function. Without them, our cells, particularly our immune cells, do not respond in a natural way.

With glycoforms, the body regulates the immune system to not overfunction, attacking the body, or to not underfunction, failing to protect the body against pathogens. Could it be that all diseases are merely a deficiency of essential sugars?

Wonderful things occur when the body is provided with glyconutrients. In lab tests, (using a standardized, stabilized blend), after just seven days, the body goes from having virtually undetectable levels of stem cells to having trillions in just one week. The body can be stimulated with nutrition to produce more stem cells than are available in all of the world that are being kept for research purposes! Stem cells, as studies indicate, go wherever needed in the body to replace tissue.

Korean researchers used stem cells to help a paralyzed woman repair spinal nerves and walk again. Researchers at Massachusetts General discovered pancreatic tissue regeneration in a diabetic patient.

Glyconutrients never cure, heal, or mitigate disease. What these nutrients do is provide the body with the building blocks that are needed to function properly and activate powerful, built-in self-healing mechanisms.

Wisely, Paracelsus, the father of pharmacology, stated in the early 1500s that "all mankind needs for good health and healing is provided in nature. The challenge to science is to find it."

In connecting good health to good nutrition, it is easy to understand why this is better news than any disease-specific drug. By activating built-in self-healing mechanisms, at the cellular level, the body does the thinking and acts appropriately. The approach of only repressing symptoms with drugs may very soon become old technology in the field of medicine.

Vital for Good Health

The body utilitizes the eight glyconutrients that are essential for cellular health by enhancing every function of the body. Ninety-eight percent of people who take enough of the eight glyconutrients in a standardized, stabilized form for at least four months have reported significant health improvements. Which of your trillions of cells may benefit?

While a supplement may be the only way to receive all the necessary glyconutrients on any given day and represents the research for optimal results, you can also make nutrition choices that contain some of the glyconutrients. Psyllium, a common fiber supplement, contains xylose. Fenugreek contains some mannose and galactose. Kelp contains fucose, xylose, mannose, galactose, and glucose. Shitake mushrooms contain n-acetylglucosamine. First milking colostrums contain all eight glyconutrients. The research is ongoing, and the jury is still out on a comprehensive list of glyconutrient content of every food.

Regardless of your health concerns, including glyconutrients in your wellness regime can be extremely beneficial for all ages. Take the time to learn how to evaluate other nutritional supplements to meet your body's glyconutritient, vitamin, mineral, amino acid, and essential fatty acid needs so that the ones that you and your loved ones take are abundantly nutritious and in a form that your body recognizes as food.

About the Author

Victoria Smith is a board-certified holistic health care practitioner through the National Association of Drugless Practitioners. She is best known for her gentle compassion and results-oriented approach to health concerns. She is the author and founder of a very popular Web site and online office, http://www.SignificantHealing.com. In general, she promotes rebalancing the body to its natural state through detoxification and nutrition, with a straightforward, easy-to-understand approach. Her monthly newsletter, "Significant Healing," is dedicated to providing people with ways to naturally transform their lifestyle over a period of time to one that supports vibrant health. Visit also http://www.SweetLifeInfo.com, or contact Victoria at Victoria@SignificantHealing.com, (859) 801-1730.

101

Simple Solutions for Recovering Your Health and Extending Your Life Span

Chris Smith

Food is perhaps the most important cornerstone of health recovery and longevity, with an amazing power to nourish, protect, and heal your body. Improper nutrition, however, will promote the acceleration of disease and aging in many ways, including calcification, acidosis, oxidation, insulin resistance, immunodeficiency, and excitotoxicity. Unfortunately, the typical North American diet promotes all of these processes, leading to serious and widespread health problems in the United States and elsewhere.

Let me share with you four simple and accessible solutions to the above problems that have positively impacted my own health. I found that by eating organic whole foods and taking quality nutritional supplements, it is possible to counteract these processes and experience remarkable improvements in one's health. During my search for ways to promote longevity through nutrition, I became particularly interested in the human body's requirements for certain underrated minerals, such as selenium and magnesium, as well as the multiple benefits of certain so-called superfoods, such as cruciferous vegetables and ancient grains.

The Minerals Selenium and Magnesium

Let us begin with selenium and magnesium, two essential minerals that have not received the attention they deserve. Selenium is one of the most important trace minerals for humans, yet most of us do not consume enough of it. A potent anticancer agent and antioxidant, it also counteracts premature aging, inflammation, coronary disease, and insulin resistance. It is important for protein synthesis, fat metabolism, cellular respiration, and proper thyroid functioning. Selenium boosts your immune system by stimulating white blood cells and removing heavy metals—especially mercury—from your body. It works in synergy with vitamin E to protect your body from free radical damage and is essential for producing glutathione peroxidase, another powerful antioxidant.

Selenium appears to prevent the spread of precancerous and cancerous cells. One landmark study found that consuming 200 mcg of selenium daily cut cancer mortality in half and greatly reduced rates of cancer development: 63 percent for prostate cancer, 58 percent for colorectal cancer, and 46 percent for lung cancer. Selenium may also be quite effective at preventing leukemia, breast, and ovarian cancer.

Adequate selenium intake is simple to achieve and ensures that you will experience its healthful benefits. Longevity researcher Ray Kurzweil describes selenium as one of the antioxidant "ACES," along with vitamins A, C, and E, and recommends a chemopreventive dose of 400–600 mcg daily. Adequate intake is especially crucial as you grow older, as selenium levels appear to decline with age. Selenium is found in many healthy and readily available foods, including cruciferous vegetables, Brazil nuts, garlic, onions, sweet potatoes, tomatoes, and various fruits, seeds, and grains. Yet, owing to the depleted mineral content of most soil, even organic foods may not provide you with the amount of selenium you need for optimal health. Therefore you should also take an organic (i.e., organically bound) selenium supplement, which is absorbed more readily than inorganic forms of the mineral.

Like selenium, magnesium is another important trace mineral and antioxidant that is often lacking in our bodies. It is vital to the health of your bones, muscles, heart, arteries, and neurons and is required for more than three hundred metabolic processes, including the conversion of carbohydrates and fats into energy; the production of hormones, DNA, proteins, and cells; and the activation of antioxidants and vitamins. Magnesium regulates your body's pH balance, temperature, circulation, and blood pressure; helps relax your muscles; and maintains proper lung, adrenal, and pancreatic functioning.

Higher levels of cellular magnesium appear to slow the processes of aging and the development of disease. One study associates magnesium deficiency with a 50 percent increase in the risk of sudden death by heart attack, while two other studies found that magnesium-rich foods significantly reduce colon cancer development in women. Proper magnesium intake may also help prevent diabetes, osteoporosis, fibromyalgia, chronic inflammation, and anxiety.

Magnesium is central to cell signaling and metabolism, and it normally maintains a delicate balance with calcium ions. It counteracts calcification of your cells, blood vessels, tissues, and organs—especially your brain—and thus may help prevent neurodegenerative diseases. Indeed, Alzheimer's patients often have calcium toxicity coupled with magnesium deficiency. Magnesium further promotes brain health by helping to synthesize the myelin layer surrounding your neurons, which is required for transmitting nerve impulses. It also prevents neural excitotoxicity caused by food additives like aspartame and MSG.

An astounding 80 to 90 percent of the U.S. population may be magnesium deficient, with the typical diet—high in fats and dairy—providing up to four times as much calcium as magnesium. This imbalance leads to the calcification seen in neurodegenerative and other diseases. Furthermore, coffee and alcohol drain your body of magnesium, while soft drinks decrease its absorption. Magnesium intake and absorption also tend to decrease with age.

Fortunately, it is very easy to obtain the magnesium you need to improve your health. Green leafy vegetables are a great source of this mineral, which exists in the center of the chlorophyll molecule. It is also found in a wide variety of fruits, whole grains, nuts, seeds, legumes, and other vegetables. Your daily intake should exceed 400 mg, with some specialists recommending more than one gram. As with selenium, you will most likely need to take supplements to obtain this much magnesium. Various forms of magnesium supplementation are available, including regular oral magnesium, liquid ionic magnesium, and topical magnesium oil (which absorbs well through your skin while keeping it nourished).

By simply getting enough of these two minerals through organic foods and supplements, you will reap their marvelous benefits and be well on your way toward a longer and healthier life.

The Superfoods: Cruciferous Vegetables and Ancient Grains

Let us now turn to my two favorite superfoods: cruciferous vegetables and ancient grains. We all know that vegetables are essential for proper nutrition, yet certain vegetables pack a more powerful nutritional punch than others. Cruciferous vegetables are particularly beneficial and should comprise a significant proportion of your total servings of vegetables. These sulfur-containing plants include broccoli, cauliflower, cabbage, kale, Brussels sprouts, mustard greens, and bok choy. They are packed with phytochemicals, chlorophyll, antioxidants, vitamins, minerals, and dietary fiber.

When you chew cruciferous vegetables, special plant enzymes are released that help form bioactive compounds which may be strong anticancer agents, protecting against cancers of the lung, colon, breast, and prostate. Cruciferous vegetables also help prevent acidosis by restoring your blood to a slightly alkaline state, which counteracts the development of cancer and yeast.

Slowly work your way up to several servings of cruciferous vegetables per day, with continual rotation so you don't get bored. Eat them raw as much as possible, and steam or juice the ones that seem less palatable. Buy organic for maximum nutrition and minimal chemical exposure, and seek out local varieties for maximum freshness.

The so-called ancient grains are also referred to as superfoods due to their impressive nutritional profiles. Quinoa, amaranth, and millet are particularly ideal because, unlike other grains, they are alkaline forming. The cultivation of quinoa, technically a fruit, stretches back at least five thousand years in South America and was called the "Mother Grain" by the Incas. Also not a true grain, amaranth is over eight thousand years old and was revered by the Aztecs. Millet is at least seven thousand years old, with at least six thousand varieties. It is easily digestible and is the only true grain that retains its alkalinity after cooking.

Ancient grains can replace the refined, glutenous grains in your diet, helping prevent the development of insulin resistance and diabetes. Your body quickly converts wheat-based foods such as pasta, breads, and cereals into simple sugars, causing spikes in blood sugar and insulin. Furthermore, the wheat gluten protein itself may bind to insulin receptors, which has caused weight gain and insulin resistance in animal studies.

A combination of quinoa, amaranth, and millet will provide you with phytosterols, dietary fiber, balanced protein, vitamins A, C, and E, most B-complex vitamins, magnesium, calcium, potassium, phosphorus, iron, zinc, copper, manganese, and folate, all of which play important roles in improving and maintaining your health. Whole, organic ancient grains are now widely available in many forms at health food stores and some supermarkets.

Integration

Together, these four simple solutions will detoxify your body, provide essential nutrients, boost your immunity, prevent diseases from developing, and slow your biological aging.

About the Author

Chris Smith is the cofounder and president of Extend Your Lifespan Corp, a new company developing an online health recovery and longevity program that is centered on nutrition. Chris graduated with honors from Stanford University with a BA in psychology. While an undergrad, he investigated the neurobiology of anticipatory states and taught a course on quantum theology, the convergence of science and spirituality. His experience includes performing sleep research at Stanford School of Medicine and managing a neuroanatomical mapping project at Artificial Development Inc. Visit his Web site at http://www.extendyourlifespan.com.

ABOUT SELFGROWTH.COM

SelfGrowth.com is an Internet super-site for self-improvement and personal growth. It is part of a network of websites owned and operated by Self Improvement Online, Inc., a privately held New Jersey–based Internet company.

Our company's mission is to provide our Web site guests with high-quality self improvement and natural health information, with the one simple goal in mind: making their lives better. We provide information on topics ranging from goal setting and stress management to natural health and alternative medicine.

If you want to get a sense for our website's visibility on the Internet, you can start by going to Google, Yahoo, America Online, Lycos, or just about any search engine on the 'Net and typing the words "self-improvement." SelfGrowth.com consistently comes up as the top or one of the top Web sites for self-improvement.

OTHER FACTS ABOUT THE SITE:

SelfGrowth.com offers a wealth of information on self-improvement. Our site:

- Publishes nine informative newsletters on self-improvement, personal growth, and natural health that go out to over 950,000 subscribers.
- Offers over 4,000 unique articles from more than 1,100 experts.
- Links to over 5,000 Web sites in an organized directory.
- Features an updated self-improvement store and event calendar.
- Gets visitors from over 100 countries.

CONTACT INFORMATION

ADDRESS: Self Improvement Online, Inc.
20 Arie Drive
Marlboro, New Jersey 07746
PHONE: (732) 761–9930
E-MAIL: webmaster@selfgrowth.com
WEB SITE: www.selfgrowth.com